Village and Colony Asylums in Britain, Ireland and Germany, 1880-1914

Environmental approaches to patient treatment in Edwardian institutions for the insane

Gillian Allmond

BAR BRITISH SERIES 665 | 2021

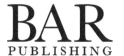

Published in 2021 by
BAR Publishing, Oxford

BAR British Series 665

Village and Colony Asylums in Britain, Ireland and Germany, 1880–1914

ISBN 978 1 4073 5758 4 paperback
ISBN 978 1 4073 5759 1 e-format

DOI https://doi.org/10.30861/9781407357584

A catalogue record for this book is available from the British Library

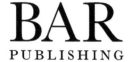

BAR titles are available from:

BAR Publishing
122 Banbury Rd, Oxford, OX2 7BP, UK
EMAIL   info@barpublishing.com
PHONE   +44 (0)1865 310431
FAX   +44 (0)1865 316916
www.barpublishing.com

Of Related Interest

État sanitaire entre Ancien Régime et révolution industrielle
Étude paléoépidemiologique de deux populations provençales
Marie Perrin

Oxford, BAR Publishing, 2021   BAR International Series **3030**

The Outcast Dead
Historical and archaeological evidence for the effect of the New Poor Law
on the health and diet of London's post-medieval poor
Brittney K. Shields Wilford

Oxford, BAR Publishing, 2018   BAR British Series **634**

Social Dimensions of Medieval Disease and Disability
Edited by Sally Crawford and Christina Lee

Oxford, BAR Publishing, 2014   BAR International Series **2668**

Bodies of Knowledge: Cultural Interpretations of Illness and
Medicine in Medieval Europe
Edited by Sally Crawford and Christina Lee

Oxford, BAR Publishing, 2010   BAR International Series **2170**

Acknowledgements

I have been supported by many people in the journey to bring this research to fruition. It takes a village to raise a child, and a lengthy research project such as this cannot be undertaken successfully without the help of colleagues, and the forbearance, at least(!), of friends and family. This book began life as my PhD thesis and I would like to thank my supervisor Dr Mark Gardiner, who encouraged me to pursue further research and whose guidance and experience was of inestimable value. He gently reigned in my excesses, for which I am grateful. Even through the difficult days, he made our meetings enjoyable and the research journey a pleasant one—I always came out of our discussions buzzing with enthusiasm and ideas. I would also like to thank members of staff at Queen's University, Belfast for their support and ideas, particularly Professor Audrey Horning and Professor Keith Lilley. Carol Dunlop, the subject librarian at QUB went the extra mile in getting access to material for me, and Libby Mulqueeny's careful drawings are a big improvement on the originals. Max Meulendijks directed me to some very helpful sources and Brian Johnston, Siobhan McDermott and Lorraine Barry were generous with their time in assisting me to use ArcGIS successfully. All the members of the lunch club, especially Wills McNeilly, Marco Aquino Lopez and Caroline McGrath, deserve thanks for being humorous and supportive when and where it was needed.

The original research on which this book is based was made possible by a studentship and research grant from the former Department for Employment and Learning, Northern Ireland. My fieldwork was also enabled by generous grants from other sources, namely: Society of Antiquaries of Scotland, Scottish Society of the History of Medicine, Royal Historical Society, German History Society, Society for the Social History of Medicine and a prize from my department at Queen's University, the 75th Anniversary Fieldwork Award.

Archive research was assisted by many helpful and thorough members of staff, particularly the following: at the Public Record Office of Northern Ireland (Lorraine Bourke), Edinburgh University (Louise Williams), the National Records of Scotland (Jennifer Ozers), Historic Environment Scotland (Joe Waterfield), Aberdeen University (Fiona Watson and Fiona Musk), Aberdeen Central Library (David Oswald), the Mitchell Library in Glasgow (Alistair Tough), Hertfordshire Archives and Local Studies (Aurora Sampson), and Lancashire County Archives (Victoria McCann).

My visits to the sites were assisted by the security staff at Bangour Village, by Michael Regan in estates at Dykebar, by Raymond Hamilton and Cormac McDaid at Knockbracken (Purdysburn), who also gave me access to the extensive collection of original plans and by Katrin Schreiter and Mario Kulisch at Alt Scherbitz who opened the fascinating Traditionskabinett for me. Residents of Kingseat were tolerant of my strange activities and some even invited me in to measure ceiling heights and window sizes, for which I am very grateful.

Some aspects of this study have appeared in print previously, in particular, parts of Chapter 6 which appeared as 'The outer darkness of madness: an Edwardian Winter Garden at Purdysburn asylum for the insane poor', in: M. Dowd and R. Hensey, eds. The Archaeology of Darkness, published by Oxbow Books of Oxford. Parts of Chapter 8 were published in a paper that appeared in *History of Psychiatry*, 'Liberty and the Individual: the colony asylum in Scotland and England', Volume 28, Issue 1, pages 29 to 43.

More recently, I have benefitted from the encouragement of Professor Eileen Murphy and Dr Colm Donnelly to publish my thesis and the careful and patient support of BAR Publishing, particularly Dr Ruth Fisher.

Most thanks must go to my long-suffering family members, near and far, particularly Finn and Pierse, who were taken along on many asylum and archive visits and were amazingly cheerful throughout. While preparing this study, I thought often of my grandmother, Elizabeth Millar McArthur Allmond who spent many months in the former Argyll and Bute asylum in the 1950s and whose story helped me to appreciate that mental illness can be frightening but mentally ill people deserve our compassion and not our fear.

Contents

List of Figures

List of Tables

Abbreviations

ACDLB	Aberdeen City District Lunacy Board
BDLA	Belfast District Lunatic Asylum Management Committee
EDLB	Edinburgh District Lunacy Board
ELC	English Lunacy Commissioners
GPI	General Paralysis of the Insane (tertiary stage of syphilis)
ILC	Irish Lunacy Commissioners
JMS	Journal of Mental Science
LAB	Lancashire Asylums Board
RDLB	Renfrew District Lunacy Board
SLC	Scottish Lunacy Commissioners

Note: For simplicity's sake, archive reference numbers have not been given in the text for asylum annual reports or minutes, which are identified by the name of asylum and date only. Archive reference numbers for these are listed in the bibliography.

Glossary of Terms

Architrave	*Mouldings* framing a window or doorway
Ashlar	Masonry consisting of blocks of accurately cut, dressed and finished stone
Baroque	Theatrical and exuberant architectural style featuring flowing curves and complex geometries
Bartizan	A small turret supported by corbels projecting from an angle at the top of a wall.
Bay (structural)	Vertical divisions of the exterior of a building, marked by windows
Bay (window)	A projecting, curved or angular (canted), window
Bellcote	A framework on a roof from which a bell is hung
Classical architecture	A revival of Greek and Roman styles, characterised by symmetry and the use of *pediments* and *orders*
Colony asylum	Asylum plan based on dispersed buildings, without corridor connections, distributed across a rural site
Cornice	Any projecting *moulding* at the top of a wall or arch, or along the edges of a *pediment*
Corridor asylum	Asylum plan based on wings composed of long corridors with rows of cells leading off
Course	A continuous layer of stones or bricks in a wall
Cupola	A small dome crowning a roof or turret
Drip mould	A *moulding* positioned to throw off rainwater and prevent it from running down the building
Eaves	Underpart of a sloping roof overhanging a wall
Elevation	External faces of a building, or drawings thereof
Elliptical-headed arch	An arch of which the upper part forms the outline of an ellipse
Finial	Formal ornament at the top of a *gable* or spire
Frieze	Horizontal band below a *cornice*
Gable	Wall of a building that closes the end of a pitched roof, (usually) forming a triangle
Gablet	Small *gable*-shaped feature
Galleting	Small stones inserted into mortar, usually for decorative purposes
Gothic	A revival of medieval architecture, characterised by pointed arches and asymmetrical massing
Leaf (door)	The part of the door that folds and is hung on hinges
Modillion	A series of small brackets supporting a *cornice*
Moulding	A continuous projection with a contoured profile, often marking the meeting of ceiling and walls. Egg-and-dart *moulding* is a classical ornament composed of ovoid elements separated by pointed forms. Cavetto is a convex *moulding*, about a quarter circle in section
Mullions	Stone verticals dividing window apertures
Oculus	A circular opening in a wall or pediment
Order	A column composed of base, shaft, capital and entablature

Oriel	*Bay window* supported by brackets or corbels
Panopticon	An institution characterised by a central observation tower surrounded by cells, first proposed by English philosopher Jeremy Bentham
Pavilion asylum	Asylum plan characterised by separate blocks arranged symmetrically with connecting corridors
Pediment	A low-pitched *gable*, often surmounting *classical* columns
Plinth	Projecting base course of a wall
Quoins	Stones used to emphasise the external corners of a building
Radial plan	An institutional plan composed of a central hub with corridors radiating from it, as in the spokes of a wheel.
Re-entrant angle	Two walls meeting at an internal angle
Reveals (window)	Sides of the wall aperture in which a window is set
Segregate system	Alternative term for a *colony asylum*
Stugged	Stonework featuring small deliberately-created indentations
Villa colony	Term used for Purdysburn *colony asylum* in Ireland
Villa system	Alternative term for a *colony asylum*
Village asylum	Usual term used for a *colony asylum* in Scotland
Wallhead dormer	A type of roof window that rises through the eaves, characteristic of Scottish architecture,

Architectural definitions derived from Curl, J S and Wilson, S *The Oxford Dictionary of Architecture* (2015) Oxford: Oxford University Press and Fleming, J, Honour, H and Pevsner, N *The Penguin Dictionary of Architecture and Landscape Architecture* (1999) London: Penguin Books.

Introduction

'There they stand, isolated, majestic, imperious, brooded over by the gigantic water-tower and chimney combined, rising unmistakable and daunting out of the countryside–the asylums which our forefathers built with such immense solidity to express the notions of their day. Do not for a moment underestimate their powers of resistance to our assault.' (Powell, 1961)

Enoch Powell, right-wing libertarian and Minister of Health, prefigured the first wave of closures of mental hospitals in 1961 in his well-known 'Water Towers' speech, in which he emphasised the material presence of asylum buildings within the landscape, although it was to be another two decades before the closures began. The asylum, and later mental hospital, had been the dominant approach to care for the mentally ill for more than a century by this stage. Trenchant critiques of psychiatry and the asylum system were launched by Goffman, Foucault and Szasz the same year, and have been continued by historians and others in the past half century. These point to the asylum system as a failure, and accuse asylum authorities of ultimately building 'warehouses' and 'museums of madness' merely with the object of sequestering society's unwanted out of sight, as cheaply as possible (Foucault, 1961; Goffman, 1961; Szasz, 1961; Scull, 1979).

Within this overarching context a considerable scholarship has been produced on the architecture and spaces of asylums. The establishment and early development of the asylum system has been seen as a 'golden age' of asylum construction, in which hopes were high that therapeutic environments could bring about cures in large numbers of the suffering. The later period of asylum building, has been described as an era of 'therapeutic pessimism', following the inexorable increase of numbers of insane, which is thought to have fatally undermined any belief in the restorative powers of the asylum. Perhaps as a result of the historiographical assertion that asylums of this period had merely become ways to house economically ever larger numbers of the mentally ill, some developments in asylum architecture and layouts have not received the attention they deserve. Across Europe and America, and in Britain and Ireland, the later decades of the nineteenth century saw both a trend to segregate asylum accommodation into separate buildings, and a further, associated trend, to situate these segregated buildings on expansive 'colony' sites in rural areas, where patients were set to work as much as they were able. There was considerable variation in how far these trends were adopted in each jurisdiction. In Germany and Scotland, however, the 'segregated system' was universal for new building after 1900, the latter taking its inspiration from the former, and particularly the earliest example of the

colony asylum at Alt Scherbitz, which was a model for asylums around the world.

The colony asylum exhibits several important differences from the traditional asylum style. Firstly, it was usually located at a far remove from centres of population, in contrast to earlier asylums that tended to be within easy reach of an urban centre. Secondly, its segregated character gave an unprecedented freedom in the way buildings were distributed around the site. Thirdly, the smaller size of buildings allowed for them to resemble ordinary dwelling houses, in architecture, layouts and decoration/furnishing.

This raises several interesting questions about the nature of asylum accommodation at this period and whether or not they can truly be compared to 'warehouses'. But this study seeks to go beyond the implications of such buildings for the asylum project and to ask how we should see such experiments in relation to the rise of the middle classes in this period and burgeoning environmentalism taking new forms in utopian projects, such as the garden city. Also prominent in this period are changing concepts of gender and fears of racial degeneration associated with urban slums, which provide a historically-situated context for such changes in asylum accommodation. Asylum buildings were part of emerging medical and social discourses, having symbolic power and meaning beyond the intentions of the asylum builders. Textual evidence is examined in this study for the implied, the understated and the allusive traces of attitudes and beliefs concerning the poor and the insane, in order to connect asylum materiality to concepts and ideas that formed part of culture at this period.

The colony asylum is a stage of development in the history of institutions for the mentally ill that has as yet received limited attention in the prolific literature on insanity and there has been no detailed assessment of the extant material evidence relating to this asylum type in Scotland and Ireland. The archaeology of institutions, a relatively new area of study, has produced very little published work on asylums for the mentally ill, and none relating to this particular asylum type.

For the purposes of this study, six asylum sites were selected as case studies. Having determined that, within Britain and Ireland, the colony asylum layout was most enthusiastically adopted in Scotland, the three public asylums that were built here after 1900, Bangour, Dykebar and Kingseat were made the core of the study. These were supplemented by a colony asylum in the north of Ireland, Purdysburn, and the German asylum that provided the inspiration for the Scottish and Irish examples, Alt Scherbitz. A traditional-style asylum, built in Lancashire, was included in the study as a point of comparison.

This study sets out to analyse the colony asylum in order to determine how its appearance as a material phenomenon of the Asylum Age is connected to cultural change, both in terms of medical thinking and also more widely. The analysis also uncovers how the colony asylum expressed cultural difference, in terms of differences in the way society was conceptualised in Scotland and in England.

A primary aim of the study is to trace the historical development of the colony asylum in Scotland and Ireland in the period up to World War One, by identifying the unique characteristics of the this asylum layout in relation to earlier asylum types and by exploring the reasons why colony asylums were built in Ireland and Scotland in this period but not in England. The colony asylum is positioned within the context of utopian communities, such as labour colonies and the garden city.

A second aim is to analyse the layouts, built form, interior spaces and furnishings of the colony asylum in relation to themes suggested by contemporary literature and archives. The study identifies how a concern with hygiene, particularly light and ventilation, is expressed in the way the buildings have been constructed and laid out and further identifies the ways in which the buildings were rendered 'home-like' both architecturally and in terms of layouts and furnishings, and the tensions introduced to this aspiration by the requirements of the institution. This analysis reveals how the material culture of the colony asylum was influenced by contemporary understandings of mental health and therapeutic care

A third aim is to determine what the architecture and interiors of the colony asylum can tell us about contemporary attitudes to environment, class, poverty and health, both mental and physical. This aim challenges a historiographical orthodoxy which holds that asylums of the early twentieth century were built as 'warehouses' to sequester the unwanted. The tools of discourse analysis are used to connect the materiality of the asylum with wider cultural issues such as degenerationism and antipathy to urbanism and industrialization. The study identifies the ways in which the environment of the asylum attempted to address the problem of poverty and madness by providing idealised bourgeois domestic spaces.

The following sections critically examine the background to the study of institutions within historical archaeology and consider how archaeologists have approached the study of asylums, in particular. A survey of the study of asylum environments across disciplines is followed by a summary of recent thinking in buildings archaeology and buildings theory, leading to the positioning of this study within previous scholarship and an assessment of the methodological strategies used.

1.1. Archaeology of institutions

The archaeology of institutions, defined by Baugher (2009:5) as organisations that 'control people's behaviour and daily life', can be said to have been established in the early and mid-twentieth century with the excavation of Spanish missions in the United States (Farnsworth and Williams, 1992; Thomas, 1993; McEwan, 2002; Orser, 2002). The last fifteen years has seen a flowering of the archaeology of institutions which has begun to range across sites as diverse as almshouses, asylums, prisons, reformatories and schools. A shift in focus has taken place from early studies which consisted largely of uncovering building footprints for the purposes of historical preservation to a diverse range of research questions encompassing 'class, inequality, gender, race, ethnicity and ideology' (Baugher, 2009: 7). Archaeological work on institutional sites can be divided roughly into the almshouses and poorhouses dating from the pre-industrial era on one hand, and nineteenth and twentieth-century asylums, psychiatyric hospitals and prisons on the other. The latter are often categorised together as differing qualitatively from the institutional sites that preceded them. Work on pre-industrial institutions for the poor has raised questions about whether living conditions were as severe as might have been predicted. Food remains have pointed to a varied diet (Baugher, 2001: 188) and artefacts to a comfortable, if frugal, lifestyle, which has been contrasted to the 'mean-spirited' conditions that were thought to prevail in the nineteenth century (Cotter, Roberts and Parrington, 1993; Baugher, 2001; Huey, 2001).

Some authors have identified a change in attitude towards the lower classes in the nineteenth century, in which the poor became morally culpable for their plight and could be reformed by placing in what Goffman later termed a 'total institution' (Goffman, 1961). This era is characterised by what has been called a 'carceral enthusiasm' in which ever-rising numbers of the poor and marginal were catered for in institutions. Three published works, Beisaw and Gibb's collection of papers on institutional life (Beisaw and Gibb, 2009): Casella's (2007) summary of archaeological work on institutions and a related collection of papers on internment (Myers and Moshenska, 2011) have sought to give an overview of institutional life in the nineteenth and twentieth centuries by drawing together the research to date. Casella (2007), in particular, connects institutions through time and space and asks broad questions relating to why society (with an emphasis on American society) incarcerates in the present. Although much of the historical context she identifies is useful, the attempt to draw together a multiplicity of sites through common themes may have worked against a deeper understanding of sites, such as asylums for the mentally ill which are not easily encompassed within the prison model. Although Casella acknowledges that 'institutions exist not only to detain, but also to teach, heal, accommodate and inspire', she ultimately reads the archaeology as a commentary on how individuals endure disciplinary control through various strategies of coping and resistance (Casella, 2007: 75).

Casella and others are highly influenced by two theorists, who emerge in a large majority of published work on institutions, using their work in particular ways. Goffman's work on the 'total institution' is used for its exploration of the ways in which inmates are subordinated through being stripped of their individuality and the range of responses to this, withdrawing, challenging or accepting their confinement (Goffman, 1961). Foucault's work on the institutionalisation of the individual, is used mainly for its focus on surveillance as the means of producing disciplined bodies. Archaeologists of institutions do not usually engage with Foucault's broader approach to governmentality, which culminates in *Discipline and Punish* with the colony institution of Mettray wherein were superimposed the 'coercive technologies' relating to family life, the army, the workshop and the prison within increasingly individualised spaces. Foucault suggests that disciplinary regimes were subject to 'descending individualisation', the least powerful in society being the most subject to classification and tabulation (Foucault, 1977: 193, 200-209, 293-297).

Critics of these approaches, which appear to deny or minimise the agency of individuals, have sought to introduce feminist perspectives, evidence of resistance and of the heterarchy of power. A common theme in the archaeology of institutions has been the examination of artefactual evidence in order to determine whether inmates were well or badly treated, whether the artefactual evidence corroborates or disproves the documentary evidence, or whether it shows that individuals resisted or subverted their confinement. Buildings are often not extant, or do not form a significant part of the study. For example, an excavation of Walnut Street Prison in Philadelphia, found among other artefacts bone dice that have been interpreted as prohibited gaming activities that formed part of inmate coping and exchange strategies (Cotter *et al.*, 1988; Casella, 2007: 87). Feister's excavation of a nineteenth-century orphanage found the toys which were recovered spoke of a relatively benign regime that did not fit with preconceived ideas (Feister, 2009). Artefacts obtained at Industrial Indian School sites (Lindauer, 1996), such as dinner plates with bifacially flaked rims, worked with traditional technologies, can be seen as a form of cultural resistance. Buildings are occasionally included in the narrative of resistance, as at Old Rhode Island Penitentiary, where changes to the built environment were made including a rebuild after an act of arson (Garman 2005). Some studies have found evidence which reinforces the expectation that institutions were places of harsh treatment and poor living conditions, such as Cook's (1991) analysis of skeletons at the Uxbridge Almshouse burial ground. This study uncovered pathological conditions arising from work requirements in the asylum, while a similar study at Cook County Poor Farm, Illinois found evidence of cavities, gum disease, bone trauma and periostitis linked to health, diet and hygiene conditions at the institution (Cook, 1991; Grauer, McNamara and Houdek, 1998).

On the whole, archaeological studies of institutions take as their starting point the expectation that the material practices of these sites are informed principally by the attempt of institutional authorities to maintain control over inmates/patients. Inmates/patients submit to or resist this control producing artefactual evidence which either conforms with or challenges an expectation of an environment which is harsh and oppressive. This concentration on underlying power dynamics can work to detach the archaeology from its historical and cultural context by focussing on essentially ahistorical, structural dimensions of meaning. While power relations are no doubt essential to an understanding of institutions, there are many dimensions of meaning, that do not fall within a simple dichotomy of powerful and subordinated.

For example, built remains are difficult to fit into the dialectic of control and resistance that informs much institutional archaeology. Unless adaptations have been made as a result of inmate resistance (Spencer-Wood and Baugher, 2001; Thomas, 2013) buildings can be seen straightforwardly as symbols of, and mechanisms for control, rather than repositories of layers of meaning. Furthermore, the analysis of institutions for the mentally ill is informed by a very contemporary (i.e. late twentieth and early twenty-first century) understanding of the asylum project as a failure, an understanding which is itself a product of cultural change fed by the work of Foucault and Goffman, among others. Scholarship sometimes chooses to appraise institutions for how 'institutional' they are, or how effectively they were resisted, in our own terms, rather than as cultural artefacts, informed by values and aspirations that are not self-evident but need to be deliberately uncovered. Institutions, in common with other archaeological remains of the historical era, have been seen overwhelmingly as part of the historical development of capitalism, a means of managing the economically unproductive and those threatening to social order.

Some writers have sought to develop a more nuanced approach towards institutions and De Cunzo's study of the Magdalen Asylum of Philadelphia (1995) is worthy of note in this regard. De Cunzo reads the history and archaeology of the asylum as an interplay between the objectives and desires held by the asylum authorities and the 'fallen' women occupants. The asylum was designed to reform wayward women through labour and cultivate a 'purified feminine identity' (Casella 2007: 119). However, the attempt to instil guilt and foster redemption in the inmates was largely a failed exercise, the women making use of the institution for their own ends as a place of refuge and respite from difficult circumstances in the outside world. De Cunzo emphasises the rituals of asylum life which were intended to mark women's rejection from society, transformation and re-integration as moral citizens. Drawing on anthropological understandings of pollution, cultural context is interrogated in order to uncover the values informing a contemporary understanding of poverty, disease and immorality. 'Philadelphians connected bodily and moral contagion. As epidemics raged through the city, the 'fallen' woman, carrier of sexually-transmitted disease, symbolized contamination and pollution that must be checked' (De Cunzo 1995: 131). The material remains of the asylum are explicitly connected to contemporary ideology, 'Plain, functional furnishings and dress curbed ostentation and aspirations above one's social and economic place, even as refined dinner and tea wares signified the principles of pious consumption—the beauties of moral purity and its embodiment, nature' (De Cunzo 1995: 126).

Spencer-Wood (2009) brings a gendered perspective to the archaeology of institutions through research which addresses the institutionalisation of women as 'systematic patriarchal control of women's bodies and their sexuality'. She puts forward a Marxist analysis that women's unpaid domestic labour was essential to the operation of institutions and was exploited for profit. The Foucauldian concept of 'docile bodies' is countered with the argument that women developed strategies of resistance both individually and collectively and were able to negotiate to improve their situation in ways which can not only be seen as resistance but also as 'self-empowering actions driven by goals such as freedom to control one's own life and identity'. American colonial women were also social agents, creating new organizations and charitable institutions. Spencer-Wood points to a contemporary gender ideology which considered women as 'innately more pious, pure and moral than men because of the separation of women's domestic sphere from men's capitalist sphere' (Spencer-Wood, 2001: 106).

De Cunzo and Spencer-Wood both situate their research within a cultural context that gives specific historical meaning to ideas such as 'womanhood' and 'morality'. However, neither of these writers seeks to attach cultural meanings to buildings themselves, instead making use of these ideas as the wider historical background against which their sites are situated and as informing the symbolic resonance of artefacts and spaces.

While American archaeology has often focussed on the artefacts associated with institutions, rather than the buildings themselves, and is dominated by excavation as a methodology, scholars from the UK have had comparatively more to say about buildings, beginning as in the US with investigations into almshouses (Fennelly and Newman, 2016). Recent work has built on ideas of power/control/resistance to consider other social and cultural modes such as Improvement and Reform, while also considering the ways in which buildings and environments reflect ideologies including public policy, and symbolise cultural values (Springate, 2017). Workhouses have become another theme, beginning with Lucas's examination of the changing use of workhouse buildings in Southampton and culminating in Charlotte Newman's recent examination of the use and adaptation of workhouses in West Yorkshire

and Liz Thomas's assessment of the changing moral geometry of Ulster asylums (Lucas, 1999; Newman, 2010, 2013a, 2013b, Thomas, 2013, 2017). Newman interprets the choice of workhouse location on the outskirts of towns as 'removing paupers to the margins of society', while within towns they served as a reminder of 'dominance and authority' (Newman, 2010: 148-149). Building style is also linked to dominance, authority and order, while the spaces and architecture of the buildings are seen as implementing strategies of surveillance, segregation and specialisation, which were subject to change over time and across the region. Liz Thomas emphasises themes of uniformity, discipline and classification in Ulster workhouses, while uncovering the ways in which resistance to the authority of Commissioners by both Guardians and inmates led to buildings being altered and used in unintended ways, including the gradual movement of children within workhouse schemes to a more privileged position reflecting their gradual idealisation within society. The archaeology of internment camps, prisoner of war camps, concentration camps and other material phenomena associated with wartime has been another strong theme in the UK and Europe, emphasising issues of power and control (Myers and Moshenska, 2011; Mytum and Carr, 2012; Carr, Jasinski and Theune, 2017). An understanding of the cultural context of these sites has started to bridge the gap between macro-scale social theory and micro-scale enumeration of artefacts and buildings.

1.2. Archaeology of the asylum

Several archaeologists have written on the historical background to asylums for the insane and their place within the archaeology of institutions, emphasising the potential of archaeology's focus on materiality to offer a perspective on 'individual bodily encounters with institutional life' (Casella 2007; Casella 2009:27 Beisaw & Gibb 2009; Spencer-Wood & Baugher 2001). However, there has been comparatively little detailed investigation of asylum sites to date by archaeologists. Until the 2000s, there were no published archaeological studies of asylum environments i.e. studies that used archaeological method, such as site visits, building survey or the study of artefacts. Work by Piddock and Longhurst, examines sites in Australia, with some reference to English asylums, while Fennelly and Newman are the authors of published work relating to Britain and Ireland (Piddock, 2001, 2007, 2011, 2016, Longhurst, 2011, 2015, 2017; Fennelly, 2014, 2019; Newman, 2015). Piddock's (2007) work on lunatic asylums in South Australia and Tasmania takes as its essential premise the existence of an 'ideal' asylum in terms of types of room and standard of accommodation, conceived, and to some extent, practised in Britain. Piddock finds that the asylums that were built in South Australia do not conform to the 'ideal' in many important respects and seeks to explain this by reference to several factors; economic constraints, ignorance of the literature and practice in Britain and social perceptions of insanity as caused by intemperance and vice (a belief, incidentally, which was equally held in Britain at the time). She takes the ideal/reality approach familiar to archaeologists, in which archaeology provides a challenge to the picture drawn by historical documents but her work does not generally explore the significance of the ideals, concluding that the asylum was intended to be therapeutic but that the reality was somewhat different (Piddock, 2016). Piddock's use of analytical techniques to assess asylum buildings is rare, and welcome, and the identification of a contemporary discourse around the 'ideal' asylum is well founded, but it is not clear that the Australian authorities would have built the 'ideal' English asylum under any circumstances.

Longhurst (2011; 2015; 2017) makes a comparison of four institutions for the mentally ill in New South Wales, to some extent building on the work of Piddock but adding a dimension of change through time. Longhurst follows Piddock in analysing the difference between psychiatric ideals and the way asylums were actually built, but takes this further by looking at the ways asylum management coped with this dissonance over time through strategies of tolerance, mitigation and finally abandonment. Authorities responded to this dissonance by modifying the buildings, with closure of the institution taking place at a point where the non-correspondence between ideas and reality could no longer be tolerated or mitigated against. Again, the focus is on what 'should' have been built, rather than what was built. This position is dependent on an understanding of contemporary psychiatric discourse as singular and uncontested. This is not borne out by reference to contemporary debates which continually betray uncertainty, controversy and a consciousness of mental illness as poorly understood.

Newman's (2015) study is unusual in that it makes use of a collection of architectural fragments retained from a private Georgian madhouse, relating these fragments to the image the proprietors wished to represent of 'respectability, benevolence and improvement' (Newman 2015: 160). Newman notes that standards of decoration were high and a concerted effort was made to provide an environment that would have been familiar in taste and comfort to the patients. Katherine Fennelly's (2014) study explores the soundscapes of asylums, situating the asylum project within a drive towards urban and social improvement during the nineteenth century. Fennelly reconstructs historical asylum soundscapes from documentary sources, in a partly phenomenological study which speculates on the impressions noises such as keys turning in locks may have made on patients. Fennelly deals in some detail with patient classification, which was a means of separating noisy from quiet patients and with such features as vaulted ceilings which would have acted to reduce noise. Following archaeological method, Fennelly uses the position of rooms within the asylum buildings as a form of primary evidence, rather than relying solely on documentary sources.

Fennelly has questioned the bracketing together of differing types of institution, such as asylums and prisons, and advocates for the heterogeneity of institutional sites,

particularly in her monograph on the archaeology of Georgian asylums in England and Ireland, which explores aspects of spatial organisation and movement within asylum buildings. (Fennelly 2019: 155). Fennelly and Newman propose multiple research methodologies for the analysis of institutional buildings in order to uncover 'individual institutional practices that reflect the local economic, social and political environment' (Fennelly and Newman, 2016: 187). Archaeologists are well-placed, it is argued, to comment on the lives of those left out of the historical record, using material evidence to reconstruct everyday lives.

The totality of archaeological scholarship around institutions shows an emphasis on exposing mismatches of various kinds; between the historical record and the lived experience of inmates, between the 'total' institution and resistance/insubordination, between the 'ideal' and the reality. Although, no doubt productive, these approaches can be seen as relegating archaeology to the position of 'handmaiden' with regard to historical disciplines (Hume, 1964), where archaeology concerns itself largely with the material 'gaps' that no other discipline can fill. In order to understand the material culture of institutions it is necessary to understand material and discursive practices as intimately informing one another, rather than acting in opposition to each other. This entails an appreciation of the material world as culturally situated and symbolically resonant and means that we must explicitly uncover the meanings and values associated with materiality in the past, rather than bringing a contemporary understanding to our analysis. One of the most significant impediments to our understanding of institutions for the mentally ill is the contemporary view of the asylum as a failed experiment, an understanding which pre-judges the outcome of our analyses and fails to credit the historical impulse behind their creation. A focus on power relations in a narrow sense, deriving from a number of influential theoreticians, encourages us to reflect backwards with a modern sensibility and find what we seek. A more integrated archaeology of institutions must aim to uncover the historically-situated, culturally contextualised meaning of institutions for the mentally ill, encompassing issues of therapeutic care, enlightenment aspiration and improving zeal. Asylum scholarship in other disciplines has both continued some of the themes seen within historical archaeology and added a greater focus on documentary sources. The contributions of some of the major scholars in the areas of historical geography, architectural history, social history and landscape history are considered below.

1.3. Other scholarship relating to asylum environments

The critical study of the architecture, interiors and physical environment of asylums can be said to have initially been stimulated by Foucault's 'Madness and Civilization', and his 'Discipline and Punish' (Foucault, 1965, 1977). It is often Foucault's work on prisons, rather than his earlier work on the history of madness, that has been of interest to scholars of asylum materiality, particularly his analysis of Bentham's 'ideal' disciplinary structure, the panopticon. By this and other architectural means, 'docile bodies' are produced by rendering inmates visible but unaware of whether or not they are being watched. Hence, argues Foucault, a state is induced in the inmate, 'of conscious and permanent visibility that assures the automatic functioning of power' (Foucault 1977: 201). Scholars of the asylum have also been engaged by Foucault's rejection of Whiggish accounts of asylum history, and his recasting of asylum reform in the early nineteenth century as 'an insidious instrument of bourgeois social control' (Brown 1980: 105). Although Foucault's historical analysis of institutional confinement has been questioned (notably by Porter 1990; Sedgwick 1981), his reading of architecture in terms of surveillance and control continues to be influential.

The study of asylum architecture began, following Foucault, with the attempt to connect buildings and spaces with wider social themes, particularly power and sequestration of those deemed socially problematic. Thompson & Goldin (1975) identify the main determinant in asylum design as 'supervision and control', and consider the progression in asylum design from the cells and chains of Bethlem to the classified, hygienic spaces of Derby Asylum (1851) through this lens, which sees the forms of surveillance and restriction modified according to progressing medical discourses. Several important studies published in the 1980s continued these themes. Andrew Scull, perhaps the leading scholar of Victorian asylum history, attributes the sequestering of the insane to the advent of a mature capitalist economy in which the unproductive became a burden. Scull has suggested a number of underlying reasons for the commitment to public asylums, including the emergence of a psychiatric profession who were anxious to further themselves by distinguishing the insane as a distinct category who could only be cared for in an institutional setting (Scull 1993:41). Scull implies that the continual assertion by alienists that patients could not be cured at home, but must be removed to an institution, formed part of a strategy to consolidate their jurisdiction over mental illness (Scull 1993: 136). Enumerating the arguments of contemporary critics (for example, that the company of other mad people was detrimental to the well-being of patients and that the routines of the asylum were infantilising), Scull suggests that the asylum project was 'a venture which was misconceived from the start' (Scull 1993: 142). Asylums were a means of preserving order by removing the insane from society, the buildings becoming ever larger in order to benefit from economies of scale. He sees classification of space within asylums as a means of control through creating a reward system. Scull is willing to acknowledge an early utopianism in the asylum project but refers to later Victorian asylums as 'warehouses for the unwanted', that were architecturally 'bald and monotonous', a further excuse for isolating the mad in asylums, at this period, being the acceptance of hereditary explanations for their illness, which meant that they should not be allowed to reproduce. Asylum buildings

and environments, for Scull, are little more than the means of sequestering and controlling the insane as cheaply as possible (Scull 1980: 26; Scull 2015: 223).

Tom Brown looks at the history of the Canadian mental health system through the asylum at Toronto, and tries to balance the 'social control' theory of asylum development with a perspective that credits the intentions of the asylum builders. He finds that the asylum environment was explicitly chosen to be therapeutic. The asylum buildings were to be small in size, warm and well-ventilated with spacious rooms and as home-like as possible, with a benign father-figure in the medical superintendent at the centre (literally and figuratively), and with patient classification that would ensure protection for calmer from more disruptive patients. This ideal ultimately failed to deliver in practice, however. The heating and ventilation systems did not function, the physical size of the building made it 'intimidating and alienating' and difficult to negotiate for staff and patients, producing an environment that was 'frightening, dis-orienting, and ultimately overwhelming' (Brown 1980: 123). Brown does not connect his analysis specifically to discourses of power and surveillance, but states that the physical environment of the asylum, failed to function even in the terms of medical discourses of the day, falling short of the great hopes that were held out for them. Donnelly (1983) continues to emphasise the asylum as a therapeutic instrument, that managed inmates and replaced the 'mechanical restraint' of an earlier era. Donnelly contrasts the semblance of liberty offered by an asylum with the reality of security and restraint, emphasising surveillance, classification and segregation within asylum buildings.

A geographical approach to asylum spaces is taken by Chris Philo (1989), who questions the Foucauldian concept of panoptic surveillance through segregation within asylum buildings, pointing out that as the asylum project proceeded panoptic styles fell out of favour and patients tended to be, in fact, aggregated together in large dormitories and dayrooms. In the latter decades of the nineteenth century, there was considerable argument over the best type of plan for asylums, but surveillance was rarely made a significant factor and segregation of patients in internal accommodation was avoided. The factors Philo pinpoints as of concern to asylum builders, were economy, ease of construction, accessibility, ventilation, fire risk and home surroundings. Philo concludes, however, that Foucauldian panopticism could exist independently of strictly panoptic layouts and that despite the intention to reform/cure the insane, the consequence of withdrawing the mentally ill to institutions was 'to produce and then continually reproduce a population designated as different, deviant and dangerous by a 'mainstream' society' (Philo 1989: 284).

The following decade saw two major studies of hospitals in the field of architectural history by Taylor (1991) and Richardson (Richardson *et al.*, 1998), both of which have substantial chapters on asylums/mental hospitals in

England and Wales. These studies take a similar approach in choosing outstanding examples of asylum architecture and judging the success of buildings in both architectural and functional terms, while tracing the development of asylum architecture from an 'evolutionary' standpoint. Although the Richardson volume, in particular, is based on a Historic England survey of asylum buildings, only selected buildings are covered by both studies, and so it is difficult to judge how typical the examples are that have been chosen, or the range of asylum types that were being built in any particular time period. Plans and elevations (and some photographic evidence) together with contemporary published material are the sources used, and the study of asylums is progressed by considering some of the ways in which the asylum paralleled hospital development, for instance, in the way in which pavilions were adopted in the later nineteenth century.

Thomas Markus (1993) again concentrates on control and segregation in the planning and construction of asylum buildings, noting the attempt that was made to remove penal features from such structures but concluding that as the nineteenth century wore on, 'buildings became surveillance-oriented, larger, more crowded and Spartan—in fact, carceral' (Markus 1993: 140). He notes that public buildings are not only outcomes of contemporary ideas but also formative of them, however, it is unclear in what sense this is meant since his reading of asylum history is fairly conventional (Markus 1993: 132-133).

Markus Reuber (1996) concentrates on asylum buildings in Ireland for his study of asylum development, which sees the architecture of asylums moving through stages from isolation and classification to the development of a 'curative society' in the colony asylum at Purdysburn. Using plans and published contemporary material, Reuber considers the development of asylums mainly within the terms of the asylum builders themselves.

Barry Edginton published a number of papers in the 1990s and 2000s relating largely to the architecture of the York Retreat, an asylum that was highly influential for the history of the treatment of the mentally ill (see Chapter 2). Edginton concentrates on order and discipline as features of the asylum environment and the ways in which observation and classification were facilitated by the York Retreat. Edginton also emphasises the role of the surrounding landscape as calming and elevating. However, he relies a great deal on secondary materials and on contemporary published material rather than primary records, photographs or plans for his assessment of buildings and environments, therefore running the danger of replicating the viewpoints and ideology of the asylum builders.

Leonard Smith (1999) takes a slightly different approach in focussing on the dichotomy between the façade of the asylum which he associates with the impression of cure, and the internal arrangements which he associates with custody and prison-like features, once more associating the reality of asylum with power and control. Smith makes use of a full range of primary and secondary written sources, but no plans are shown and he makes only general references to architecture and environment.

A study of Severalls asylum (opened 1913) carried out by Diana Gittins (1998) differs markedly from previous work in that she makes extensive use of oral history, garnered from interviews with patients and staff. Gittins adds to the historiographical orthodoxy, that asylums were intended to be therapeutic and healthy, particularly in terms of situation and that they were at the same time sites of constraint, categorisation and control, by demonstrating that there were a range of responses and behaviours associated with asylum life. From abusive staff to those who treated patients with great kindness, from patients who remember their time at Severalls with horror and those who recalled it with gratitude. Gittins uses an anthropological approach to show that spatial division and classification in the asylum worked not only in terms of gender, class and diagnosis, but also to separate the insane from the sane. The laundry building, for example, was organised to separate men's, women's, staff and officers' laundry, through fears of the 'polluting powers of the mad and of madness, and, in particular, the polluting potential of fluids and water in relation to them' (Gittins 1998: 21-24).

Since 2000, there have been three important general studies of asylums in the field of architectural history, by Catherine Stevenson, Carla Yanni and Alison Darragh and a collection of papers on the subject of built environments and spaces. Stevenson's (2000) work concentrates largely on the architecture and interiors of Bethlem hospital and other contemporary institutions for the insane in the eighteenth century. The asylum is seen as fulfilling a range of requirements, aesthetic, therapeutic and functional, with an emphasis on the change from 'palatial' architecture to more sober, therapeutic styles as Bethlem underwent phases of rebuilding. Stevenson considers the 'magnificence' of the charitable institutions that were a striking feature of eighteenth-century welfare provision, Bethlem being described as 'for many years the only building which looked like a palace in London'(Stevenson 2000: 33). The beginnings are noted of a significant tension between 'charitable display' in which the magnificence of buildings manifested the wealth and compassion of the patrons and the feeling that ostentatiousness was antithetical to charity, demonstrating that too much money had been spent on buildings rather than charitable care. Allied to this was the feeling that 'architecture should inspire an emotional tone appropriate to the building's function' and therefore decorative exuberance was unsuitable (Stevenson 2000: 103).

Yanni (2007) deals with the American public asylum in its period of establishment and full flowering from 1770 to 1894, focussing largely on the popular Kirkbride plan of pavilions stepped back in echelon and the 'cottage plan' of segregated buildings, which partially succeeded it. Yanni emphasises the attention to light, air, landscapes and other features of curative environments.

An anthology published the same year and edited by Leslie Topp, James Moran and Jonathan Andrews (Topp, 2007) brings together a number of architectural and spatial studies from major scholars in the field such as Leonard Smith, Barry Edginton, Chris Philo and Jeremy Taylor. pioneering volume of collected essays about the built environment of asylums, constitutes a 'state of the discipline' marker point. The introduction to the volume opined that the historiography of asylums had not done justice to the history of psychiatric spaces and that interdisciplinary studies could have much to offer, nuancing earlier studies on asylum materiality.

Asylum landscapes and layouts were the subject of several studies after 2000, the major contributors being, Sarah Rutherford (2003;2004;2005), Clare Hickman (2005; 2009; 2013) and Leslie Topp (Topp and Wieber, 2009; Topp, 2017). Rutherford and Hickman both concentrated on the designed landscapes surrounding asylums and their perceived therapeutic properties. Rutherford showed how asylum landscapes were modelled on country house estates, while airing courts often resembled domestic town gardens. Rutherford also considers architectural styles of buildings and their layouts as part of the designed landscape. She concludes that the landscapes of asylums should be seen as part of an 'environmental discipline of the poor' (Rutherford, 2004).

Hickman's work emphasises the ways in which asylum landscapes participated in a general discourse of 'nature' as healthful, tranquilising and beneficial to the psyche during the Victorian period and earlier. Leslie Topp's work on asylums of the Austro-Hungarian empire in the late nineteenth and early twentieth century has constituted the most analytical scholarship on the layouts of colony-style asylums within their landscapes. Topp concludes that the 'freedom' discursively implied within the colony form, and the distribution of buildings across a rural estate, was belied by the reality of involuntary confinement and, in fact, constituted a response to anti-psychiatry movements and an engagement with early modernism (Topp, 2017).

Two scholars focussed, at least partly, on the spatial location of asylums, Chris Philo on asylums in England and Wales and Kim Ross on asylums in Scotland. Philo (2004) discusses the factors influencing the location of asylums, in particular, whether or not they were sited in more rural areas, or nearer to urban centres. Philo teases apart the complexity of discourses in this period and sees increasing ruralisation of asylums as a meeting of medical and moral approaches to the treatment of the insane in which rural areas were seen as healthier and better able to offer the picturesque views and cheerful prospects which could soothe the mind. However, he concludes that as somatic and hereditary explanations for madness became more prevalent towards the end of the nineteenth century, environment became downgraded as a cause of insanity.

Ross's unpublished thesis (2014) concentrates on the 'affective power' of asylums across different scales from site and situation to grounds and buildings. Ross perceives the spatial location of Scottish asylums as drawing together moral, medical and hygienic dimensions that favoured rural sites, and in contrast to Philo, points to a renewed faith in environments as therapeutic towards the end of the nineteenth century.

The last fifteen years has seen a response to the 'material turn' in historiography in the form of an increased interest in the interiors and furnishings of asylums. The principle scholars in this area have been Mary Guyatt, whose 2004 chapter appears to have first stimulated this area, and Jane Hamlett (Hamlett 2015; Hoskins & Hamlett 2012). Guyatt stresses that late Victorian and Edwardian asylum interiors were homely and comfortable and considerable thought was given to the correct way to furnish and decorate because of the increasing recognition that many patients would spend their lifetimes in an asylum. Hamlett's work traces the development of asylum interiors from spaces that derived their domestic feel from their organisation as a household under a patriarch in the early years of the asylum system to the gradual building of environments that resembled middle-class homes in the second half of the nineteenth century. By the end of the nineteenth century she finds that concerns with hygiene began to militate against the domesticity of interiors at English asylums.

Overall, it can be seen that studies of asylum environments have fallen into six main categories, namely: 1) architecture of asylum buildings, 2) internal building layouts, 3) spatial location of buildings, 4) spatial distribution of buildings on a site, 5) landscapes and grounds, 6) interior decoration and furnishings. Studies have appeared in several disciplines, most commonly, history, architectural history, historical geography and historical archaeology. Many scholars have contributed in more than one area, but there has been a tendency for each discipline to concentrate on one of these areas. For example, the spatial location of asylums relative to urban centres has largely been tackled by geographers, and the architecture of asylums by architectural historians. Each discipline also tends to favour a distinct theoretical approach, with geographers engaging more with Foucauldian analyses of spatial forms and architectural historians with typology and aesthetics.

A number of themes cut across the asylum scholarship to date. Asylums are treated as a reform project in which the asylum was, at least in the early stages of the asylum construction programme, informed by ideals that sought to make buildings and spaces therapeutic and aesthetically pleasing as well as functional living spaces for numbers of patients. Many authors focus on how asylums fell short of the ideals and were compromised by the need to sequester and control, and most agree that the ideals broke down, in any case, towards the end of the nineteenth century. Themes for investigation have been asylum location, classification and segregation, measures for control and surveillance and hygiene and therapy, but few asylum studies have analysed building sites/topography, building interiors and building architecture at a level of detail that

Table 1. Selected Scholarship to date relating to asylum buildings and environments.

Scholar	Year	Location and period of study	Sources (PR= Primary records PPM= Primary published material)	Discipline	Methodology	Interpretation of asylum environments
Dieter Jetter	1971-1981	Europe (1780-1840)	PPM, plans	History	Typological	Asylums as reform project
John D Thompson & Grace Goldin	1975	Europe (c1650-c1850)	PPM, plans, elevations	Architectural History	Typological	Asylums as reform project
Andrew Scull	1977-2015	England and Wales (c1800-c1900)	PR, PPM, plans	History	Documentary research, building analysis	Asylums initially conceived as utopias but ultimately become warehouses for the unwanted
Tom Brown	1980	Canada (1792-1910)	PR, PPM, photographs, plans	History	Documentary research, building analysis	Asylums idealised therapeutic spaces that failed to live up to ideal in practice
Thomas A Markus	1982-1993	Scotland and Europe (1780-c1850)	PPM, plans, elevations	Architectural History	Spatial analysis diagrams and contemporary commentary analysis	Asylums as reform project
Michael Donnelly	1983	Britain (1790-1850)	PPM, plans	History	Analysis of buildings and contemporary commentary	Asylums as reform project
Chris Philo	1987-2004	England and Wales (c1250- 1870)	PPM, plans	Historical Geography	Analysis of buildings and contemporary commentary	Spatial location of asylums with reference to rural/urban dyad, spatial organisation within and of asylum buildings
Harriet Richardson	1988-2010	Scotland (1729-c1970) England and Wales (1660-1948)	PR, PPM, plans, elevations, photographs	Architectural History	Typological	Development of asylum types over time, emphasis on architecturally outstanding buildings
Jeremy Taylor	1991-1995	England and Wales (1840-1914)	PPM, plans, elevations, photographs	Architectural History	Typological	Development of asylum types over time, emphasis on architecturally outstanding buildings
Markus Reuber	1994-1999	Ireland (1600-1922)	PR, PPM, plans, elevations, photographs	History	Typological	Development of asylum types in relation to ideas about treatment
Barry Edginton	1994-1999	England (1792-1914)	PR, PPM, plans, elevations, photographs	History	Analysis of buildings in relation to medical discourses	Influence of 'moral treatment' on asylum design
Christine Stevenson	1997-2000	England (1660-1815)	PPM, plans, elevations	Architectural History	Analysis of buildings in relation to social and cultural discourses	Asylum architecture and spaces informed by a variety of concerns: aesthetic, therapeutic and functional
Leslie Topp	1997-2017	Austro-Hungarian Empire (1890-1914)	PR, PPM, plans, elevations, photographs	Architectural History	Documentary research, building analysis	Asylums as embodiments of socio-medical values such as freedom and progress.
Diana Gittins	1998	England (1913-1997)	PR, PPM, interviews, plans, elevations, photographs	History	Oral history and building analysis	Asylums are responded to in varying ways, both positively and negatively, by patients and staff.
Leonard D Smith	1999-2007	England (1750-1820)	PR,PPM, elevations	History	Documentary research	Asylums had impressive façades with more prison-like facilities behind
Johann Louw and Sally Swartz	2001-2007	South Africa (c1850-c1920)	PR, PPM, plans elevations	History	Documentary research, building analysis	Asylum spaces as expressions of therapeutic ideas, colonial discourses and white/black segregation
Susan Piddock	2001-2016	Britain and Australia (1800-1880)	PR, PPM, site visits, plans, elevations, photographs	Historical Archaeology	Documentary research, building analysis	Asylums often fail to correspond to psychiatric ideals

9

Scholar	Year	Location and period of study	Sources (PR= Primary records PPM= Primary published material)	Discipline	Methodology	Interpretation of asylum environments
Svein Atle Skålevåg	2002	Norway (1820-1920)	PPM, plans, elevations	History	Analysis of buildings and contemporary discourses	Asylums as therapeutic, reflecting changing ideals in psychiatry from moral to somatic treatment
Carla Yanni	2003-2007	United States (1770-1900)	PR,PPM, plans and elevations, photographs	Architectural History	Analysis of buildings and contemporary discourses	Asylums as therapeutic environments, developing over time
Sarah Rutherford	2003-2008	England (1808-1914)	PR, PPM, maps, plans	Landscape History	Analysis of landscapes and building layouts	Asylums (buildings and grounds) as designed landscapes of a therapeutic nature.
Mary Guyatt	2004	England (1880-1914)	PPM, photographs	History	Analysis of interiors and contemporary discourses	Asylum interiors as homely and calming
Clare Hickman	2005-2013	England (1800-1860)	PR, PPM, photographs	Landscape History	Analysis of contemporary discourses	Asylum landscapes as therapeutic.
Elizabeth Malcolm	2009	Australia (1850-1890)	PPM, plans, photographs, elevations	History	Analysis of contemporary discourses	Kew asylum as well meant but out of date and inadequate in practice
Alison Darragh	2011	Scotland (1781-1930)	PR, PPM, plans, maps, photographs	Architectural history	Typological	Asylums as therapeutic environments, development of designs over time.
Peta Longhurst	2011-2017	Australia (1835-2003)	PPM, plans, photographs, site visits	Historical Archaeology	Analysis of buildings and contemporary discourses	Asylums fail to live up to psychiatric ideals due to factors such as economics. Dissonance is responded to by tolerance, mitigation and finally abandonment.
Katherine Fennelly	2012-2019	England and Ireland (1808-c1850)	PR, PPM, site visits, plans, photographs	Historical Archaeology	Analysis of buildings and documentary records to reconstruct soundscapes	Sound control in asylums related to paternalistic, moral ideas of insanity and reform
Jane Hamlett	2013-2015	England (1845-1914)	PR, PPM, plans, photographs	History	Documentary research and analysis of contemporary discourses	Emotional role of environment in the creation of a 'home' and modifying behaviour
Juliet L H Foster	2013	England	Secondary Sources	Psychology	Literature Review	Asylum buildings as a source for understanding changing attitudes towards mental health
Kim A Ross	2014	Scotland	PR, PPM, site visits, plans, photographs	Historical Geography	Documentary research and analysis of contemporary discourses	Asylums as engineered environments producing docile subjects. Evolution of siting and design over time.
Rebecca McLaughlan	2014-2016	New Zealand	PR, PPM, site visits, plans, photos	History	Documentary and building analysis	Asylums a compromised attempt to meet needs of mentally ill
Charlotte Newman	2015	England	Artefacts, plans, photographs	Historical Archaeology	Analysis of artefacts and contemporary discourses	Private madhouse shows material evidence of a high quality interior, spaces also show evidence of control

would enable the claims made by asylum authorities to be tested. Most asylum studies rely heavily on contemporary published and documentary evidence to which the sites and buildings provide support, rather than the reverse, in which sites and buildings are given priority. Scholarship relating to the study of buildings, and built environments more broadly, are assessed in the following section, as this constitutes a critique of some of the approaches usually taken.

1.4. Buildings archaeology and buildings theory

Buildings archaeology is a relatively new sub-discipline within the field of archaeology,[1] that has appropriated the analysis of upstanding buildings as a legitimate field of archaeological enquiry. Buildings archaeology began with a concern for the accurate and meaningful recording of upstanding structures, but was always interdisciplinary in nature, drawing on architectural history, social and cultural history and folk-life studies among others (Johnson 2010:10-11; Arnold et al. 2006). As a discipline it has shifted rapidly from a purely descriptive mode to include an emphasis on interpretation (Newman 2010: 2), placing buildings in their craft and design tradition, but also contextualising them socially and culturally (Leech, 2006). The recognition that buildings survey can only ever be partial and subjective and must therefore be informed by an understanding of meaning and significance has been critical to the development of the discipline (Giles, 2014).

Several scholars outside the field of archaeology have sought to address the shortcomings of other disciplines in relation to the understanding of buildings as socially and historically located structures. The work of French cultural theorists, Bourdieu, Foucault and Lefebvre has been influential. They have made links between the spatial and the conceptual, be it Bourdieu's structuralist division of domestic space according to North African cosmology, Foucault's use of the 'panopticon' as metaphor for the mechanism of power or Lefebvre's concept of the reproduction of society through the social production of urban space (Bourdieu, 1970, Lefebvre, 1991). All these approaches are heavily influenced by Marxist theory and are subject to criticism, not only because they apparently minimise agency, but also because they tend to suppress mid-level cultural phenomena, as discussed below. Giddens' 'denial of structure' has been critiqued for its **over**-emphasis of human agency, however (Storper, 1985). Thomas Gieryn has suggested that neither agency nor structure dominate in social reproduction, and we should see buildings, not as the objects of human agency but as in themselves agents of social reproduction, with which we are involved in a 'recursive relationship of mutual constitution and presupposition'(Gieryn 2002: 36). In other words, the social meaning of buildings extends beyond what was intended, and this is not to minimise the

intention but also to recognise that built space constrains social and cultural interaction. Buildings may hide as much as they reveal, including 'the many possibilities that did not get built, as they bury the interests, politics and power that shaped the one design that did' (Gieryn 2002: 39). Gieryn concludes that buildings analysis 'must respect the double reality of buildings, as structures structuring agency but never beyond the potential restructuring by human agents'(Gieryn 2002: 41). Gieryn identifies three ways in which buildings structure social action, by making material 'demands and expectations' that society must submit to in order to satisfy their own needs and wants; by 'concealing the politics and interests inherent in their design behind interpretative registers that focus on instrumental efficiency, cost or possibly aesthetics'; and by stabilizing social action due to the cost and difficulty of subsequent alterations (Gieryn 2002: 43-44). Gieryn's concept of 'interpretative flexibility' reminds us that the meaning of buildings is 'contingent and variable' and is not to be thought of as fully determined by the designers or the attributes of the building itself. However, Gieryn's case study makes plain the ahistorical nature of his sociological understanding, which is detached from the cultural context of architecture and science. William Whyte (2006) takes further the question of buildings and meaning, with a more historically-situated interpretation of 'architecture as evidence'. Whyte notes that buildings are frequently likened to texts to be 'read' as a code or language, but suggests instead that we should think of buildings as comprising a series of transpositions whose meaning changes over time and must be translated. He notes that buildings have been widely understood to be meaningful in a way that goes beyond structure and function and which articulates ideas, emotions, beliefs and social and cultural values. Buildings are frequently seen to embody meaning by expressing the 'spirit of the age' in which they were built. However, their complexity makes any methodology for 'reading' them elusive. Buildings are functional, ornamental, symbolic. They are three-dimensional art forms, which must obey the laws of physics and stand rather than fall, carrying out the practical purpose for which they were built. Further the historian or archaeologist of buildings has access to a range of sources beyond the building itself, including primary and secondary written sources and representations of the building in drawings, maps, plans and photographs, all of which raise methodological issues. Whyte asks how historians can be sure 'that they are accurately interpreting the subject' and are not in fact projecting on to architecture the meanings they expect to find. The metaphor of language has, he argues, been used to imply that built forms are straightforwardly legible in a way which is not justified (Whyte 2006: 165-7). The way they are interpreted will change 'through time and among cultures' and therefore historians must 'study buildings within their context, examining how they relate both to their immediate environment and to their wider culture' and noting how they were received by contemporaries and used by those they were built for. This 'diversity of focus' together with the 'multidimensionality of buildings' means that architecture cannot be compared to a text but should

---

[1] The first academic volume on the topic was published in 1994 (Wood and Chitty, 1994), the first Masters' degree in the subject was established in York c2000, and the Buildings Archaeology Group was reformed as a special interest group of the Institute for Archaeologists in 2003.

rather be seen as an idea translated to plan, drawing and then building. These are a series of genres with differing conventions and specific logics. These genres are linked by a 'series of transpositions', which 'shape each artefact, and inevitably influence he final product of the process, the building itself'. Whyte suggests that historians use 'every possible piece of evidence' to explore the evolution of the building with an awareness of the logic of each genre and the changes and transformations that occur between genres, leading to a multiplicity of meanings.

The privileging of textual over material sources that is seen in much historical work has been questioned by Andrew Ballantyne, who suggests that buildings, because costly and time-consuming to produce, can be a better guide to the value-system of a society than words: 'What people say they care about, in their conversation or in their books, is one kind of evidence for the system of values in a society, but a better guide to what they really believe is to look at how they act [i.e what they build]' (Ballantyne 2006: 37). Furthermore, buildings as material objects and works of art, can be resonant in a multiplicity of ways that can be harder to find in texts, particularly the kind of texts that are produced by scientists, managers and administrators and form the bulk of historical primary sources.

1.5. Approach taken in this study

Several disciplines and sub-disciplines have taken on the study of asylums, their culture and materiality, including archaeology, architectural history, medical and social history and historical geography. It has been argued here that the potential for the study of asylum buildings to inform our understanding of their social context and, equally, the potential of their social context to inform our understanding of asylum buildings has, so far, been under-explored. A positioning of asylums with prisons and workhouses as emblems of control within the progress of industrial capitalism has only limited explanatory power in assessing these buildings. Other broad socio-cultural movements may be at least as important to an analysis of asylum buildings, such as changes in attitudes to insanity and personal liberty associated with the Enlightenment, and the moral, intellectual and physical betterment of the self and of the environment associated with what has been termed the 'Age of Improvement'. With regard to the latter concept, Sarah Tarlow has pointed to the reductionism of the historical archaeology of capitalism, which seeks to reduce all human practices to the 'exercise, legitimation, manipulation or rejection of power relationships of inequality'. Tarlow suggests that there are other concepts which are at least as significant in shaping the material world, such as beliefs, aspirations and cultural values (Tarlow 2007: 9).

This study argues that asylum buildings should be seen not only in the context of providing a solution to the problem of unproductive, undisciplined bodies, but that the discursive construction of asylums as an enlightenment project, tending towards increased liberty and therapeutic care for the insane, can be further elaborated as an explanatory paradigm. The 'improvement' of the working classes through specific types of constructed environment should also be taken into account when analysing asylum buildings. All these macro-level concepts can be historically situated within the late-nineteenth-century/early-twentieth-century historical moment, in which concepts of degeneration, leading to the nascent pseudo-science of eugenics together with a resurgent environmentalism, were strongly influential on the types of buildings and landscapes that were deemed suitable for the insane poor. This study also proposes local variations in asylum building schemes, suggesting that the colony asylums built in Scotland and the north of Ireland differed substantively from those deemed suitable south of the border, due to cultural variations that are not explicable in terms of an appeal only to 'capitalism' or 'enlightenment' as explanatory contexts.

The analysis of asylum plans and elevations has generally been founded upon an interest in the topics of surveillance, sequestering of the insane, rural surroundings, classification/segregation of patients and the part played by hygienic considerations such as light and air in asylum buildings. Architecture and layouts have generally not been analysed in any systematic way, however, with heavy reliance being placed on written sources for interpreting the character of the asylum environment and what should be considered significant. Buildings and environments are not usually given primacy as evidence, but act to support the documentary record. This means that the interpretation of environments tends to rely on a rationale which is internal to medical discourses and either adopts or critiques the point of view of the asylum builders. Attitudes and allusions which are betrayed or suggested by material culture and written sources but not explicitly stated, are not generally explored. Later work has addressed these issues to some extent. Stevenson, in particular, makes sensitive assessments of asylum architecture which allude to how forms are linked to their social and cultural context. Hamlett has suggested that asylum interiors should be seen in the context of the development of middle-class interiors in which objects were often treated as having a moralising character, thus connecting the material world of the asylum to the society in which they were situated. However, the literature is often driven by the conflict and interplay between medical discourse (micro scale) and structures of power (macro scale) without giving sufficient consideration to the meso scale of asylum materiality as an embodiment of social and cultural trends as these change over time.

Studies of asylum environments are often based on a few example institutions, especially those relating to English asylums, which account for the majority of the scholarship. It is challenging, therefore, to position example institutions within a broader framework, where they can be understood as more or less typical of each period and to make generalisations about how asylums developed over the nineteenth century, particularly whether or not their interior environments became more or less 'domestic' or 'hygienic'.

Hamlett has suggested that cultural history is now moving away from a 'supposed dichotomy between representation and reality' and is instead exploring the reach of such representations and how they affect materiality and practices' (Hamlett 2015: 15). This is very pertinent for the study of asylums, which has tended to rely on a supposed 'failure' of the asylum in practice to live up to the intentions and ideals proposed at mid nineteenth century.

Asylum environments did not achieve the rates of cure that were proposed, and regimes which were supposed to be gentle and caring were apt to become abusive and neglectful. However, asylum culture and materiality can also be interpreted in its own terms, as a product of and a contributor to medical and other discourses and an authentic representation of those discourses. If asylums do not adhere to the prescriptions in contemporary psychiatric literature, we must consider what influences and motivations **did** influence their construction, whether explicit or implicit.

This study starts from the assumption that buildings have a multiplicity of meanings and that at least some of these meanings can be accessed, by the historical archaeologist, using the evidence of the building itself, its architectural style, layout and interior spaces, as well as its positioning in the landscape and relative to other structures. The historical archaeologist also makes use of primary sources relating to the building, such as elevations and plans; sources relating to the architects, builders and other authorities engaged in the construction and published sources which convey the cultural context in which the building is situated, but the buildings and environments themselves are given considerable weight in any interpretation. Materiality may offer a validation for one discourse over another, where competing viewpoints exist, and can give weight to an opinion that may be difficult to discern within documentary materials. Additionally, the material world sometimes betrays attitudes that cannot be easily expressed verbally, are contradictory, or alternatively so entrenched that they are no longer apparent to the holder.

'Meaning' in the context of buildings can be seen as the connotations of building structure, style, layouts, spaces and siting that go beyond the physical description of parts and connect the building to contemporary culture by defining what they represent. For example, a window, may have a literal meaning as a (usually glazed) opening in a wall that admits light and/or air. However, it may also express or represent a multitude of further aspects of contemporary culture that are not unconnected to its physical form but situate it as a product of its particular time and place. The style, size and shape of the window and its positioning relative to others may indicate a concern with architectural fashion, its size and orientation may also suggest a concern with the therapeutic qualities of light and air. The style and size of windows may symbolize a connection with the

domestic rather than the carceral as conceived at a certain time period. It may also represent, through the admission of light, a commitment to therapeutic care on the part of asylum authorities and a public assertion of a particular asylum as a space of humane treatment.

Fundamental to the understanding of culture, as it relates to materiality in the past, is that it is *particular* to a certain place in the world and to a certain period of history, and that therefore present day understandings of insanity, and poverty cannot be transposed backwards in time and must be redefined by reference to contemporary cultural artefacts. This study also argues that the culture of asylum building and management (if not the subsequent inhabitation of the asylum) is particular to a certain class stratum, namely the educated middle classes composed of architects, doctors, councillors and others and is largely limited to the male gender, being informed by these partial perspectives. This study does not attempt to reconstruct patients' perspectives through their voices, which are very much subdued due to the nature of surviving evidence relating to the asylum project, but neither are patients absent from this account. Patients are here seen as culturally constructed through the discursive (material and textual) practices of the Asylum Age,[2] and this is inescapable, however their voices may be or not be recorded.

The powered nature of institutional care underwrites this approach to interpreting the asylum. The materiality of asylum remains form part of a construction by asylum authorities through whom wider cultural forces take shape, the material remains expressing and representing a concept of asylum inhabitants, which, it is argued, constituted them in relation to late-nineteenth-century concepts of domesticity, individuality, hygiene and degeneration. The emphases in buildings and layouts, supported by documentary and contemporary published materials constitutes the patient as a defined presence, subject to ideological definition.

1.6. Methodology

Early scholars of the asylum environment, made use of plans, elevations and published contemporary materials, such as books, journal articles and parliamentary papers. Several early studies relied primarily upon contemporary published material, but later work has made increasing use of primary records including asylum minutes, reports and photographs. Site visits did not form part of the methodology used, until the systematic surveys of the 1990s and the advent of archaeological studies after 2000. The recording of buildings through site visits is generally not made a central part of the research, where such visits have occurred, often due to the fact that many asylum buildings are still in use as psychiatric facilities or have been repurposed. A few scholars have

---

[2] The Asylum Age is here used as a shorthand for the era of large-scale institutionalisation of the insane, commencing in the early to mid-nineteenth century across Europe and peaking in the 1950s.

used unusual methodologies, such as spatial analysis diagrams (Markus, 1993), oral history (Gittins, 1998) and artefactual analysis (Newman, 2015). The latter two clearly depend on the availability of and access to artefacts and informants. Markus's spatial analysis diagrams were not used in this study, as the buildings in this study are of a relatively simple character and ground plans were felt to be sufficient to show spatial relationships and access points.

An analytical approach to the material evidence is used in this study, combined with evidence drawn from primary unpublished sources and from contemporary published materials. Using this evidence, asylum buildings are situated within a particular cultural historical moment, as part of the broader context of the development of industrial capitalism, and of Enlightenment theories of liberty, individuality and improvement, but making a finer grained reading of the material evidence which also connects it to concerns particular to the period c1900, namely, degenerationism and environmentalism.

1.6.1. Material evidence

Choice of Sites

The sites chosen for study were:

- Purdysburn Villa Colony, Belfast, Northern Ireland
- Kingseat Asylum, Aberdeen, Scotland
- Bangour Village Asylum, Edinburgh, Scotland
- Dykebar Asylum, Renfrewshire, Scotland
- Whalley Asylum, Preston, Lancashire
- Alt Scherbitz Asylum, Leipzig, Germany

The sites in Ireland and Scotland were selected as the only examples of general colony asylums that were constructed in Britain and Ireland in the period before the First World War. Although some institutions were built on colony lines in England, as discussed in Chapter 2, these were usually charitable enterprises or built by Poor Law Guardians and catered only for a distinct sub-set of the asylum population, either epileptics or the cognitively impaired. Only one colony asylum was built by an asylum authority, (Ewell Epileptic Colony) and this was exclusively for epileptics. It was only in Scotland and the north of Ireland that the village or colony model was adopted for a general asylum population, and indeed in Scotland, the village was the only type of asylum that was built after the mid-1890s. The more enthusiastic adoption of the village model in Scotland, particularly, appears to have been a development that was distinct from the more cautious and tailored approach in England, and English colonies were therefore excluded from the study.

All the asylums chosen were public asylums for the insane poor built under the relevant legislation for each jurisdiction. Crichton Royal Lunatic Asylum, a charitable asylum near Dumfries, built a 'Third House', along colony lines in order to house their pauper patients during the period covered by this study. It was decided not to include this institution in the study because of the charitable nature of the asylum's administration which raised issues that set it apart from the public asylums at the core of the study. In addition, the colony was built on a pre-existing site, which meant that the location could not be analysed in the same way as the other sites.

Alt Scherbitz asylum, near Leipzig in Saxony was chosen as the earliest colony asylum in Europe and the model which Aberdeen and Bangour Village explicitly claimed to follow, architects and asylum authorities from Scotland, including the Lunacy Commissioner, having visited Alt Scherbitz from 1897 onwards. Although the influence of Alt Scherbitz on Purdysburn is not explicitly credited in asylum records, a local medical journal stated that Alt Scherbitz was the example being followed at Purdysburn (*Belfast Health Journal*, May 1901). The Scottish-trained medical superintendent of Purdysburn, William Graham, appears to have borrowed the term 'Villa Colony' from a Lancashire report which describes Alt Scherbitz and this was the term used at Purdysburn (and nowhere else) to describe the new asylum form (*Report of a Lancashire deputation*, 1900). Although other colony asylums existed in Germany by this period, Alt Scherbitz was the first and most influential. It is considered here, therefore, as the primary continental influence on Scottish and Irish colony asylums.

As discussed in Chapter 2, the majority of typological asylum studies do not take a comprehensive approach to sites and buildings, making comparison between asylum sites challenging. Because of this, it was decided to include in the study a traditional asylum built in Lancashire in the pre-war period, for the purposes of comparison. Whalley was chosen particularly because it was the result of a lengthy struggle within the Lancashire Asylums Board, many of whom wanted to build a colony asylum, and who were eventually over-ruled after some years, an asylum along more traditional lines being constructed instead. The decision-making process that took place with regard to Whalley clarifies some of the resistance to the colony system in England, and is included for comparison with Scotland. The overall layout used at Whalley was not typical of asylums constructed in England at this period, in fact, was comparatively old-fashioned, but the use of pavilions *was* typical and individual pavilions have been analysed as a comparator with asylum villas of the colony layout. Only further analytical study of asylum sites can clarify whether pavilions varied widely from site to site across England and Scotland.

Buildings – Desk Survey

The focus of the study is asylum buildings rather than landscapes. However, buildings are considered in their setting in terms of where the sites are situated and how buildings are distributed on the site. The location of all public asylums in Ireland and Scotland was determined and an approximate distance was plotted for each site from the nearest centre of habitation. This was then compared with all other asylum sites in Ireland and Scotland (1815-1914) in order to establish changes over time in the positioning of asylum sites relative to urban centres. Using ARCGIS and datasets obtained from Land and Property Services (Ireland), and EDINA Digimap (Scotland and England) a relief map was constructed for each site, allowing the position of each building relative to the detailed contour pattern of each site to be determined. Historic map evidence was used to analyse the layout and distribution of buildings on each site relative to other major features and to each other. Map evidence was used to compare asylum sites with other types of settlement form such as the garden city.

Buildings - Field Survey

Field survey was informed by an understanding, suggested by contemporary literature and secondary sources, of what were likely to have been important considerations in building construction. The focus was therefore on the following building features:

- Building size and dimensions
- Architectural style and ornamentation externally and internally
- Building materials, externally and internally
- Ventilation features such as ventilation grilles and turrets
- Lighting, size of windows and presence or absence of internal glazing
- Height of rooms and cubic area of internal space
- Layout of rooms internally

Although access was available to techniques such as photogrammetry and laser scanning, it was decided that less time-consuming and potentially disruptive techniques were more suitable, given such issues as the sensitivity of the sites (where still in use by psychiatric patients, or where the sites have been converted into housing) and the poor condition of many of the buildings. All of the required information was therefore obtained through direct observation, photography and measurement. In many cases, due either to the condition of the buildings or their occupancy, it was not possible to access interiors.

- Photographs were taken of all elevations, individual features and interior rooms where possible
- Measurements were taken of exterior wall lengths and heights, window and door sizes, ceiling heights and room sizes (where possible)
- Notes were taken on the phenomenology of the sites, vistas from various points and views through windows.

The data thus obtained was analysed in terms of two major principles:

- Function – how were the buildings constructed in order to perform their purpose both as homes for the mentally ill and as therapeutic environments?

- Implicit meanings – how could the building spaces, layouts and architecture be seen as connected to contemporary cultural values?

1.6.2. Textual and other non-material sources

The wider social and cultural context for the buildings was examined through the use of textual and other non-material sources, with the aim of exploring the connections of asylum buildings with concepts of:

- Insanity: how it was conceived of, dealt with and/or treated
- Class difference: how the poor were constructed through medical and other discourses
- Social utopianism: the connection of the asylum project with utopian social movements such as the labour colony and the garden city

Primary Records

For each asylum site a wealth of primary records was consulted, as set out in Table 2.

These primary records provided important data for site and building biographies, building construction and furnishings, building functions, and attitudes of architects, management committees and medical staff to the buildings, patients and staff.

Contemporary published material

A significant source of information for this study was a variety of contemporary published material which may be organised into the following categories:

- Government reports – The separate lunacy administrations of England and Wales, Scotland and Ireland produced separate annual reports, allowing approaches to be compared across jurisdictions. Reports of general government enquiries into insanity and the 'feeble minded' were also useful.
- Contemporary newspapers and journals – including national and local newspapers, and architectural journals.
- Medical Journals – particularly the *Journal of Mental Science, British Medical Journal* and *The Lancet*
- Longer contemporary works on medical topics, architecture and social and cultural themes

Published material was approached from both a quantitative and a qualitative perspective. Digital searches of books and journals established the frequency of occurrence of important terms, and the ways in which they were used and understood. Published material was qualitatively analysed as part of the relevant discourse. In other words, it is assumed that textual material is part of institutional (e.g. medical, class etc) attempts to constitute human subjects whether these be the insane, the working classes or any other group or class. A discursive approach

Table 2. Primary records consulted.

Site	Item	Where held
Purdysburn	Original plans of asylum buildings	Knockbracken Healthcare Park Estates Dept
	Asylum Annual Reports	Queen's University Belfast (QUB) Medical Library
	Management Committee Minutes	Public Record Office of Northern Ireland (PRONI)I
	Miscellaneous brochures, photographs etc	PRONI
Kingseat	Asylum Annual Reports	NHS Grampian Archives, University of Aberdeen
	ACDLB Minutes	Aberdeen Central Library
	Site photographs	Historic Environment Scotland
	Garden city archives	Herts Archives and Local Studies; Garden City Collection, Letchworth
Bangour Village	Asylum Annual Reports	Lothian Health Services Archive, University of Edinburgh
	EDLB Minutes	Lothian Health Services Archive, University of Edinburgh
	Site photographs	Historic Environment Scotland
	Historic photographs	Lothian Health Services Archive, University of Edinburgh
	Plans	National Records of Scotland
Dykebar	Asylum Annual Reports	NHS Greater Glasgow and Clyde Archives, Mitchell Library, Glasgow
	Renfrew District Lunacy Board Minutes	NHS Greater Glasgow and Clyde Archives, Mitchell Library, Glasgow
	Site photographs	Historic Environment Scotland
Alt Scherbitz	Site photographs and maps	Altscherbitz Traditionskabinett
Whalley	Lancashire Asylum Board Minutes	Lancashire Archives, Preston
	Plans	Lancashire Archives, Preston
General Background	Contemporary publications on madness, architecture and cultural and social movements	QUB Medical Library, British Library, Wellcome Library, RIBA Library, Linenhall Library, archive.org

to texts is sceptical about their claims to truth and assumes that the way we think and act is structured by them. It assumes that texts (and indeed images) can be analysed for their use of words or other representations in constructing a particular social world (Rose 2011: 136). For example, characterisations of the insane poor as 'animal-like' or lacking in individuality are a part of a discursive formation which entails certain kinds of practices in addressing the 'problems' that have been discursively created. Sources were analysed using the methodology outlined by Gillian Rose, which sets out the following steps:

1. looking at your sources with fresh eyes
2. immersing yourself in your sources
3. identifying key themes in your sources
4. examining their effects of truth
5. paying attention to their complexity and contradictions
6. looking for the invisible as well as the visible
7. paying attention to details (Rose 2011: 158)

Having identified contemporary discourses, links were made to asylum materiality, while recognising that the 'meaning' of any text or building is unlikely to be amenable to linear, correlative strategies which connect, for example, the specific shape and size of windows to ideas such as 'health', 'surveillance' or 'economy'.

Discourse analysis acknowledges the complexity of the connections between material practices and texts and the tendency of both words and built structures to be resonant, evocative and discursively powerful.

1.7. Discussion and conclusion

The methodology was chosen in order to achieve several objectives. A systematic, analytical approach was taken to the physical evidence, namely buildings and their setting, with due weight given to material remains. This allows some of the claims made by medical discourses to be assessed against what was constructed and how it was constructed, noting the precise ways in which medical priorities were enacted. Although archaeological method, in terms of site visits and analysis of materiality, is the means of investigation chosen, this study is interdisciplinary in the sense that previous scholarship from many disciplines has been built upon, and, in particular, a spatial awareness familiar to historical geographers has been vital for the understanding of spatial location and layouts. The firm grounding given by assessment of buildings through site visits, which allows the authenticity of photographic and documentary representations of asylum buildings to be assessed, and the gaps in these representations to be filled, is used as a starting point for the evaluation of the ways in which asylum environments are connected both to medical discourses and to wider social currents. Documentary and contemporary published evidence has been used in order to seek and pinpoint links to broad cultural trends such as Enlightenment approaches to insanity, individual liberty and Improvement and to particular early twentieth-century manifestations of movements such as degenerationism and environmentalism. But buildings themselves are also considered as part of medical and social discourses relative to the poor insane. In this sense, buildings are not only functional, but also symbolic and representational, and these two aspects frequently overlap and intertwine. An assessment of buildings in the field is of particular use in assessing historiographical claims that asylums were built as warehouses for the unwanted. These claims depend on the assumption that asylum authorities glossed over the true nature of asylum accommodation and that therefore documentary sources must be viewed with some suspicion as self-serving. An assessment of the material nature of asylum accommodation allows these claims to be tested.

The analysis of medical discourses entirely through published and documentary material tends to lead to an understanding of psychiatric thought at this period as uniform and monolithic. The appearance of substantial regional differences in the type and styles of asylum being built is a starting point for an awareness of potential local variations in discourses relating to the insane poor. Although segregation of accommodation is understood to be a feature of asylum evolution during the early twentieth century, site visits provide a much more immediate and direct means, than the study of plans and elevations, of understanding the effect that was intended by asylum builders. However, the effects and uses of asylum buildings as cultural objects cannot solely be attributed to intentions and a synthesis of material and documentary evidence is used to access more implicit meanings of architecture and spaces. Materiality is seen here as representing discourses of various kinds, going far beyond the medical, and adding a deeper dimension to a textual study of the early twentieth-century moment in the social organisation of the insane poor.

2

Historical Background

This chapter outlines the establishment and development of large-scale institutionalisation of the insane during the course of the nineteenth and early twentieth centuries by making use of existing scholarship supplemented by primary sources, where necessary. Each jurisdiction, England and Wales, Ireland, Scotland and Germany is treated separately, beginning with an assessment of pre-asylum treatment of the insane, followed by an outline of the progression of asylum provision across each country. The introduction of colony asylums is identified in each jurisdiction, and this is further elaborated by two final sections, the first of which considers colonisation of the poor as a nineteenth-century phenomenon with its roots in utopian communities and Improvement ideology; the second section examining contemporary medical understandings of insanity.

2.1. Introduction

It is generally agreed, that across Europe before the Enlightenment, the insane were treated within institutions in ways that ran the gamut from neglect to physical violence. Assumed to be insensitive to their surroundings, accounts abound of individuals who were kept in unlit, unheated and filthy cells, if institutionalised; or beaten and taunted, if at liberty. Enlightenment reformers reported conditions that seemed increasingly shocking as awareness and sympathy grew for the plight of a social grouping that were characterised as uniquely deserving and badly treated (Thompson & Goldin 1975: 53). More enlightened care of the insane is usually dated to the end of the eighteenth century and, in particular, the work of Vincenzo Chiarugi in Italy, Pinel in Paris, the Tukes in England and the Romantic psychiatry movement in Germany, headed by Johann Reil (Porter 1996: 291-2). Pinel, in particular, has achieved a mythic significance for the history of psychiatry. His alleged 'striking off the chains' of patients during the revolutionary period in France is allegorical both for the treatment of the insane and for the establishment of popular freedom and enlightened thought in general (Weiner, 1994). At the Salpetrière (for women) and the Bicêtre (for men), accommodation was organised into ranges of small cells or 'loges' which opened onto a communal courtyard, and in which close attention was paid to ventilation, and heating was provided in winter. Pinel was one of the first to advocate for moral authority rather than 'mechanical restraint' and physical coercion in the treatment of the insane, and to develop a system for placing patients in dedicated areas of the institution according to the nature of their condition (Thompson & Goldin 1975: 56-9). The reform movement called for humane, regulated, institutional provision for the insane, particularly the insane poor, and legislation was subsequently enacted to establish networks of public asylums across Europe, starting with Ireland in

1821. France and Switzerland followed suit (1838), then England and Wales (1845), Norway (1848) and Belgium (1850) (Reuber 1994:70). Other European countries, such as Germany, did not enact legislation but nevertheless began to provide networks of institutions for the insane poor during the early to mid-nineteenth century.

2.2. England and Wales

The most comprehensive survey of English hospital and asylum architecture has been that of the former Royal Commission on the Historical Monuments of England which carried out a survey of hospital buildings in England and Wales between 1991 and 1995 including many of the asylums listed in Table 3. The Survey's primary records now form part of the archives of English Heritage (National Monuments Register). However, the published report of the survey (Richardson et al., 1998), covers only selected examples of asylum buildings and it is difficult to draw firm conclusions from this about what was usual for the asylum movement as a whole, or exceptional for individual sites. The following account, therefore, is based on a number of sources both primary and secondary. Among primary sources, Lunacy Commissioners' Reports are critical for detailed statistical information and a record of architectural changes. A desk-based survey of the maps, photographs and plans, where available, has been carried out for several asylums in order to assess the nature of asylum architecture at a number of key sites and periods. A number of secondary sources were particularly helpful, notably Jeremy Taylor's survey of hospital and asylum architecture in England, although this is also selective in its approach (Taylor, 1991; Richardson et al., 1998). Some online sources have also been useful, particularly Historic England's listed buildings sites (https://historicengland. co.uk and www.pastscape.org.uk), the Middlesex University-hosted asylums index (www.studymore.co.uk) and the County Asylums site (www.countyasylums.co.uk).

2.2.1. Institutional care of the insane prior to public asylums

As elsewhere, the insane poor in England and Wales were usually not differentiated from other types of social undesirable in the period prior to the end of the eighteenth century. The vast majority were not incarcerated in any kind of institution, while prisons, poorhouses and infirmaries provided accommodation for those who were exceptionally needy or troublesome (Scull 1993:2). However, England was the home of one of the first charitable institutions dedicated to the care of the insane, which became a model for buildings across Britain and Ireland, and beyond, Bethlehem Hospital in London (later known as Bethlem, and colloquially as Bedlam) (Andrews *et al.*, 1997).

Bethlem Hospital was founded as a priory in 1247 and the insane were confined there from at least the early fifteenth century, but the building which became influential for asylum architecture was constructed in 1676 to designs by Robert Hooke, and was rebuilt to a broadly similar plan in 1815 (Taylor 1991: 134) (Figures 2-1, 2-2). The Bethlem of 1815 resembled many other types of large public and

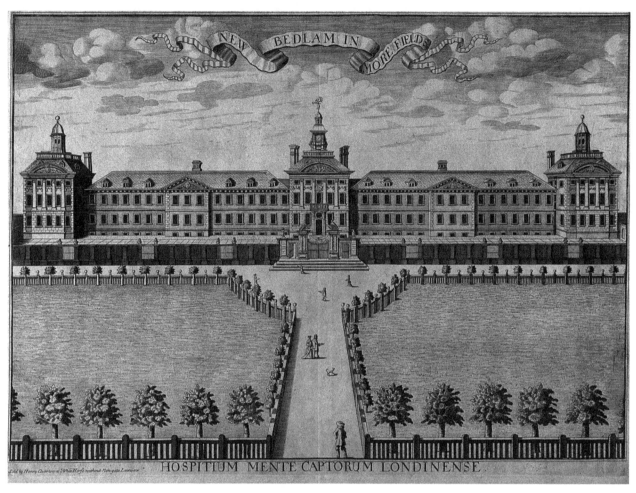

Figure 2-1. The hospital of Bethlem [Bedlam] at Moorfields (built c1676): the entrance façade. Engraving by A Soly. Source: Wellcome Collection Attribution 4.0 International (CC BY 4.0).

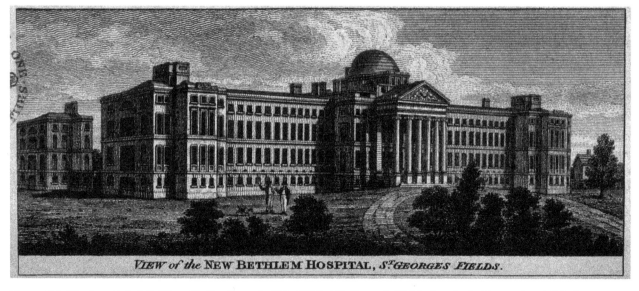

Figure 2-2. The hospital of Bethlem [Bedlam] as rebuilt in 1815 at St George's Fields, Lambeth. Engraving, 1816. Source: Wellcome Collection Attribution 4.0 International (CC BY 4.0).

private building at the period, from barracks to palaces, with a wide and dominating, multi-bay public façade focussed on a classical central block with projecting bays terminating each wing. The architectural function of the exterior was to demonstrate the wealth and charity of those who had contributed towards its construction and maintenance (Stevenson, 1997). The interior of the building was structured around a lengthy corridor or gallery which provided the means of exercising in bad weather. Patients were accommodated in small rooms or cells, and dayrooms were provided at the end of each corridor. Exterior spaces were divided into walled 'airing grounds' where patients could take the air and the central block provided rooms for the superintendent, medical staff and 'keepers'. Accommodation was strictly divided along gender lines with no access to the female accommodation

except through the central block (Yanni, 2007: 17-20). This 'corridor' model of asylum was to provide, with some exceptions, the principal model of asylum architecture throughout England, Wales, Scotland and Ireland until c1870, although it was often modified by the arrangement of corridors into a U or H shape or punctuated by a series of cross-wings.

Other early dedicated asylums for the insane were the Bethel Hospital in Norwich (1713), the Manchester Royal Lunatic Hospital (1763), Newcastle (1769), St Luke's in London (1751, rebuilt in 1786) (Figure 2-3), York (Bootham Park) asylum (1777), Liverpool (1792), Leicester (1794), Hereford (1799), St Thomas's Hospital, Exeter (1801) and Nottingham (1812) (Figure 2-4). The majority of these charitable establishments were for less than 100 patients,

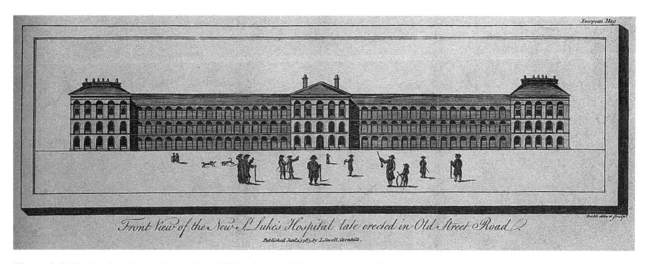

Figure 2-3. Nottingham Lunatic Asylum (1812). Source: Blackner, John (1815) *The History of Nottingham from the earliest antiquity to the present time.*

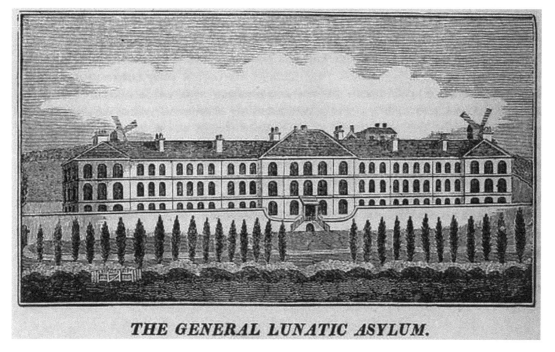

Figure 2-4. St Luke's Hospital, Cripplegate, London (built 1751, rebuilt 1786). Engraving by W. Deeble, 1785. Source: Wellcome Collection Attribution 4.0 International (CC BY 4.0).

and often adopted the same classical style and corridor plan as Bethlem (Figure 2-2). Many insane poor continued to be incarcerated in prisons, cared for in workhouses or infirmaries. From the seventeenth century onwards private madhouses began to be established and from 1774 they were required to be licensed, providing by this time the majority of accommodation for the insane. However, reformers became increasingly critical of the way that the insane were housed. For example, John Howard enumerated the lunatics held in prisons and campaigned for them to have separate and more suitable accommodation relative to convicted criminals (Howard, 1791). There were a total of 50 licensed private establishments in 1800, none of which, at first required medical supervision for patients, although following a series of Acts from the 1820s, this became a requirement. Private asylums ranged in size from a handful of patients to c200 and catered for pauper as well as wealthier patients, the former being maintained by the parish (Porter 2002: 95-97). By far the most influential private asylum for the insane was the Retreat at York, built in 1796 by the Quaker William Tuke (Figure 2-5). The Quaker community had been distressed at the death of a Friend in unexplained circumstances at the asylum in York

and set out to provide a more enlightened form of care, centred on the improving influence of a 'Moral Governor', and basing the regime around the ideal of family care in a 'domestic' residence (Edginton, 1997). Although the Retreat was a relatively small establishment constructed for around 30 patients, it also followed the corridor plan, with patient sleeping and dayrooms provided each side of a main corridor, and walled airing courts to the rear (Figure 2-6). Externally, however, it was understated relative to other asylums of the period, resembling a large middle-class dwelling house. The Retreat provided the model for enlightened psychiatric care at this period, and together with Pinel, the Tukes were invoked continually throughout the nineteenth century as the forefathers of a new chapter in the treatment of the insane. By the period of this study, none of the early asylums cited above accepted pauper patients, receiving only paying clients in premises that were generally smaller in scale than the county asylums. A handful of charitable asylums were built after the county asylum system was begun, but these also received only paying patients by the end of the century (E.g. Lincoln (1820), Oxford (1826)) (ELC Report, 1910: 258-265).

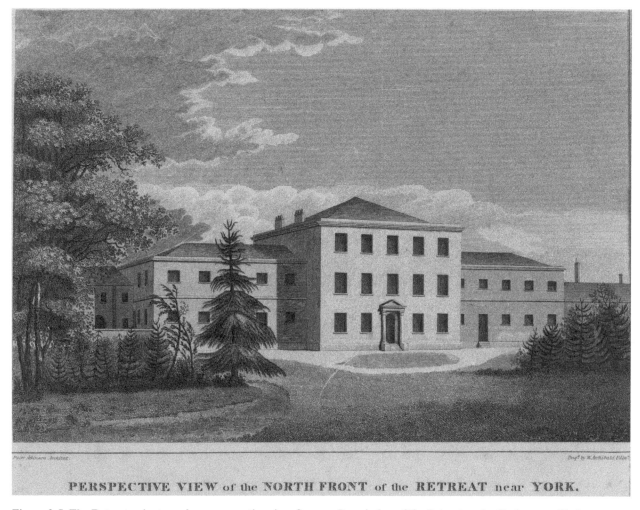

PERSPECTIVE VIEW of the NORTH FRONT of the RETREAT near YORK.

Figure 2-5. The Retreat private asylum, perspective view. Source: *Description of the Retreat, an institution near York, for insane persons of the Society of Friends: containing an account of its origin and progress, the modes of treatment, and a statement of cases.* **By Samuel Tuke. With an elevation and plans of the building. Wellcome Collection Attribution 4.0 International (CC BY 4.0).**

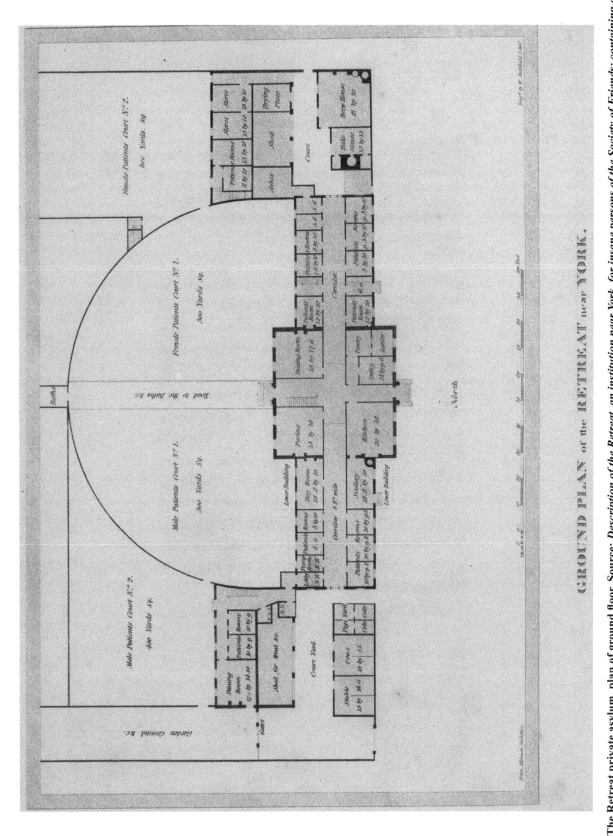

Figure 2-6. The Retreat private asylum, plan of ground floor. Source: *Description of the Retreat, an institution near York, for insane persons of the Society of Friends: containing an account of its origin and progress, the modes of treatment, and a statement of cases.* **By Samuel Tuke. With an elevation and plans of the building. Wellcome Collection Attribution 4.0 International (CC BY 4.0).**

23

2.2.2. Establishment of public asylum system

Following criticism of the conditions obtaining for the insane in existing accommodation, a 'permissive' Act of 1808 allowed justices to collect funds for the establishment of asylums and the care of the insane but only 15-17 county asylums were built as a consequence (Jones 1993: 60-64; Taylor 1991: 134; Edginton 1997: 92).[1] The Act specified that the site chosen for an asylum should be 'an airy and healthy situation, with a good supply of water, and which may afford the probability of the vicinity of constant medical assistance', but there were otherwise no direct specifications for asylum construction (Scull 1993: 88). A second County Asylums Act of 1845 made the provision of asylums compulsory. Some early asylums were financed by a combination of charitable donations and support by the rates, e.g. Nottingham, Stafford, Gloucester and Leicester, but this early tendency lapsed and later asylums were entirely publicly/rate funded (www.studymore. co.uk). The earliest county asylum to be built, Bedford, was demolished in the 1860s, and the earliest county asylums in Nottingham and Leicester had been taken out of service by 1910. Otherwise, most asylums built during the nineteenth century remained in use into the early decades of the twentieth century during a period of huge expansion in patient numbers—in the most severe cases, asylums that had originally been built for c100 were accommodating around eight to ten times that number by 1910 (e.g. Chester, Cornwall, Lancaster)(ELC Report 1910: 258-265). The expansion was managed by a combination of extension of existing buildings and the construction of several county asylums in some larger counties. For example, Yorkshire had five asylums, Lancashire built a total of six county asylums and London County Council constructed nine asylums, in the period up to 1915 (Board of Control Report 1916: 48). In addition, county borough asylums were constructed in the later decades of the nineteenth century in many counties with large urban centres. The tendency for asylum buildings to grow in size over time can make the interpretation of sites problematic, as the integrity of original designs can be compromised by later additions, and a variety of different styles and layouts may exist on a single site. When identifying the plan form of asylums, therefore, the assessments here are based on the earliest design. In some cases a clear plan form also emerges for later extensions but this is not always the case where later extension has been piecemeal (See Table 3). The majority of asylums of the first period of construction (1808 to 1845) were built to the corridor plan and were classical in the earlier period, moving to gothic later. For example, Lancaster's classical, pedimented central block and attached giant order, is surrounded by wings forming an enclosing U-shape, and represents a modification of the Bethlem style of asylum (Taylor, 1991: 134) (Figure 4-16). At the end of this period, gothic styles were more popular, as it became clear that asylums were likely to be added to over time (the gothic style being seen as more suited to gradual accretion). Shrewsbury Asylum is typical of this trend (Figure 2-7). However, several of the county asylums built in this period also show features which are likely to

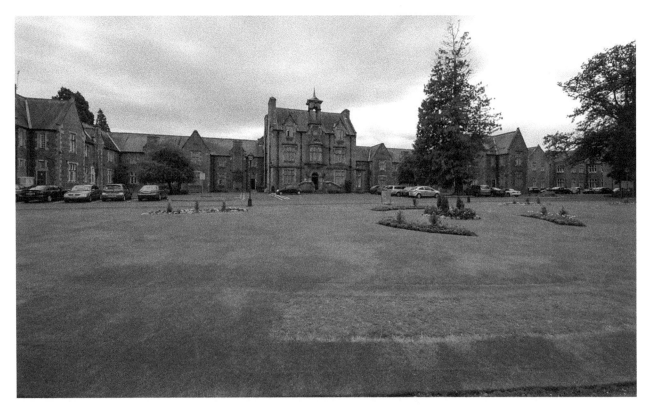

Figure 2-7. Shrewsbury Asylum (built 1845). Source: www.countyasylums.co.uk, reproduced with permission.

---

[1] The scholars cited differ as to the exact number of asylums built under the County Asylums Act (1808)

have been influenced by 'Moral treatment' as a form of asylum care. 'Panoptic' features emphasise the authority of the Moral Governor by placing him architecturally at the centre of the asylum regime and allowing his benign authority to be felt across the asylum structure (Edginton, 1997). Wakefield (1818), for example, featured panoptic hubs on each side of the central administration block from which patient corridors could be observed (Figure 2-8). A similar arrangement was in place at Hanwell (1831), where the central administration block had panoptic features and also featured panoptic hubs terminating each wing. Two asylums in the south-west, the Cornwall (1818) and Devon (1846) county asylums, were designed on a radial plan. Cornwall, the earlier of the two, presented six corridors attached to a central hub, but this was criticised by the architect for Devon asylum (Charles Fowler) who pointed out that the close connection of wings with the centre inhibited the circulation of air and the admission of light. The design also meant that all access to wards had to take place through the centre, which was therefore cut into by passages. His solution was to provide a circulating corridor in order to access wards without passing through the centre, diminishing the panoptic nature of the administration block but retaining its central significance to the plan (Figure 2-9). The compact nature of Fowler's design meant that wards were much more closely related to the centre than was the case in some corridor asylums, such as Hanwell, where dinners had to be delivered by horse and cart (Taylor 1991: 136-7). However, John Conolly, whose influential work on asylum construction, was published shortly after the opening of Devon County Asylum, criticised the early asylums for their resemblance to prisons, and advised that 'the external aspect of an asylum should be more cheerful than imposing, more resembling a well-built hospital than a place of seclusion or imprisonment'(Conolly 1847: 14). Although criticising his own place of work, Hanwell, for the unfavourable impression on newcomers made by the view into the panoptic centre as they arrived, he also comments favourably upon Hanwell's linear design, which allows full access to light and air. Following Conolly's publication and his emphasis on reducing the appearance of a prison in asylum architecture, radial and panoptic

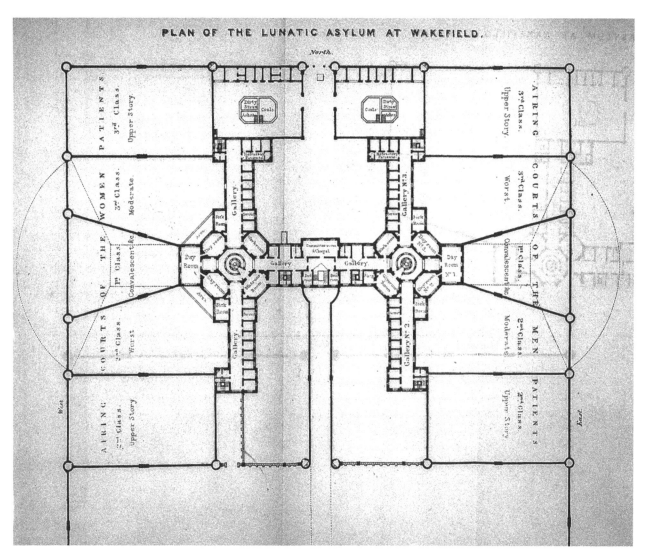

Figure 2-8. Wakefield Asylum built 1818. Source: *On the construction and management of hospitals for the insane; with a particular notice of the institution at Siegburg.* **By Dr.Maximilian Jacobi. Translated by John Kitching. With introductory observations, &c., by Samuel Tuke. Wellcome Collection Attribution 4.0 International (CC BY 4.0).**

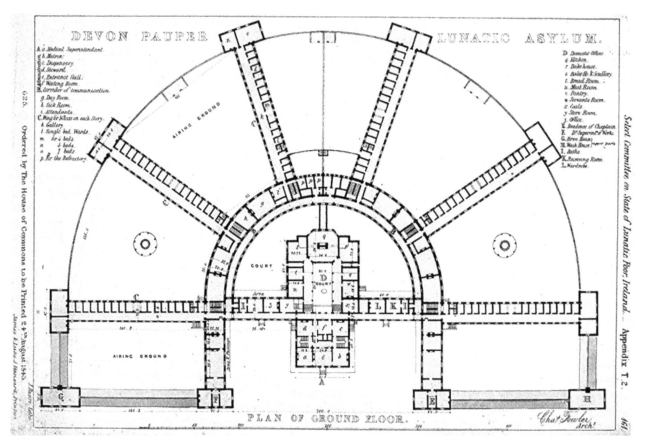

Figure 2-9. Devon County Lunatic Asylum ground floor plan. Source: *Select Committee of House of Lords on State of Lunatic Poor in Ireland* **(1843) Appendix T. Image from ProQuest's House of Commons Parliamentary Papers. Permission provided by ProQuest LLC**

designs fell out of favour. Radial designs had been common for prison architecture since the late eighteenth century and the radial plan for prisons continued to be popular well into the nineteenth century, giving it an irrevocable association with the carceral, in addition to its other perceived disadvantages (Evans, 1982:146). It should be noted that it is John Conolly's name that is associated with the doctrine of 'non-restraint' that, after mid-century, was taken to be a guiding principle of asylum care. This stipulated that 'mechanical' means for restraining patients should be avoided, an orderly and disciplined asylum ideally replacing the need to shackle or confine (Suzuki, 1995).[2]

The County Asylums Act of 1845 made the provision of county asylums compulsory, and brought them under the inspection of the Commissioners of Lunacy, who also approved asylum designs. The Act stimulated a much more extensive phase of asylum building and over 40 were built in the period up to 1875, almost entirely to corridor plans. The vast majority in the period 1845–1875 were built for between 100 and 500 patients. A very few larger asylums were built in the late 1860s and early

1870s (Surrey (1867, for 650), Chester (1871, for 640), York (West Riding) (1872, for 752), Lancaster (1873, for 1,000) and Kent (1875, for 905), but the largest and most expensive asylum to be built for some years was Colney Hatch, the asylum for Middlesex. Colney Hatch was built in 1851 for 1,255 patients to an Italianate style by Samuel Daukes and was a visitor attraction in the year of the Great Exhibition, proclaimed for its size and modernity (Taylor 1991:138). The building was constructed on the corridor principle but the wards were effectively separated into self-contained units connected by a corridor which ran externally to the front of the building, allowing the staff to access all wards and to reach the upper floors by means of regularly placed stair towers (Figure 2-10). This allowed a large number of patients to be efficiently categorised. The 'dayrooms' or ward corridors faced southwards with dining space provided in an alcove and patients' sleeping accommodation was divided into one-third single rooms and two-thirds four- to five-bed dormitories (Taylor 1991: 138). Another influential design which opened the same year, was Derby County Asylum for 360 patients (Figure 2-11). This asylum was identified by John Conolly as an ideal type, due in part to the arrangement of corridors and cross wings which meant that each ward was connected with the centre without the necessity of passing through the other wards. Corridor plans which had initially taken a simple linear form henceforward began to become increasingly complex with a variety of interconnecting

---

[2] According to Andrew Scull, it was actually Robert Gardiner Hill at Lincoln Lunatic Hospital who introduced the principle of non-restraint into the everyday running of the asylum in the late 1830s (Scull, 1985). However, Conolly has become irrevocably associated with the idea, due to his monograph on the subject published in 1856 (Conolly, 1856).

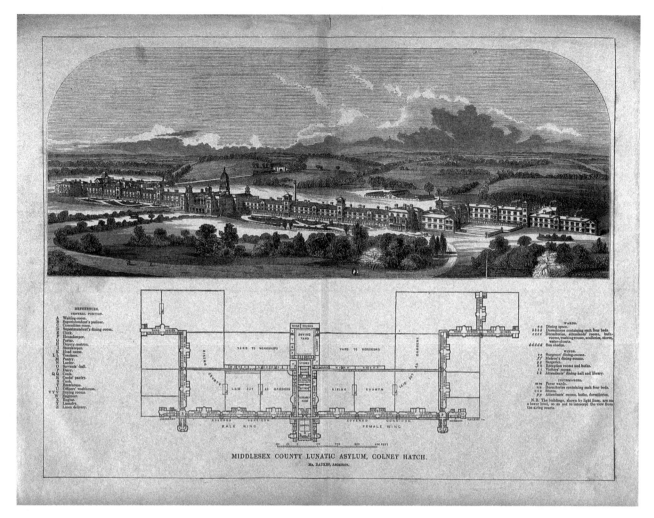

Figure 2-10. Middlesex County Lunatic Asylum, Colney Hatch: bird's eye view with detailed floor plan and key. Wood engraving by Laing after Daukes. Wellcome Collection Attribution 4.0 International (CC BY 4.0).

ranges, as in the Essex Asylum at Brentwood (1853) (Figure 2-12).

In 1856 the Commissioners issued 'Suggestions and Instructions' to guide architects in their asylum designs which suggested various potential economies in asylum provision including separate (and cheaper) accommodation for the orderly chronic, the introduction of third storeys of dormitories and the use of open fires and stoves rather than complex heating or ventilating systems. In addition, the Commissioners recommended the building of detached blocks for working and convalescing patients which, it was hoped, would give them greater freedom, self-respect and self-control leading to more rapid cure (ELC 1856: 26-28). By 1867, detached blocks are noted at Kent, Devon, Chester, Prestwich, Nottingham, Glamorgan and Wakefield, generally in connection with the laundry (female) or workshops (male) (ELC 1867: 71). Detached blocks constituted a different style of accommodation within the asylum and were often set at a distance. For example, a detached block at the Cheshire County Asylum was built in 1860 as a miniaturised version of the corridor layout with two bay-fronted dayrooms either side of a central corridor and a similar plan was used for

the detached block at Wakefield (Figures 2-13, 2-14). These blocks were generally for 100 patients and more, and were sometimes connected to the main building by means of a covered corridor. They provided a simple method of increasing accommodation at the sorely pressed county asylums.[3] In the 1870s, the tendency to enlarge asylums by the addition of detached blocks began to be incorporated into the construction of new asylums which were built from the start as a series of detached blocks connected by corridors. Another influence at this period was the adoption of detached pavilions in hospital design in order to contain the spread of disease (Taylor, 1991:5-8). The earliest pavilion asylums were two institutions for 'imbeciles' at Leavesden and Caterham (also later adapted for Banstead (1877) and Whalley (1915) (Figure 2-15). These were built by the Metropolitan Asylums Board for 1500 patients each, and opened in 1870 to designs by Giles

---

[3] Smaller scale accommodation for up to c30 patients in the form of 'cottages' in asylum grounds is also often mentioned in Commissioners' reports. Asylum cottages performed a range of functions, but were most frequently used to provide separate accommodation for private patients, or for pauper patients who were farm/garden workers or alternatively were used as 'cottage hospitals' for infectious patients. Cottages never constituted more than a tiny fraction of county asylum accommodation, however.

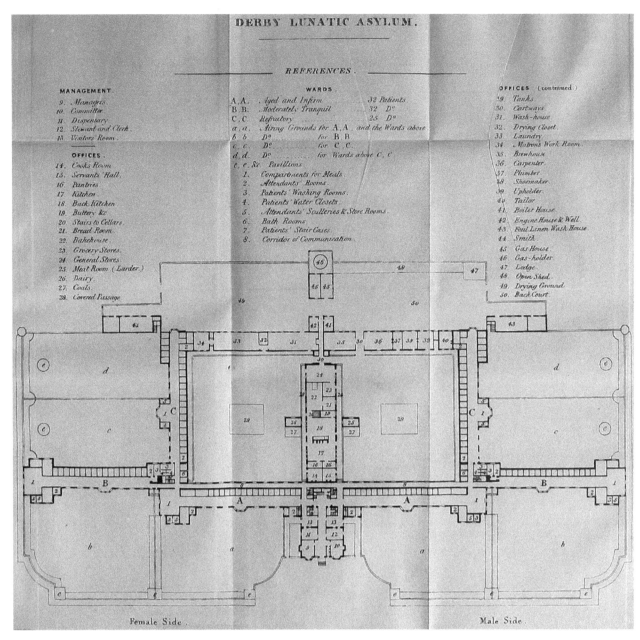

Figure 2-11. Derby County Lunatic Asylum ground floor plan. Source: Conolly, J (1847) *The construction and government of lunatic asylums and hospitals for the insane.*

& Biven. They comprised two identical rows of three-storey pavilions, with administration and service buildings running along the centre. From this point, pavilion asylums became the norm, gradually eclipsing the corridor plan. Initially, pavilions were arranged in a number of different configurations, linear, as at Leavesden, horseshoe (Whittingham 1873), radial horseshoe (Cane Hill 1883) and circular (Prestwich Annexe 1884)(Figures 2-16, 2-17, 2-18). Revised 'Suggestions and Instructions' drawn up by the Lunacy Commissioners in 1870, specified a quarter acre of land for each patient, and separate accommodation for at least three classes of patient, with uninterrupted views of the country and free access to sun and air, with principal rooms having a southern aspect. Rooms were to be no less than 12 feet high with 50 superficial feet for each patient in dormitories and 40 in dayrooms. With numbers of patients relentlessly increasing, (London

asylums reached the size of over 2,000 patients, and Lancashire and Yorkshire each built one asylum on this scale, although outside London, new asylums for 300-400 patients were still common), fulfilling the Commissioners' requirements became problematic. The solution designed for Gloucester in 1884 (although the asylum was never completed as designed) was a 'broad arrow'[4] layout, with the pavilions stepped outwards in echelon so that blocks had freer access to daylight, air and views. This broad arrow design, however, was only adopted in one other full-size asylum, namely Yorkshire's West Riding at Menston. The design was felt to increase the distance between the centre and farthest points, rendering supervision more

---

[4] The terms 'broad arrow', 'compact arrow' and 'dual pavilion' derive from an unpublished 2004 study by Cracknell, summarised at http://studymore.org.uk/asyarc.htm.

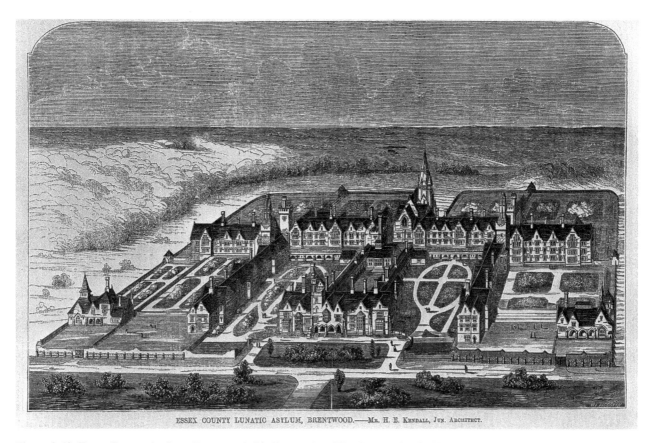

Figure 2-12. Essex County Asylum, Brentwood. Bird's eye view. Wood engraving by W E Hodgkin, 1857, after H.E. Kendall. Source: The Builder, 16th May 1875, p. 275. Wellcome Collection Attribution 4.0 International (CC BY 4.0).

difficult (Taylor 1991:152) (Figure 2-19). Under the Local Government Act of 1889, responsibility for asylums passed from committees of justices to the county and county borough councils. Asylum construction speeded up and a new asylum type became almost universal in the period before the war, the compact arrow. The best-known example of this type, opened at Claybury in 1893, was one of the larger asylums, built for 2,000 patients to designs by G T Hine (Figure 2-20). Hine subsequently, and as a consequence of his Claybury design, became the foremost asylum architect of the late nineteenth and early twentieth centuries. The design modified the broad arrow, so that pavilions hugged the corridors and rendered the distances between centre and outskirts shorter. Claybury was a particularly large asylum, but the compact arrow plan was nonetheless adopted for almost all subsequent asylums. The colony at Ewell, and a late dual pavilion at Whalley in Lancashire were exceptions to this rule.

2.2.3. Colony asylums in England

The tendency to add 'detached blocks' or 'cottages' to asylum sites for working/convalescing patients from c1860 has been alluded to above. A survey of the *Journal of Mental Science* for the period 1880-1910 and of Lunacy Commissioners Reports (1868-1910) suggests that the addition of 'villas' (implying buildings of domestic scale, perhaps somewhere between the 'detached block' and the 'cottage' in size) to pre-existing traditional public asylums in order to provide accommodation for private patients was

relatively common. Villas for pauper patients also became more usual in the later years of the nineteenth and early twentieth centuries. Villas were built at Northumberland, Sunderland, Durham, Manor (Epsom), Banstead, Napsbury, Colney Hatch, Wiltshire, Nottingham City and Portsmouth (villas here were inspired by Kingseat, Aberdeen)(Taylor 1991:152; *JMS* 1901, 47(197): 421-422)(Figure 2-21, 2-22).

The first asylum built in England with detached 'villas' (so-named) on the site as part of the design, rather than as an addition to a pre-existing asylum, was Bexley by GT Hine (opened 1898) (Figure 2-23). One hundred and five of the patients (of a total of 2,000) were accommodated in three villas of 35 patients each. Four subsequent compact arrow asylums (three by GT Hine) provided villa accommodation for between 5 per cent and 20 per cent of patients, likely to have been those who were able to work, i.e. Horton (1902), East Sussex (1903), Long Grove (1907) and Essex and Colchester (1913) (Figures 2-23, 2-24, 2-25, 2-26, 2-27, 2-28, 2-29).

A handful of specialist asylums for epileptics and/or the cognitively impaired were built on the 'colony' model in England in the period 1890-1914. These were largely charitable enterprises (Maghull (1888), Chalfont St Peter (1893), Lingfield (1899), David Lewis (1904), Stoke Park (1909)), or constructed under the Poor Law by Boards of Guardians (Langho (1906), Monyhull (1908), Prudhoe (1914)) (Figures 2-30, 2-31, 2-32, 2-33). Ewell epileptic

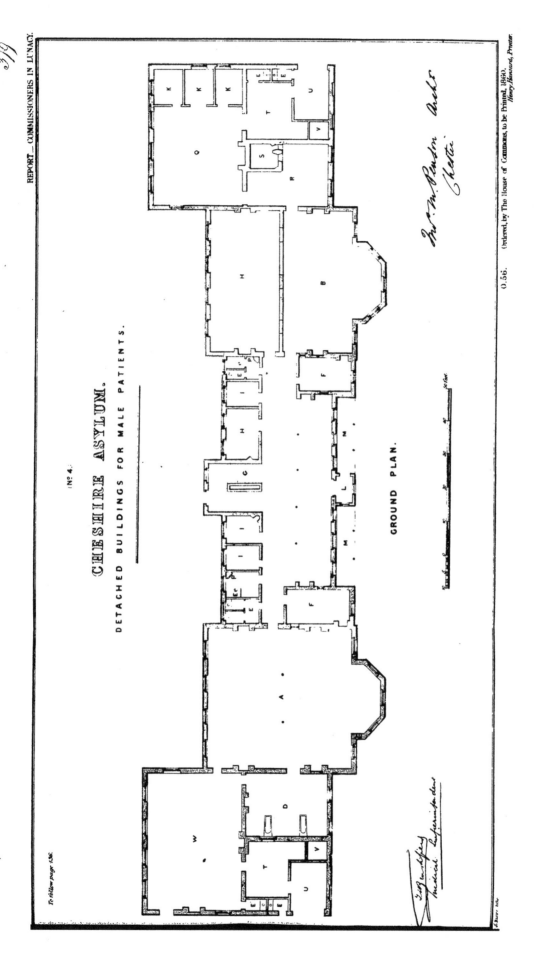

Figure 2.13. Detached block at Cheshire County Asylum, Chester, ground floor plan. Source: *Commissioners in Lunacy. Fourteenth Annual Report to Lord Chancellor,* 1860. Image from ProQuest's House of Commons Parliamentary Papers. Permission provided by ProQuest LLC.

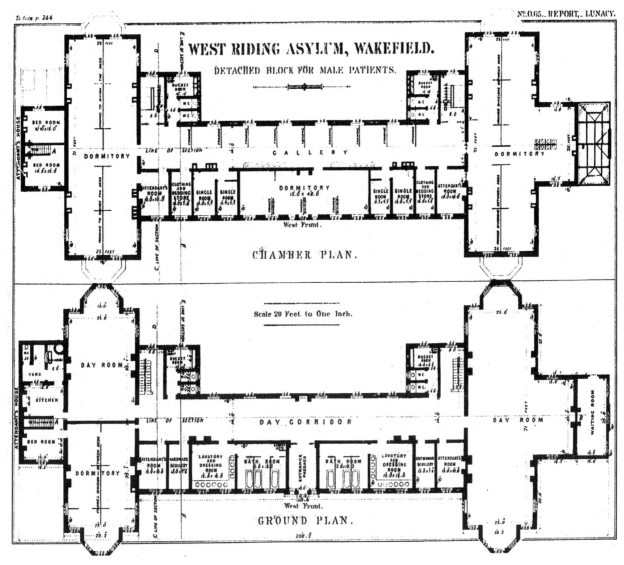

Figure 2-14. Detached block at West Riding Asylum, Wakefield. Source: *Commissioners in Lunacy, Twenty-Second Annual Report to Lord Chancellor*, 1867-8. Image from ProQuest's House of Commons Parliamentary Papers. Permission provided by ProQuest LLC.

colony near Epsom (1903) is the sole example built by an asylum authority (Figure 2-34).

Despite the accommodation of a minority of patients in detached buildings of various kinds, the tendency to asylum segregation/colonisation did not conclude with the dispersal of asylum buildings into village layouts in England as it did in Scotland and no general county or borough asylum was built on the colony model in England or Wales before the war. After 1900, therefore, the model for English asylums consisted of pavilions in a compact arrow layout connected by corridors. This layout was applied to asylums of all sizes from 200 to 2,000 patients.

2.3. Ireland

The most thorough and complete account of the development of Irish asylums is the unpublished thesis of Markus Reuber (Reuber, 1994), and his published summary which extends his analysis into the twentieth century (Reuber, 1996). The following account, therefore, is very much indebted to Reuber's work. However, many details of interest to the current study are not systematically recorded by Reuber, such as asylum size, architectural style and internal layout and recourse has been made to primary sources, particularly Commissioners' reports, maps, plans and photographs and contemporary newspaper reports of asylum construction, where necessary.

2.3.1. Institutional care of the insane poor prior to public asylums

The first public institutions in Ireland to assume care for the insane poor were monasteries, prisons and houses of correction/workhouses. However, as elsewhere in Europe, the insane were not usually differentiated from

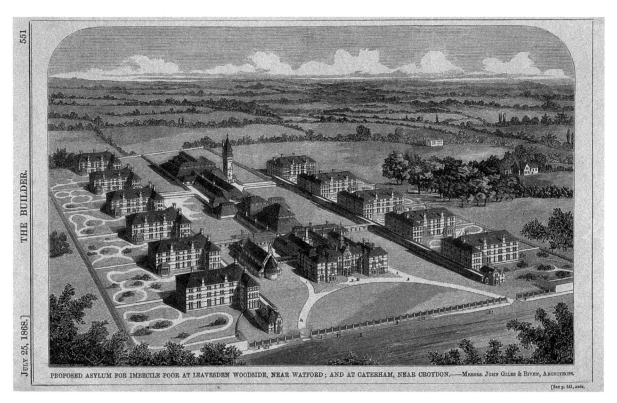

Figure 2-15. Asylum for Imbecile Poor, Leavesden and Caterham. Bird's eye view. Wood engraving by W C Smith, 1868, after J Giles & Bivan. Source: The Builder, 25th July 1868. Wellcome Collection Attribution 4.0 International (CC BY 4.0).

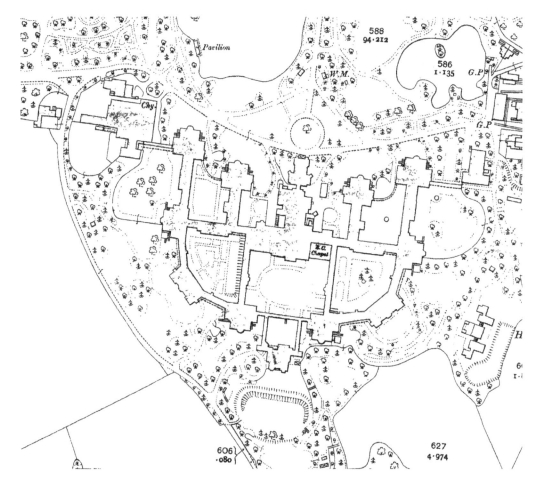

Figure 2-16. Fourth Lancashire County Asylum, Whittingham. Source: 1:2 500 County Series 1st Revision [TIFF geospatial data], Scale 1:2500, Tiles: lanc-sd5635-2, Updated: 30 November 2010, Historic, Using: EDINA Historic Digimap Service, <https://digimap.edina.ac.uk>, Downloaded: 2020-11-02 14:11:13.995. © Crown Copyright and Landmark Information Group Limited 2021. All rights reserved. 1912.

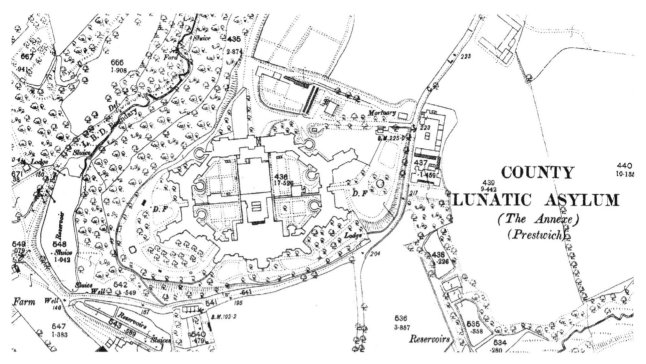

Figure 2-17. Second Lancashire County Asylum, Prestwich Annexe. Source: 1:2500 County Series 1st Edition [TIFF geospatial data], Scale 1:2500, Tiles: lanc-09609-1, Updated: 30 November 2010, Historic, Using: EDINA Historic Digimap Service, <https://digimap.edina.ac.uk>, Downloaded: 2021-04-06 14:07:19.306. . © Crown Copyright and Landmark Information Group Limited 2021. All rights reserved. 1891.

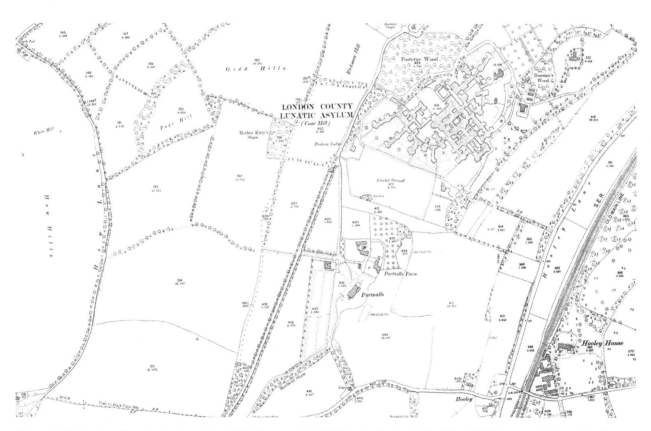

Figure 2-18. London County Asylum, Cane Hill. Source: 1:2 500 County Series 1st Revision [TIFF geospatial data], Scale 1:2500, Tiles: surr-tq2858-2, surr-tq2959-2, Updated: 30 November 2010, Historic, Using: EDINA Historic Digimap Service, <https://digimap.edina.ac.uk>, Downloaded: 2020-11-02 14:35:20.21. . © Crown Copyright and Landmark Information Group Limited 2021. All rights reserved. 1896-7.

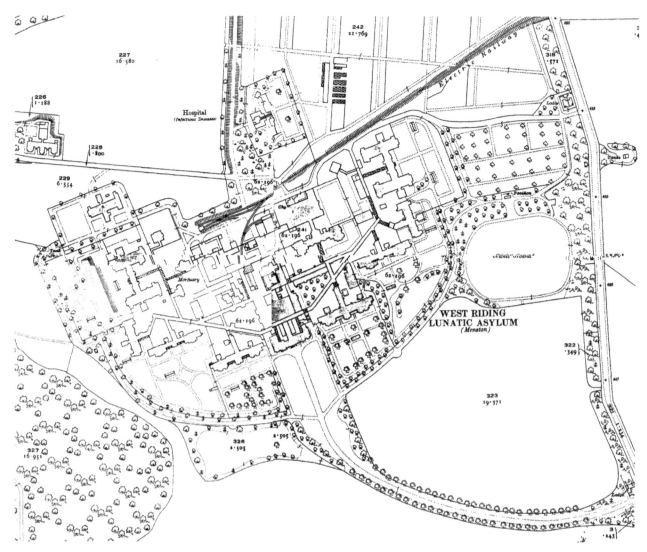

Figure 2-19. Yorkshire West Riding Asylum, Menston. Source: 1:2 500 County Series 2nd Revision [TIFF geospatial data], Scale 1:2500, Tiles: york-se1742-3,york-se1743-3, Updated: 30 November 2010, Historic, Using: **EDINA Historic Digimap Service**, <https://digimap.edina.ac.uk>, Downloaded: 2020-11-02 14:45:20.141. © Crown Copyright and Landmark Information Group Limited 2021. All rights reserved. 1921.

other classes of inmate and are likely to have been few in number, with most of those later to be categorised as insane or idiots, being cared for outside institutions. A number of 'lunatics' found their way to the House of Correction in Dublin and, following the construction of Dublin's (and indeed Ireland's) first workhouse in 1703, numbers of insane were such that it was deemed necessary to open separate quarters for lunatics. By 1729, 40 'madmen' were accommodated in a block adjacent to the infirmary in conditions that were later criticised as inhumane, chained in crowded underground cells without access to light. In 1711 accommodation in the form of cells was provided at the Royal Hospital Kilmainham for old soldiers and extended at intervals until 1849 when insane soldiers began to be sent to the Military Asylum at Yarmouth. It is likely that the only other workhouse in Ireland at this time, Cork (opened 1735) also made some provision for 'lunatics' (Reuber 1994: 17-19; Robins 1988: 45).

The first institution to be built exclusively for the care of 'lunaticks and idiots' was St Patrick's Hospital, Dublin,

constructed under the terms of a bequest from Jonathan Swift, who had formerly been a member of the Board of Governors of Bethlem Hospital in London and of the Dublin Workhouse. The hospital opened in 1757 to a classical design based on that of Bethlem, with a central administration section and wings to either side for males and females and accommodation divided into cells, the corridors serving as 'day-rooms' (Reuber, 1994: 20-31) (Figures 2-35, 2-36).

Houses of Industry were opened in various towns across Ireland (Cork, Dublin, Limerick, Waterford, Clonmel, Ennis, Kilkenny, Belfast and Wexford) in the late eighteenth and early nineteenth centuries following legislation of 1772. The insane were often among those admitted and at the Dublin House of Industry cells for lunatics were opened in 1776, rather than send the unmanageable insane to the local prison. This accommodation was gradually extended and by c1815, 92 'lunatics' were housed in 46 cells. A separate madhouse was built behind the House of Industry in Limerick in 1777 containing a combination of

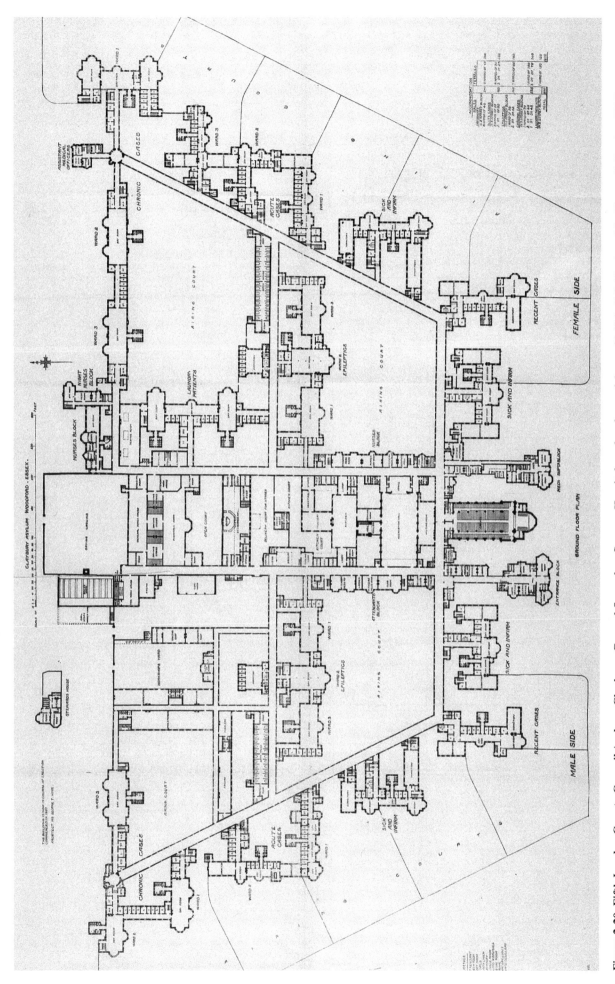

Figure 2-20. Fifth London County Council Asylum, Claybury. Ground floor plan. Source: *Hospitals and asylums of the world. Vols. 1-2,* [Asylums] by Henry C. Burdett. Wellcome Collection Attribution 4.0 International (CC BY 4.0).

Table 3. County and Borough Lunatic Asylums operational in 1910 listed in order of opening date (Source: ELC (1910): 258-265, plan forms from www.studymore.org.uk and www.thetimechamber.co.uk). Ninety-eight asylums in total (eight specialist establishments for 'idiots' and two for criminals have been excluded).

County, County Borough or Borough	Location	Number of patients in 1909/originally built for	Plan form	Date of opening	Cost of original building (£)
Norfolk	Thorpe, Norwich	992/100	Corridor	1814	34,621
Lancaster C and Stockport CB)	Lancaster Moor	2,348/150	Corridor	1816	30,000
Stafford C, Burton-on-Trent CB, Smethwick CB and Newcastle-under-Lyme B)	Stafford	881/120	Corridor	1818	29,623
York (West Riding), Bradford, Halifax, Huddersfield, Leeds, Rotherham, Sheffield and Doncaster CB	Wakefield	1,970/350	Panopticon Corridor	1818	69,250
Cornwall	Bodmin	933/100	Radial/Corridor	1820	16,019
Gloucester C and Gloucester CB	Gloucester	1,159/520 (with Barnwood)	Early Corridor	1823	131,131 (with Barnwood)
Chester C, Birkenhead CB and Stockport CB	Upton, Chester	1,019/90	Corridor (later extension Compact Arrow)	1829	25,484
Suffolk E and W	Melton, Woodbridge	829/130	Corridor (later extension Broad Arrow)	1829	26,311
London C	Hanwell	2,583/300	Panopticon Corridor	1831	103,410
Dorset	Dorchester	847/300 (with Charminster and Herrison (private))	Corridor	1832	44,290 (including Charminster and Herrison)
Kent and Gravesend B	Barning Heath, Maidstone	1,620/174	Corridor	1833	44,000
Middlesex	Wandsworth	1,233/350	Corridor	1841	68,866
Salop and Montgomery C, Shrewsbury B and Wenlock B	Bicton, Shrewsbury	805/100	Corridor	1845	16,443
Devon	Exminster	1,336/400	Radial	1846	55,849
Oxford C and Oxford CB	Littlemore, Oxford	650/270	Corridor	1846	25,140
York (North Riding)	Clifton, York	718/144	Corridor	1847	30,950
Denbigh, Anglesea, Carnarvon, Flint and Merioneth C	Denbigh	880/200	Corridor	1848	25,708
Somerset and Bath CB	Wells	814/350	Corridor	1848	42,156
Birmingham CB	Winson Green, Birmingham	638/300	Corridor	1850	61,960
Derby C	Mickleover, Derby	731/300	Corridor	1851	76,179
Lancaster C and Stockport CB	Rainhill, Liverpool	2,009/400	Corridor	1851	75,509
Lancaster C and Stockport CB	Prestwich, Manchester	2,777/500	Corridor and radial corridor annexe	1851	67,662
London C	Colney Hatch	2,229/1,255	Corridor	1851	226,290
Monmouth C	Abergavenny	937/214	Corridor	1851	29,518
Wilts	Devizes	969/286	Corridor	1851	42,451
Hants	Knowle, Fareham	1,152/400	Corridor	1852	38,291
Lincoln C, Grimsby CB, Lincoln CB	Bracebridge, Lincoln	861/250	Corridor	1852	44,394
Warwick C, Coventry CB and Warwick B	Hatton, Warwick	1,091/300	Corridor	1852	63,888
Worcester C, Dudley CB and Worcester CB	Powick, Worcester	954/202	Corridor	1852	44,743
Bucks	Stone, Aylesbury	650/200	Corridor	1853	36,026

County, County Borough or Borough	Location	Number of patients in 1909/originally built for	Plan form	Date of opening	Cost of original building (£)
Essex and Colchester B	Brentwood	1,792/450	Corridor	1853	79,000
Cambridge C, Cambridge B and Isle of Ely	Fulbourn, Cambridge	584/224	Corridor	1858	41,520
Durham C	Winterton, Ferry Hill	1,509/300	Corridor	1858	29,963
Northumberland and Tynemouth CB	Cottingwood, Morpeth	792/200	Corridor	1859	42,429
Brighton CB	Haywards Heath, Sussex	727/250	Corridor	1859	54,046
Beds, Herts and Hants	Arlesey, Hitchin	1,004/505	Corridor	1860	62,833
Bristol CB	Fishponds, Bristol	891/200	Corridor	1861	42,291
Cumberland and Westmorland	Carlisle	832/220	Corridor	1862	38,847
Dorset	Dorchester		Corridor	1863	
Glamorgan and Merthyr Tydfil CB	Bridgend	1,737/365 (with Parc Gwylit)	Corridor	1864	78,000 (with Parc Gwylit)
Stafford C, Burton-on-Trent CB, Smethwick CB and Newcastle-under-Lyme B	Burntwood, Lichfield	888/530	Corridor	1864	64,200
Carmarthen, Cardigan and Pembroke C	Carmarthen	672/250	Corridor	1865	29,195
City of London CB	Stone, Dartford	579/250	Corridor	1866	63,880
Surrey and Guildford B	Brookwood, Woking	1,389/650	Corridor	1867	75,077
Leicester CB	Humberstone, Leicester	708/300	Corridor (later extension Compact Arrow)	1869	31,858
Newcastle-on-Tyne CB	Gosforth, Newcastle-on-Tyne	843/250	Corridor (later extension Compact Arrow)	1869	47,559
Berks, Reading CB, Newbury B and New Windsor B	Moulsford, Wallingford	744/285	Corridor	1870	49,799
Ipswich CB	Ipswich	293/200	Corridor	1870	25,062
Chester C, Birkenhead CB and Stockport CB	Parkside, Macclesfield	1,053/640	Corridor	1871	133,835
Hereford C and Hereford B	Burghill, Hereford	507/371	Corridor	1871	67,049
York (East Riding)	Beverley	484/280	Corridor	1871	35,029
York (West Riding), Bradford, Halifax, Huddersfield, Leeds, Rotherham, Sheffield and Doncaster CB	Wadsley, Sheffield	1,585/752	Corridor	1872	232,886
Lancaster C and Stockport CB)	Whittingham, Preston	2,093/1,000	Radial pavilion, Corridor and Compact Arrow	1873	132,000
Kent and Gravesend B	Chartham, Canterbury	1,075/905	Corridor Pavilion	1875	211,852
Northampton C	Berrywood, Northampton	891/540	Corridor	1876	118,926
London C	Banstead Downs, Sutton	2,455/1,640	Dual Pavilion	1877	288,094
Portsmouth CB	Milton, Portsmouth	878/420	Corridor-Pavilion	1879	112,265
Norwich CB	Hellesdon, Norwich	484/320	Corridor-Pavilion	1880	62,786
Nottingham CB	Mapperley Hill, Nottingham	817/280	Corridor	1880	54,212
Birmingham CB)	Rubery Hill, near Birmingham	1,288/625	Pavilion	1882	124,246
Gloucester C and Gloucester CB	Gloucester	1,159/520 (with Barnwood)	Broad Arrow	1883	131,131 (with Barnwood)
London C	Cane Hill, Purley	2,163/1,124	Radial Pavilion	1883	236,510

County, County Borough or Borough	Location	Number of patients in 1909/originally built for	Plan form	Date of opening	Cost of original building (£)
Hull CB	De la Pole, Willerby, Hull	565/360	Corridor	1884	69,103
Exeter CB	Digbys, Heavitree	337/328	Corridor	1886	71,359
Glamorgan and Merthyr Tydfil CB	Bridgend	1,737/365 (with Angleton)	Compact Arrow	1887	78,000 (with Angleton)
York (West Riding), Bradford, Halifax, Huddersfield, Leeds, Rotherham, Sheffield and Doncaster CB)	Menston, Leeds	1,630/910	Broad Arrow	1888	300,263
Derby CB	Rowditch, Derby	351/320	Corridor	1888	46,704
Plymouth CB	Blackadon, Ivybridge	364/200	Compact Arrow	1891	50,573
London C	Claybury, Woodford	2,465/2,050	Compact Arrow	1893	483,960
Sunderland CB	Ryhope, Sunderland	387/350	Compact Arrow	1895	96,902
Isle of Wight	Whitecroft, Newport	284/318	Compact Arrow	1896	54,906
Somerset and Bath CB	Cotford, Norton Fitzwarren, Taunton	705/700	Compact Arrow	1897	169,287
Sussex W	Chichester	779/465	Compact Arrow	1897	144,945
London C	Bexley, Kent	2,157/2,000	Compact Arrow	1898	426,667
Middlesborough CB	Cleveland, Middlesbrough	425/268	Compact Arrow	1898	107,000
Herts	Hill End, St Albans	624/576	Compact Arrow	1899	177,246
London C (Manor)	Epsom	943/700	Corridor Pavilion	1899	109,513
Stafford C, Burton-on-Trent CB, Smethwick CB and Newcastle-under-Lyme B	Cheddleton, Leek	843/618	Compact Arrow	1899	242,999
West Ham CB	Goodmayes, Ilford, Essex	875/800	Compact Arrow	1901	322,149
Lancaster C and Stockport CB	Winwick, Warrington	2,075/2,050	Compact Arrow	1902	426,523
Lincoln C	Rauceby, Sleaford	380/420	Compact Arrow	1902	138,682
London C (Horton)	Epsom	2,116/2,000	Compact Arrow	1902	500,263
Nottingham C	Radcliffe-on-Trent, Nottingham	485/452	Compact Arrow	1902	147,086
Brecon and Radnor	Talgarth, Brecon	263/352	Compact Arrow	1903	123,266
London C (Ewell)	Epsom	332/326	Colony	1903	99,273
Sussex E	Hellingly	1,103/1,136	Compact Arrow	1903	369,639
Canterbury CB	St Martin's Hill, Canterbury	155/250	Compact Arrow	1903	79,187
Croydon CB	Warlingham, Whyteleafe, Surrey	475/435	Compact Arrow	1903	211,022
York (West Riding), Bradford, Halifax, Huddersfield, Leeds, Rotherham, Sheffield and Doncaster CB	Storthes Hall, Kirkburton, Huddersfield	658/2,062	Compact Arrow	1904	467,158
Middlesex	Napsbury St Albans	1,180/1,152	Compact Arrow	1905	451,290
Newport CB	Caerleon, Mon	365/368	Compact Arrow	1906	133,036
York CB	Fulford, York	365/362	Compact Arrow	1906	121,200
London C (Long Grove)	Epsom	1,997/2,013	Compact Arrow	1907	507,200
Worcester C, Dudley CB and Worcester CB	Barnsley Hall, near Bromsgrove	406/570	Compact Arrow	1907	196,200
Leicester C and Rutland	Narborough, Leicester	597/688	Compact Arrow	1908	213,065
Cardiff CB	Whitchurch, Glamorgan	684/750	Compact Arrow	1908	280,574
Surrey and Guildford B	Netherne, Merstham	Recently opened/960	Compact Arrow	1909	288,916

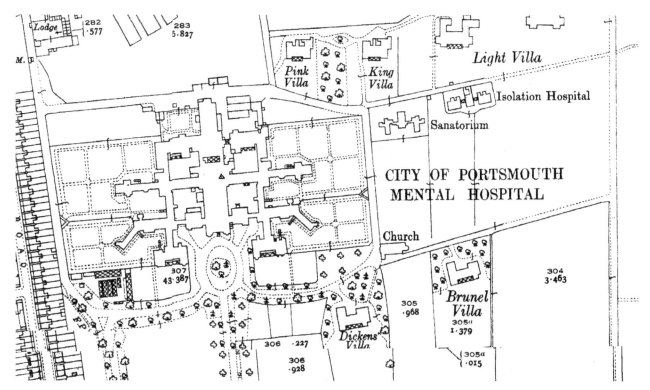

Figure 2-21. Portsmouth County Borough Asylum showing traditional pavilion asylum (opened 1879) and villas added between 1909 and 1932. Source: 1:2 500 County Series 3rd Revision [TIFF geospatial data], Scale 1:2500, Tiles: hamp-su6600-4,hamp-su6700-4,hamp-sz6699-4,hamp-sz6799-4, Updated: 30 November 2010, Historic, Using: EDINA Historic Digimap Service, <https://digimap.edina.ac.uk>, Downloaded: 2021-04-06 15:26:16.689. © Crown Copyright and Landmark Information Group Limited 2021. All rights reserved. 1932-3.

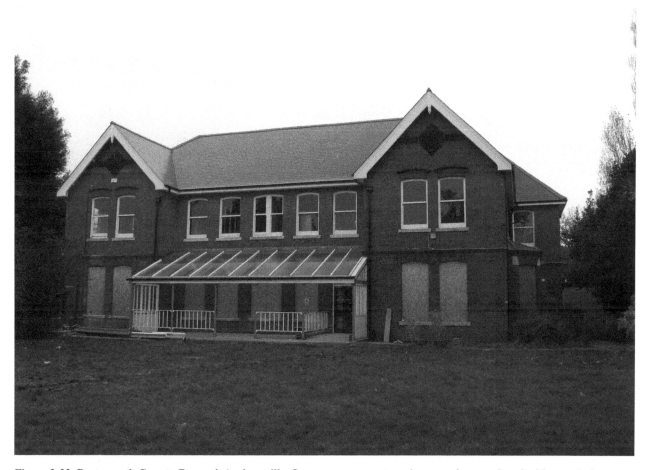

Figure 2-22. Portsmouth County Borough Asylum villa. Source: www.countyasylums.co.uk, reproduced with permission.

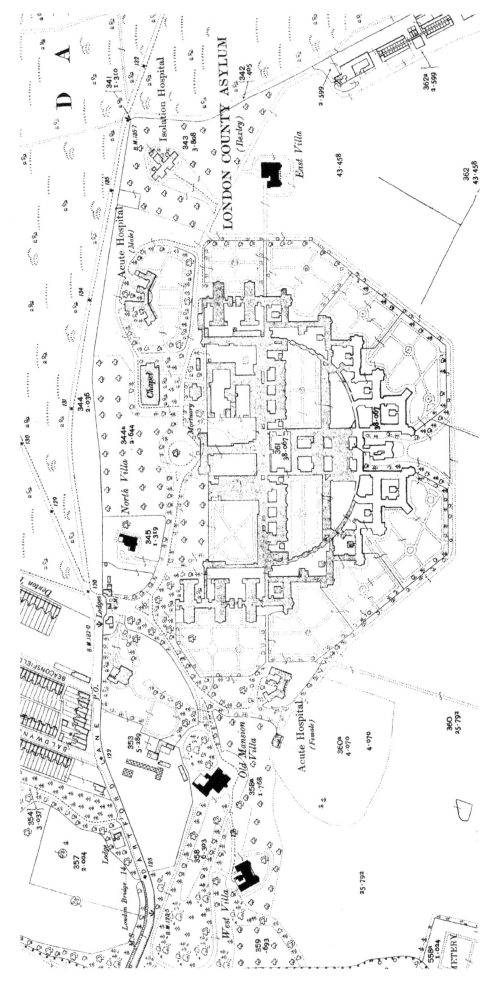

Figure 2-23. London County Council Asylum, Bexley (villas emphasised). Source: 1:2 500 County Series 2nd Revision [TIFF geospatial data]. Scale 1:2500, Tiles: kent-tq5072-3, kent-tq5172-3. Updated: 30 November 2010, Historic, Using: EDINA Historic Digimap Service, <https://digimap.edina.ac.uk>, Downloaded: 2021-04-06 16:10:53.76. © Crown Copyright and Landmark Information Group Limited 2021. All rights reserved. 1909.

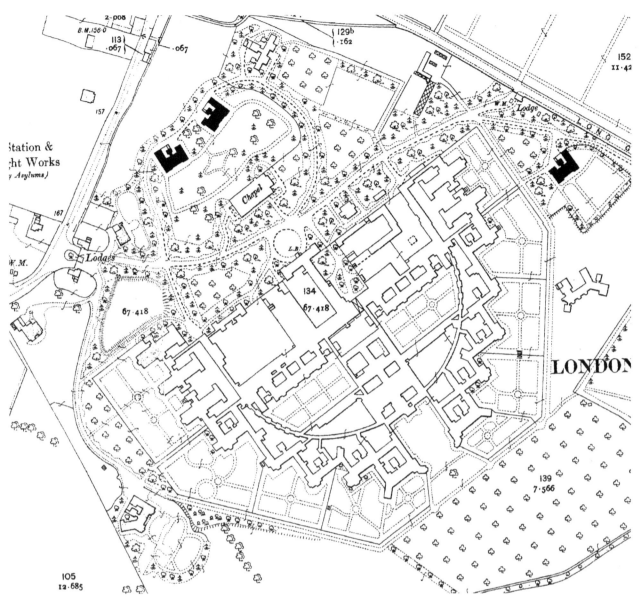

Figure 2-24. London County Council Asylum, Horton (villas emphasised). Source: 1:2 500 County Series 2nd Revision [TIFF geospatial data], Scale 1:2500, Tiles: surr-tq1961-3,surr-tq1962-3.Updated: 30 November 2010, Historic, Using: EDINA Historic Digimap Service, <https://digimap.edina.ac.uk>, Downloaded: 2021-04-06 16:32:24.525. © Crown Copyright and Landmark Information Group Limited 2021. All rights reserved. 1913.

cells and open dormitories. However, the building could not be heated and it was reported that inmates sometimes froze to death. Conditions were criticised by the English prison reformer, John Howard, and by the Inspector General of Prisons who noted that patients were chained to heavy logs. The Dublin House of Industry was similarly criticised for the dirt, noise and confusion that prevailed. At the House of Industry in Cork a lunatic department was opened in 1788 following prison reform legislation which required lunatics to be separated from criminals and a separate building for 'madmen' was completed in 1792 (Reuber, 1994: 35-41).

2.3.2. Establishment of public asylum system

Between 1804 and 1820 small, local asylums housing between 12 and 40 patients opened in Ennis, Lifford, Castlebar, Clonmel, Omagh, Islandbridge, Kilkenny,

Letterkenny and Derry, usually in pre-existing buildings and perhaps in an effort to head off the establishment of an expensive state funded system.[5] However, following criticism of provision for lunatics by reformers, and increasing overcrowding of the available accommodation, a decision was taken to provide a public asylum in Dublin, the first in Ireland, which would provide places for lunatics from the whole country. The Governors of the House of Industry were granted state funds to build Richmond Asylum to designs by Francis Johnston, architect to the Board of Works and the asylum opened in 1815 for 218 patients (Figure 2-37). The progressive physician Alexander Jackson, who had also studied in Edinburgh under William Cullen was influential for the design of the

---

[5] The closure of local asylums was recommended by parliament in 1843 because their accommodation was judged inadequate to provide supervision without restraint.

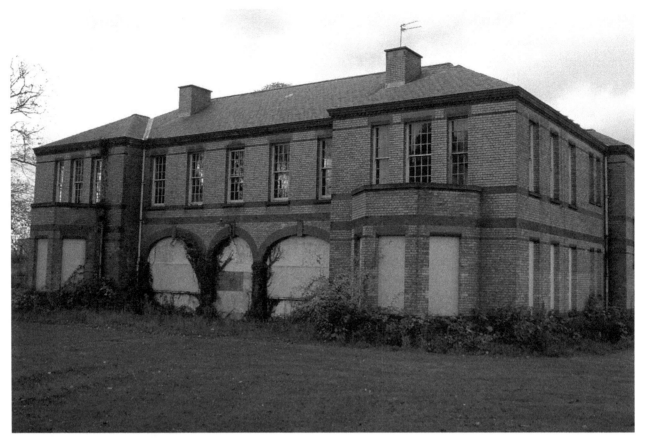

Figure 2-25. London County Council Asylum, Horton, villa for female patients (villas at Bexley asylum were identical). Source: www.countyasylums.co.uk, reproduced with permission.

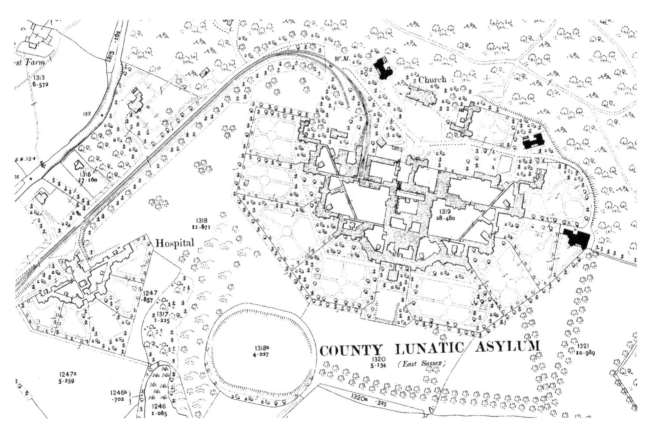

Figure 2-26. East Sussex County Asylum, Hellingly (villas emphasised, a fourth villa lies to the south, near the asylum farm). Source: 1:2 500 County Series 2nd Revision [TIFF geospatial data], Scale 1:2500, Tiles: suss-tq5912-3,suss-tq6012-3, Updated: 30 November 2010, Historic, Using: EDINA Historic Digimap Service, <https://digimap.edina.ac.uk>, Downloaded: 2021-04-06 17:05:45.961. © Crown Copyright and Landmark Information Group Limited 2021. All rights reserved. 1909-10.

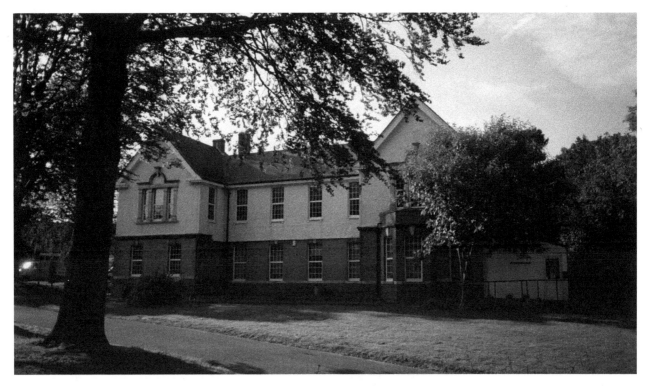

Figure 2-27. East Sussex County Asylum, Hellingly, villa for female chronic patients. Source: www.countyasylums.co.uk, reproduced with permission.

new asylum, including the division of the central courtyard into four in order to more clearly classify patients, but this early design was based largely on workhouse layouts. Jackson felt the comfort of patients was vital as an incentive to restrain themselves. He was influenced by the ideas being tried in *The Retreat* in York, known as 'moral treatment' which aimed to replace shackles and restraints with inner control through striving for the esteem of the Moral Governor. Jackson brought these ideas to Ireland and required that the environment for his patients should be pleasant and comfortable, patients should be classified and (in a departure from the situation at *The Retreat)* a qualified medical doctor should be in charge, but Jackson was ignored on this point and a medical layman was appointed resident Moral Governor. Visiting physicians advised on classification and discharge of patients and the regime in terms of diet, occupation and restraint. Jackson also required that the mentally ill be clearly separated from the 'vagrant beggars' at the House of Industry, but only patients judged 'curable' were moved to the asylum, the 'incurables' remaining at the House of Industry. The Richmond Asylum had to be extended shortly after opening and may therefore have been responsible for drawing government attention to the problem of increasing numbers of insane (Reuber, 1994: 63-70).

Ireland was the first country in Europe in which a network of publicly-funded asylums was constructed. The impetus to establish asylums in England and Ireland came out of the reform movement which had revealed shocking conditions in asylums, notably York and Bethlem. However, the passing of legislation to compel the building of asylums

in England was strongly resisted for some decades, while by contrast legislation was fairly easily passed in Ireland. Scull has suggested that this was a consequence of the 'peculiar quasi-administrative political structure English imperialism had imposed' which meant that in Ireland it was sufficient to convince the small ruling elite of the need for change, whereas local authorities in England were much more opposed to central interference (Scull 1993:45). A committee report of 1815 found that the necessity for providing for the insane was more urgent in Ireland, as there were only two public establishments and a few private houses in Dublin at this stage. The result was that, 'the pauper lunatics are allowed to wander about the country, till those who are outrageous are sent up to Dublin, in a manner shocking to humanity; while the idiots are left to go about the villages, the sport of the common people' (*Report from the Select Committee on provisions for better regulation of madhouses in England*, 1815: 4-5, 24).[6]

People suffering from mental illness were thought to be inhumanely treated outside institutions, where the insane were rumoured to be kept in holes dug in the floor of rural cabins. Institutions that were not specified for the care of the insane were also criticised, as inmates were often shackled or kept in dark, dirty conditions, although the dedicated asylums were praised for their humane care (Reuber, 1994: 73). In addition, those few asylums specifically for the insane were hopelessly overcrowded.

---

[6] The report alleged that one in five insane persons lost a limb due to the tightness of the ligature used to attach them to the back of the cart which brought them to Dublin.

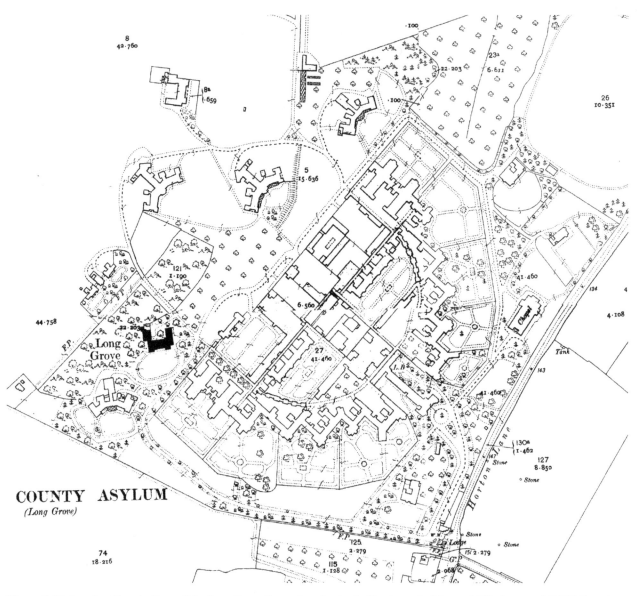

Figure 2-28. London County Council Asylum, Long Grove (emphasised villa shown in Figure 2-29). Source: 1:2 500 County Series 2nd Revision [TIFF geospatial data], Scale 1:2500, Tiles: surr-tq1962-3.Updated: 30 November 2010, Historic, Using: EDINA Historic Digimap Service, <https://digimap.edina.ac.uk>, Downloaded: 2021-04-06 16:32:24.525. © Crown Copyright and Landmark Information Group Limited 2021. All rights reserved. 1913.

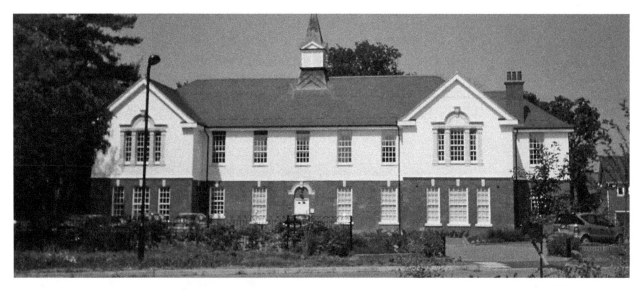

Figure 2-29. London County Council Asylum, Long Grove, villa for female chronic patients. Source: www.countyasylums. co.uk, reproduced with permission.

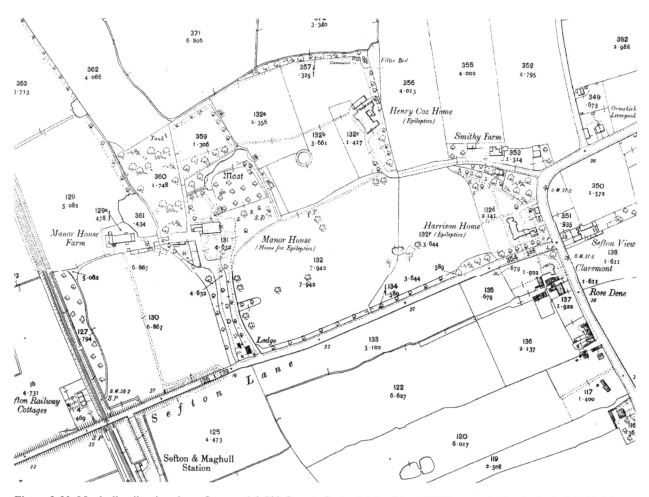

Figure 2-30. Maghull epileptic colony. Source: 1:2 500 County Series 1st Revision [TIFF geospatial data], Scale 1:2500, Tiles: lanc-sd3601-2,lanc-sd3602-2,lanc-sd3701-2,lanc-sd3702-2, Updated: 30 November 2010, Historic, Using: EDINA Historic Digimap Service, <https://digimap.edina.ac.uk>, Downloaded: 2021-04-11 13:02:34.58 © Crown Copyright and Landmark Information Group Limited 2021. All rights reserved. 1908.

A report of 1817 found that the provision for the insane poor in Ireland was wholly inadequate. It was held that 'the successful treatment of Patients depends more on the adoption of a regular system of moral treatment, than upon casual medical prescription'. Therefore patients could not be cared for outside the asylum and needed to be admitted to institutions dedicated to the care of the mentally ill (*Report from the Select Committee on the lunatic poor in Ireland*, 1817: 4).

First Phase of Construction

In 1817 an Act was passed (with minor amendments in 1820 and 1821) (57 Geo. III , c. 106, 1817; 1 Geo. IV, c. 98, 1820; 1 & 2 Geo. IV, c. 33, 1821) which allocated state funds to the construction of district lunatic asylums across Ireland to be maintained from a tax on ratepayers. Nine asylums were built, as a result, in the following counties, to designs by Francis Johnston and William Murray of the Board of Works, which consisted of two asylum types, a K-plan for 100 inmates and an X-plan for 150:

Armagh (1825) – K-plan
Limerick (1827) – X-plan (Figures 2-38, 2-39)

Belfast (1829) – K-plan (Figures 2-40, 2-41)
Londonderry (1829) – K-plan
Carlow (1831) – K-plan
Ballinasloe (1833) – X-plan
Maryborough (1833) – K-plan
Clonmel (1835) – K-plan (Clonmel was slightly smaller, for 60 inmates only)
Waterford (1835) – K-plan

The pre-existing Richmond Asylum became the District Asylum for Meath, Wicklow, Louth and Dublin in 1830. Legislation limited the size of asylums to 150 inmates, which was then thought ideal for the kind of individual treatment entailed by moral management. Also required were a peaceful situation with outdoor space and an interior design which would allow for classification and surveillance of inmates (Reuber, 1994: 74-84). The asylum was increasingly, by this time, seen as a therapeutic environment, although this was chiefly in terms of enhancing the alienist's ability to exercise 'general and constant' surveillance over the inmates and thereby influence their behaviour by means of moral management (Donnelly 1983:48). The X-plan (of which the K-plan is simply a variant) is likely to have been influenced by the

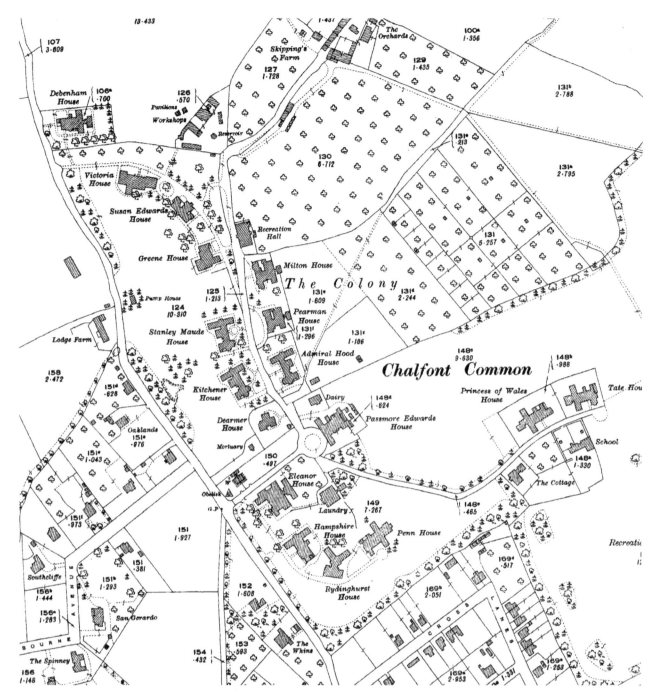

Figure 2-31. Chalfont St Peter epileptic colony. Source: 1:2 500 County Series 2nd Revision [TIFF geospatial data], Scale 1:2500, Tiles: buck-tq0092-3, Updated: 30 November 2010, Historic, Using: EDINA Historic Digimap Service, <https:// digimap.edina.ac.uk>, Downloaded: 2021-04-11 13:28:16.675 © Crown Copyright and Landmark Information Group Limited 2021. All rights reserved. 1925.

design of the Scot William Stark for the Royal Asylum for Lunatics in Glasgow, completed in 1814 (Figure 2-67, 2-68). Stark's design is thought to have borrowed its panoptic emphasis from Bentham's layout, with patients in dayrooms, corridors and airing courts visible at all times from the central octagon (although patients in cells/bedrooms were not visible). Although Bentham did envisage that his panopticon could be used as a 'madhouse', early radial asylum designs, such as those in Ireland, borrowed only the principal of centralised visual control of interior spaces, they did not fully implement Bentham's design which provided accommodation several

storeys high, arranged into circular rows. Centralised visual control seems to have been at least as much influenced by the Tuke family's emphasis on moral management, as it was by the idea of disciplinary surveillance.

Lunacy reformer, Thomas Spring Rice was also influential in developing the X-plan which was used in his home town of Limerick. It was pronounced perfectly adapted in terms of 'ventilation, light, inspection and every other particular' (*Correspondence and communication on public lunatic asylums in Ireland*, 1827: 13). According to Reuber, the X-plan allowed for better supervision than the K-plan,

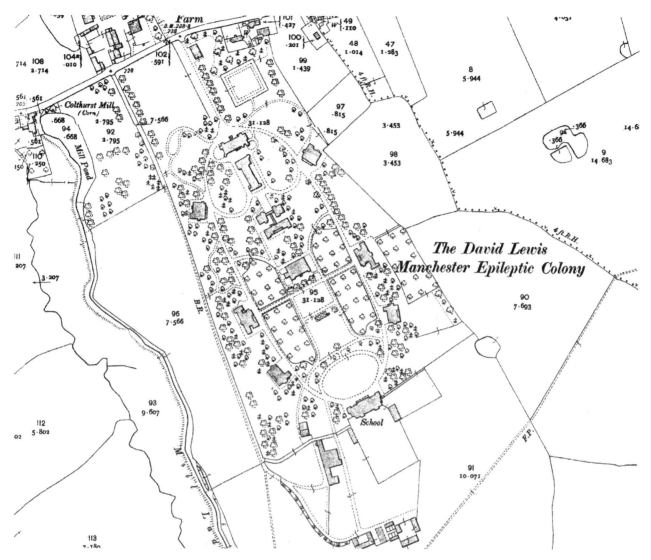

Figure 2-32. David Lewis Manchester epileptic colony. Source: 1:2500 County Series 2nd Revision [TIFF geospatial data], Scale 1:2500, Tiles: ches-sj8076-3, ches-sj8176-3 Updated: 30 November 2010, Historic, Using: EDINA Historic Digimap Service, <https://digimap.edina.ac.uk>, Downloaded: 2021-04-11 13:28:16.675 © Crown Copyright and Landmark Information Group Limited 2021. All rights reserved. 1910.

allowing for a view of corridors as well as dayrooms, and all the airing yards (Reuber, 1994: 89).

The first asylums, e.g. Richmond and Armagh, were not run by doctors but by moral governors, in the style practised by the Tukes of York, and medical practitioners were appointed as visitors. In 1848 the new Inspectors of Lunacy, after pressure from doctors, declared that only physicians would be allowed to run asylums henceforward. Inspection of lunatic asylums was initially undertaken by the Inspector General of Prisons and included in his (usually annual) report on prison accommodation. After 1842 this function was taken over by the newly-created post of Inspector of Lunacy who began to bring the district asylums under centralised control by the issuing of regulations that passed control of the asylums to medical practitioners (Reuber 1994: 127).

Numbers of insane continued to rise and some extensions were made shortly after construction, at Belfast, where

the accommodation was more than doubled (1835) and Clonmel (1842). Control of asylums decisively passed from moral managers to medical superintendents with the appointment of a doctor as the first Inspector of Lunacy. Francis White formulated the first 'General Rules for the Government of all the District Lunatic Asylums' in 1843 which specified that all treatment whether medical or moral must be the responsibility of medical practitioners and another doctor, John Nugent, joined him as an Inspector of Lunacy in 1846. They jointly ensured that only doctors were nominated for vacant posts as asylum managers and this had become universal by 1860. In 1862 the Medical Superintendent was made the highest medical authority within the asylum, other visiting doctors only being allowed to enter at his request. There was no training in psychiatric medicine (then known as 'mental science') available in Ireland at this point, but many doctors (including those of a dissenting persuasion who were not eligible to study at Trinity) would have trained in Scotland, then preeminent in medical training, where instruction in psychiatric

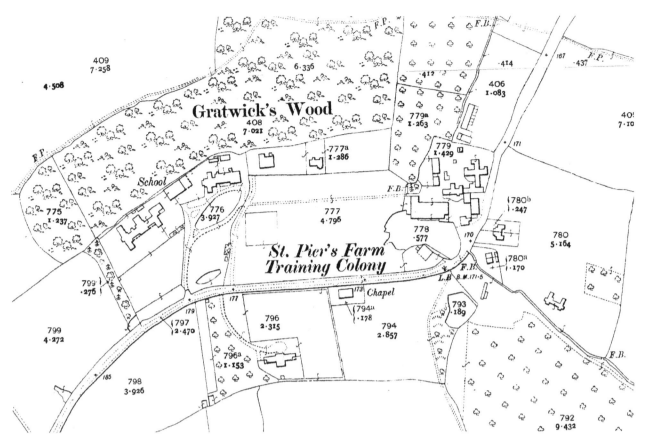

Figure 2-33. Lingfield epileptic colony, St Pier's Farm. Source: 1:2 500 County Series 2nd Revision [TIFF geospatial data], Scale 1:2500, Tiles: surr-tq4043-3, Updated: 30 November 2010, Historic, Using: EDINA Historic Digimap Service, <https://digimap.edina.ac.uk>, Downloaded: 2021-04-11 14:26:10.996 © Crown Copyright and Landmark Information Group Limited 2021. All rights reserved. 1912-13.

medicine was available. Following the assassination of a civil servant in London by the Scot Daniel McNaughtan (M'Naghten) in 1843, the provision for criminal lunatics in Ireland was investigated and judged inadequate and an institution specifically for criminal lunatics was constructed at Dundrum, opening in 1850 to designs by Jacob Owen. The asylum showed some similarities with the earlier K-plan of Francis Johnston but there was no attempt to make any part of the asylum viewable from the manager's accommodation. The main changes were the addition of a chapel, a separate hospital building and much of the sleeping accommodation was now provided in dormitories rather than cells. The Inspectors of Lunacy considered the buildings to resemble a private house with large windows, rather than the standard asylum. Both the corridors and the dayrooms were said to be cheerful and light and the wall surrounding the asylum was only 6 feet 6 in high in contrast to the usual 10 or 12 feet. This was the first asylum for the criminally insane in Britain and Ireland, Broadmoor opening 14 years later (Reuber, 1994: 132-138).

Second phase of construction

As numbers of insane continued to rise, by 1843, 2,028 patients had been admitted to asylums that had only been built for 1,220. Between 1845 and 1853 extensions were built to Richmond, Carlow, Maryborough, Limerick, Clonmel, Waterford, Belfast, Armagh and Londonderry

asylums, and a restriction on asylum size to 150 patients was lifted. New asylums were built in:

Kilkenny (1852) (160 beds) Architect: George Papworth (Figures 2-42, 2-43)
Killarney (1852) (250 beds) Architect: Thomas Deane (Figures 2-44, 2-45)
Cork (1852) (500 beds) Architect: William Atkins (Figures 2-46, 2-47)
Omagh (1853) (250 beds) Architect: William Farrell
Sligo (1855) (250 beds) Architect: William Deane Butler
Mullingar (1855) (300 beds) Architect: John Skipton Mulvany[7] (Figures 2-48, 2-49)

These asylums were all put out to public tender rather than being constructed by the Board of Works and therefore varied in plan form. However, according to Reuber, the Derby County Asylum, which was identified in 1847 by John Conolly as an ideal form, was hugely influential for this stage of asylum development in Ireland. Derby represented a modified corridor form, which was free of prison-like 'panoptic' elements but nevertheless, through the use of corridors and cross wings, allowed each ward to communicate with the centre without passing through all other wards (Reuber, 1996) (Figure 2-11). The Board

---

[7] Bed numbers in this list are from ILC Report, 1852-3; www.dia.ie and www.buildingsofireland.ie

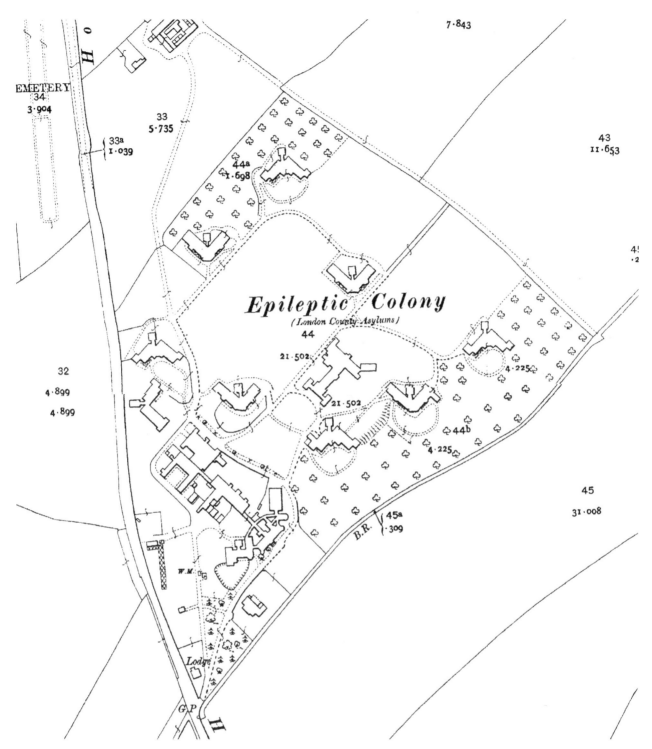

Figure 2-34. London County Council epileptic colony, Ewell. Source: 1:2 500 County Series 2nd Revision [TIFF geospatial data], Scale 1:2500, Tilessurr-tq2062-3, Updated: 30 November 2010, Historic, Using: EDINA Historic Digimap Service, <https://digimap.edina.ac.uk>, Downloaded: 2021-04-11 14:32:53.698 © Crown Copyright and Landmark Information Group Limited 2021. All rights reserved. 1913.

of Works formulated some guidance for architects in 1848, based on travel to asylums in England and Scotland and suggestions put forward by Irish asylum managers (*Sixteenth report from the Board of Public Works, Ireland, 1848*: 236*).* Architects were enjoined to remember that they were designing a hospital and not a prison and that 'the appearance of restraint and confinement' was to be as much as possible avoided while providing the necessary classification and security for patients. Walls were not to be

more that 6 ft 6 in high and windows were to be unbarred. The main front and day-rooms were to face southwards and the yards were not to be enclosed by other buildings. It was recommended that 'Gothic' style would allow more easily for additions. The rooms were to be lined with bricks but not plastered and there were to be open fireplaces in dayrooms and corridors. Dormitories (rather than cells) were not to contain more than 15 patients with at least two feet between beds and the wards were to be arranged

49

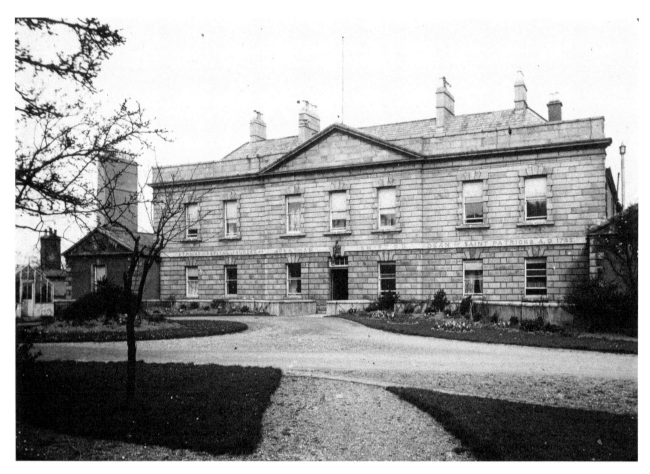

Figure 2-35. St Patrick's Hospital, Dublin. Source: NLI Mason photographic collection M31/15. Image reproduced courtesy of the National Library of Ireland.

so that the staff did not have to retrace their steps when inspecting them. Asylums were to be divided into three classes with the most difficult patients on the ground floor and the most harmless on the second floor. Windows were to be large and open at the top and could be as low as 3 feet 6 inches from the floor. The kitchen and laundry should be large enough to allow of large numbers of patients working in them. Airing yards were to be provided each side but 'tranquil' patients could use the 'pleasure-grounds'.

Asylums were largely built to these specifications, but several e.g. Killarney and Cork were criticised for their splendour and palatial appearance, despite complaints by the asylums themselves that they were underfunded and that building work was often below standard. The elevations tended, in fact, to bear a strong resemblance to the Tudor Gothic of the workhouse, which may have been a factor in the abandoning of this style in the next phase of construction. Cork, a comparatively large asylum of 500 beds, was divided into four separate blocks, linked by corridors – a central administration block, accommodation blocks for patients either side and a service block to the rear, although the linking passages were filled in before long with new construction as patient numbers grew. This arrangement makes Cork a very early example (perhaps the earliest in the Britain and Ireland) of the pavilion style that was later to become dominant in asylum design.

Third Phase of Construction

Following a commission of enquiry which found that asylums in Ireland were overcrowded, a third phase of asylums was built in the following locations (Reuber, 1996: 1185):

Letterkenny (1865) (250 beds) Architect: George Wilkinson (Figure 2-50)
Castlebar (1866) (250 beds) Architect: George Wilkinson (Figures 2-51, 2-52)
Ennis (1868) (260 beds) Architect: William Fogerty and Charles Arthur Adair (Figures 2-53, 2-54)
Enniscorthy (1868) (250 beds) Architect: James Barry Farrell and James Bell (Figures 2-55, 2-56)
Downpatrick (1869) (300 beds) Architect: Henry Smyth (Figure 2-57)
Monaghan (1869) (300 beds) Architect: John McCurdy (*Returns of the total amount of accommodation*, 1867)

The new institutions largely favoured an Italianate style, but continued with the corridor layout for the most part. Some, such as Sligo, divided the accommodation into pavilions connected by corridors in the way that had been seen at Cork. According to Reuber, this third phase of construction represented the death knell for moral management, and was influenced by the idea

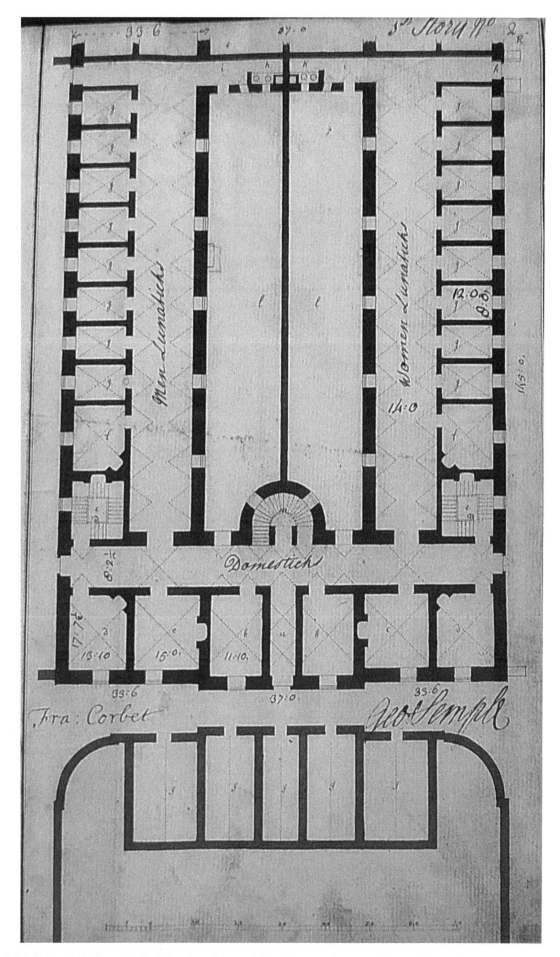

Figure 2-36. St Patrick's Hospital, Dublin, plan of ground floor. Source: Courtesy of St Patrick's University Hospital.

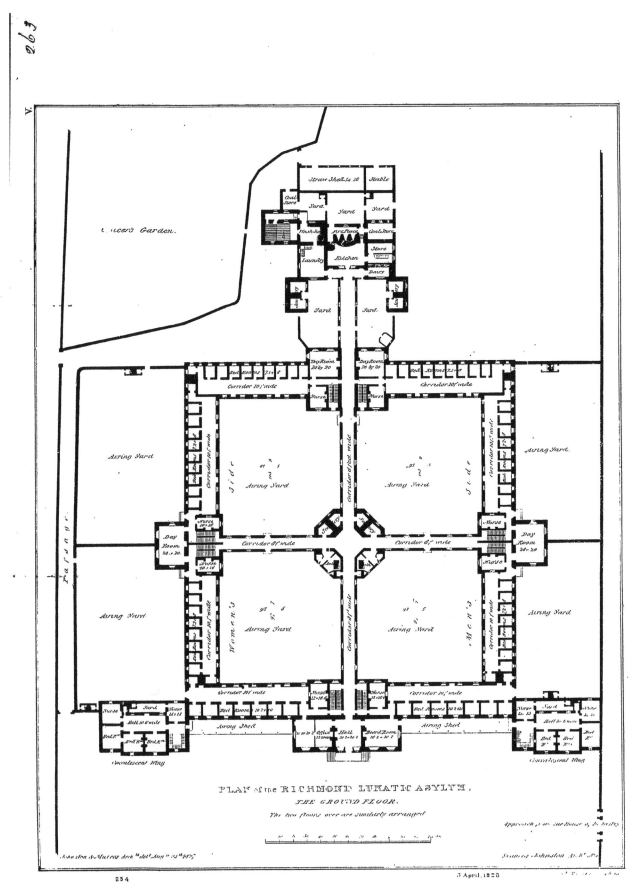

Figure 2-37. Richmond Asylum, Dublin, plan of ground floor. Source: *Correspondence and Communications on Lunatic Asylums in Ireland*, 1827. Image from ProQuest's House of Commons Parliamentary Papers. Permission provided by ProQuest LLC.

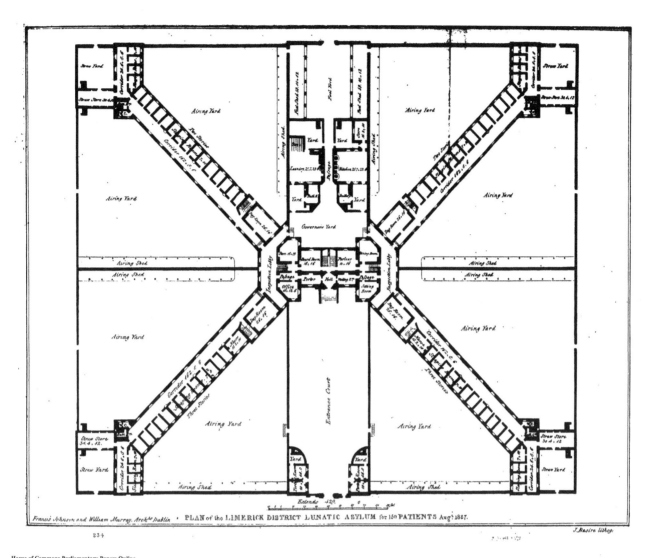

Figure 2-38. Limerick Asylum, plan of ground floor. Source: *Correspondence and Communications on Lunatic Asylums in Ireland*, **1827. Image from ProQuest's House of Commons Parliamentary Papers. Permission provided by ProQuest LLC.**

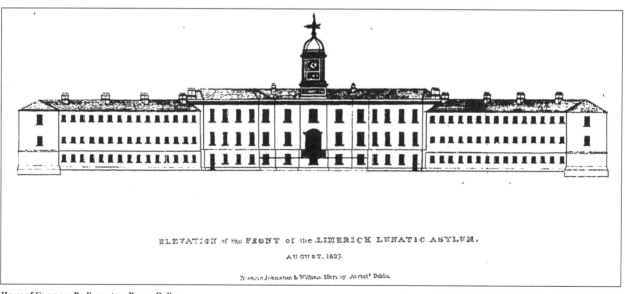

Figure 2-39. Limerick Asylum, elevation. Source: *Correspondence and Communications on Lunatic Asylums in Ireland*, **1827. Image from ProQuest's House of Commons Parliamentary Papers. Permission provided by ProQuest LLC.**

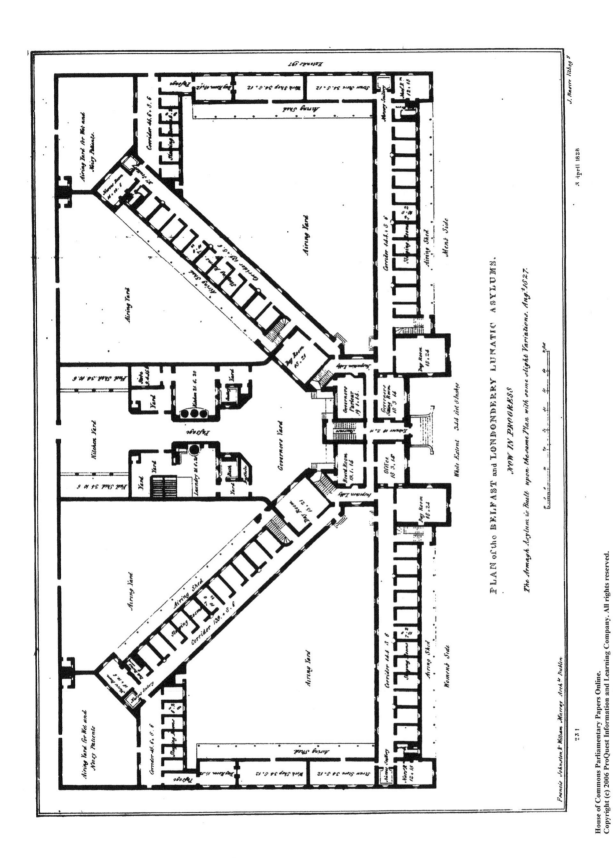

Figure 2-40. Belfast Asylum. Source: *Correspondence and Communications on Lunatic Asylums in Ireland, 1827.* Image from ProQuest's House of Commons Parliamentary Papers. Permission provided by ProQuest LLC.

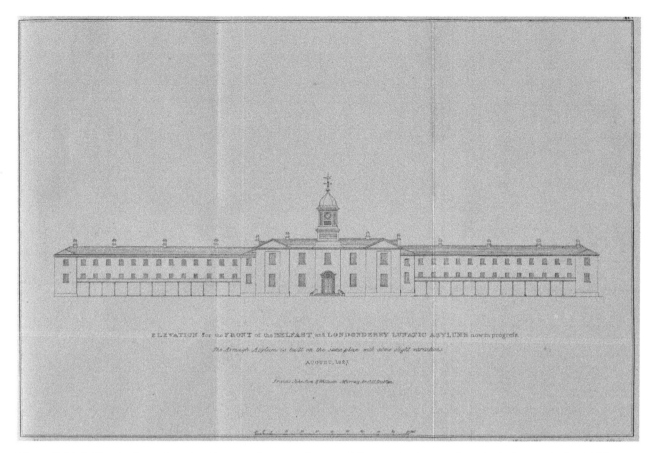

Figure 2-41. Belfast Asylum, elevation. Source: *Correspondence and Communications on Lunatic Asylums in Ireland,* **1827. Parliamentary Archives, London.**

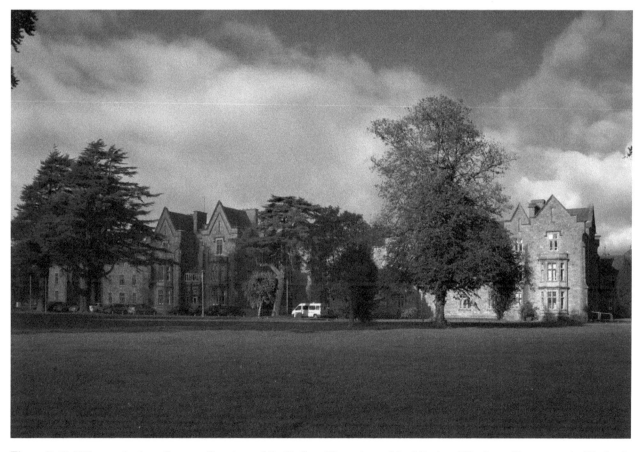

Figure 2-42. Kilkenny Asylum. Source: Courtesy of the National Inventory of Architectural Heritage, Government of Ireland.

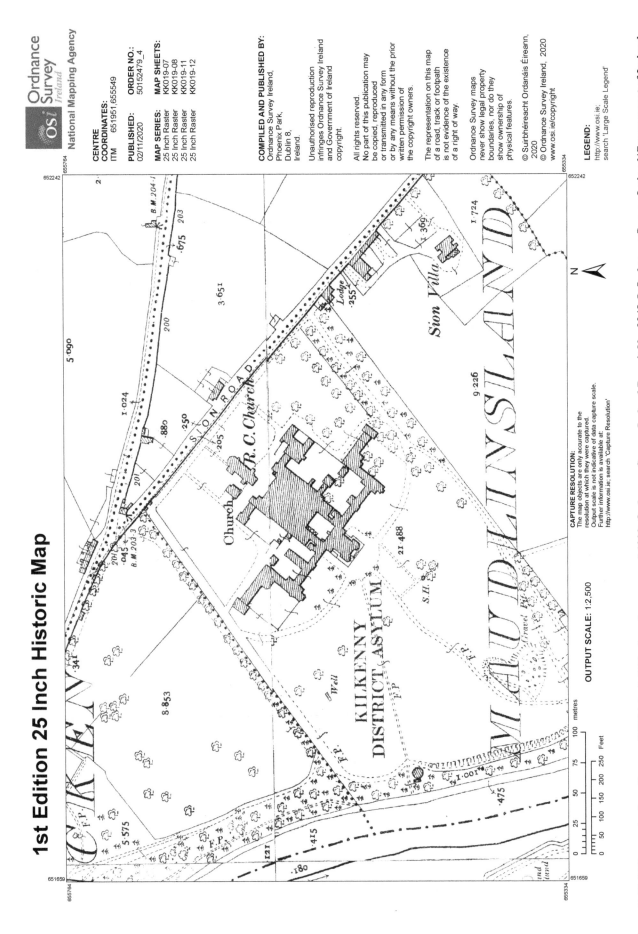

Figure 2-43. Kilkenny Asylum. Source: OSI historic 25 inch series, surveyed 1900. Ordnance Survey Ireland Permit No. 9248 © Ordnance Survey Ireland/Government of Ireland .

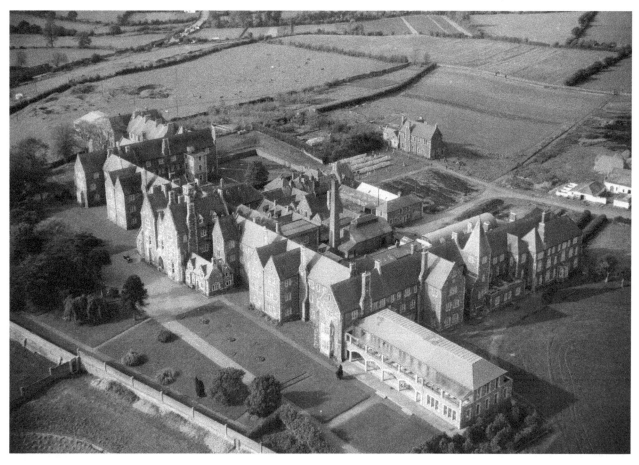

Figure 2.44. Killarney Asylum. Source: Morgan Aerial Photographic Collection NPA MOR612. Image reproduced courtesy of the National Library of Ireland.

that the association of large numbers of insane, far from producing 'turbulence and confusion' was in fact 'highly conducive to good order and quietude' (Joseph Lalor, Medical Superintendent of Richmond Asylum quoted in Reuber, 1996: 1185). However, asylum sizes and designs remained much the same as in the second phase with pavilions/wards used for patient classification, although dormitories, dayrooms and dining/recreation halls became more common (Reuber, 1996: 1185). The architect for Letterkenny and Castlebar (which were identical) was George Wilkinson who had been responsible for the standard workhouse design in Ireland, and was appointed architect to the Asylum Commissioners in 1860 (Dictionary of Irish Architects). However, his asylum design was a distinct departure from the Tudor Gothic of the workhouse and is much more imposing in style. This may have been a deliberate strategy to differentiate asylum architecture from that of the workhouse. This phase saw the introduction of features which were more domestic in nature. For instance, Fogarty, the architect at Ennis, designed an asylum which placed the dayrooms on the ground floor and the dormitories on the first floor in order to more closely replicate domestic arrangements. Criticism of the asylum as a means of treatment was headed in this period by Connolly Norman, superintendent of Richmond Asylum in Dublin, who had derived inspiration from the Scottish practice of boarding out and from what was

called the 'family care system' practised in some parts of Germany, which operated in a similar way. Norman complained that, 'the huddling together of vast crowds of people anywhere is demoralising, the crowd is apt to take its tone from the worst and not from its best elements'. He suggested that treatment in a family setting would be preferable to asylum care (quoted in Robins 1986:139).

Late Additions to Asylum System

Around the turn into the twentieth century the acute problem of overcrowding in the asylums of Ireland's two largest cities, Belfast and Dublin, stimulated firstly, the construction of a new asylum for the county of Antrim at Holywell and then new asylums for Belfast and Dublin:

Antrim, Holywell (1899) (600 beds) Architect: John Lanyon Layout: echelon or broad arrow, Style: Italianate (Figures 2-58, 2-59)

Belfast, Purdysburn (Projected for 1,000 patients, although by 1913 accommodated only c700) (1902-1913) Architects: Local: Graeme Watt & Tulloch; Consulting: George T Hine (BDLA Minutes 11th March, 1901) Layout: Villa Colony, Style: Domestic revival

Dublin, Portrane (1904) (1,200 beds) Architect: George Coppinger Ashlin. Layout: Echelon or broad arrow Style: Tudor. (*Building News*, 27th April 1900, pp.572-3) (Figures 2-60, 2-61, 2-62)

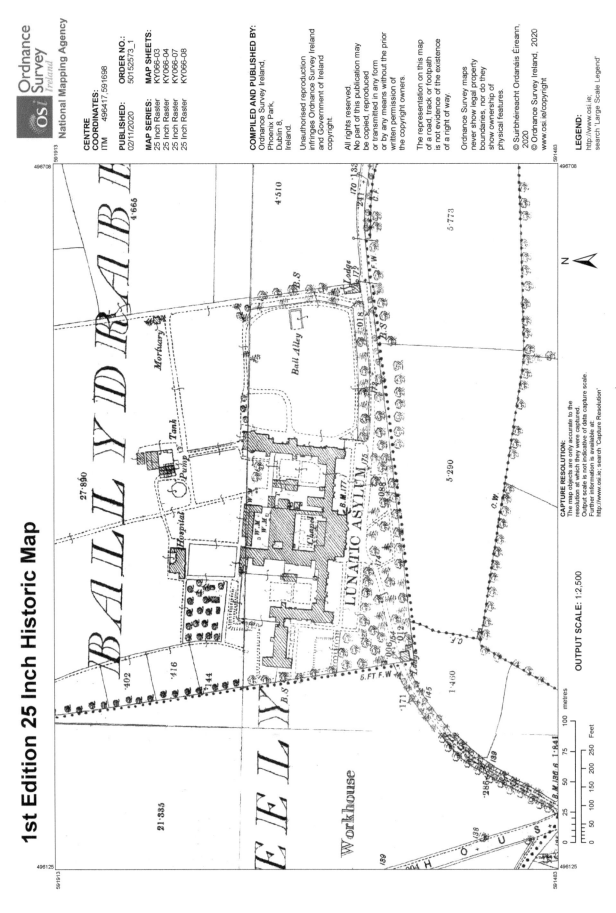

1st Edition 25 Inch Historic Map

Figure 2-45. Killarney Asylum. Source: OSI historic 25 inch series, surveyed 1894. Ordnance Survey Ireland Permit No. 9248 © Ordnance Survey Ireland/Government of Ireland.

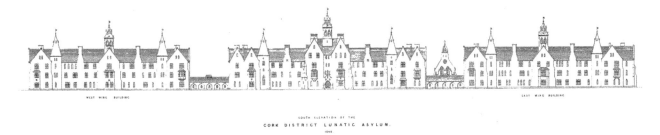

Figure 2-46. Cork Asylum, elevation. Source: *Commissioners of Public Works (Ireland), Sixteenth Report, Appendices*, **1847-8. Image from ProQuest's House of Commons Parliamentary Papers. Permission provided by ProQuest LLC.**

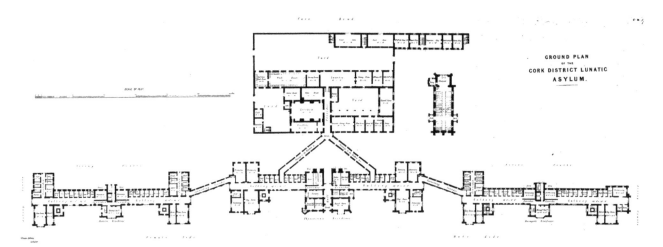

Figure 2-47. Cork Asylum, plan of ground floor. Source: *Commissioners of Public Works (Ireland), Sixteenth Report, Appendices,* **1847-8. Image from ProQuest's House of Commons Parliamentary Papers. Permission provided by ProQuest LLC.**

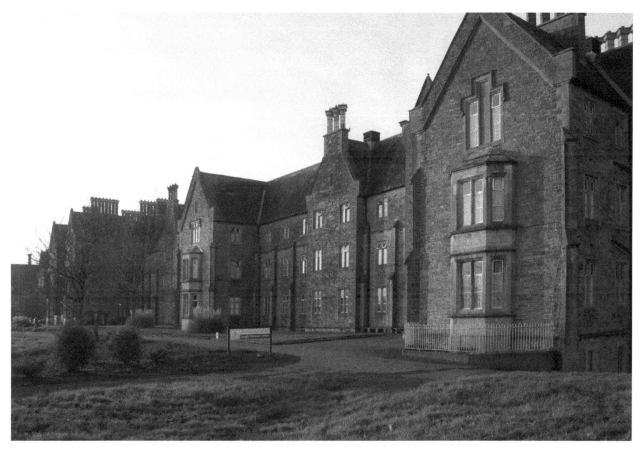

Figure 2-48. Mullingar Asylum. Source: Image reproduced courtesy of National Inventory of Architectural Heritage.

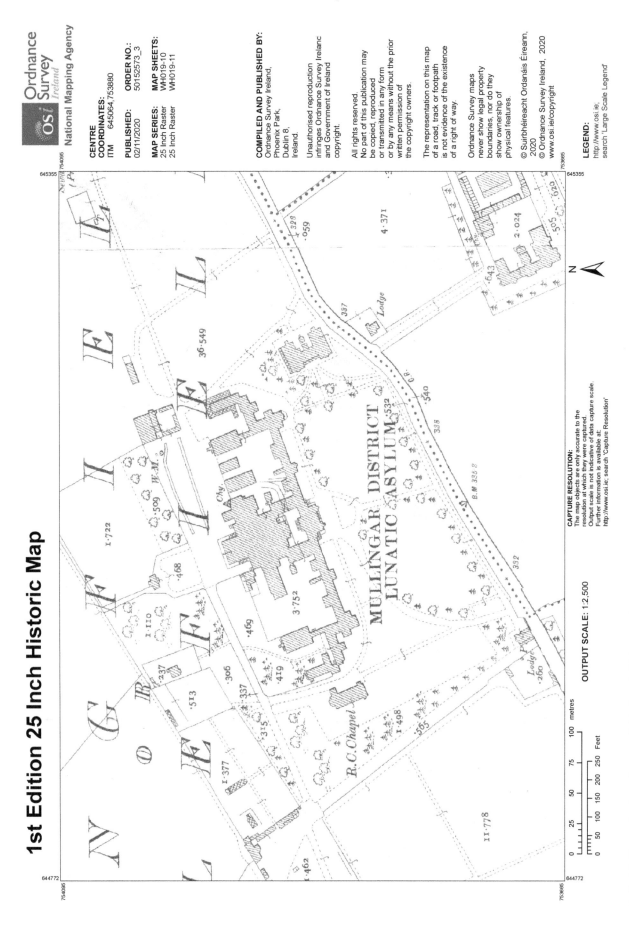

Figure 2-49. Mullingar Asylum. Source: OSI historic 25 inch series, surveyed 1911. Ordnance Survey Ireland Permit No. 9248 © Ordnance Survey Ireland/Government of Ireland.

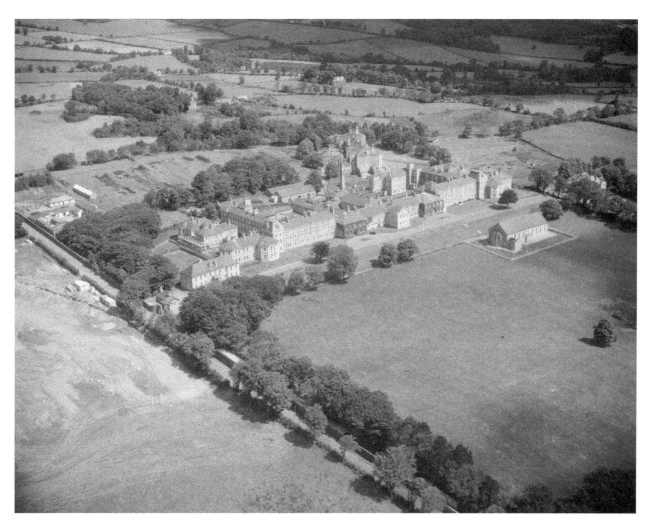

Figure 2-50. Letterkenny Asylum. Source: Morgan Aerial Photographic Collection NPA MOR254. Image reproduced courtesy of the National Library of Ireland.

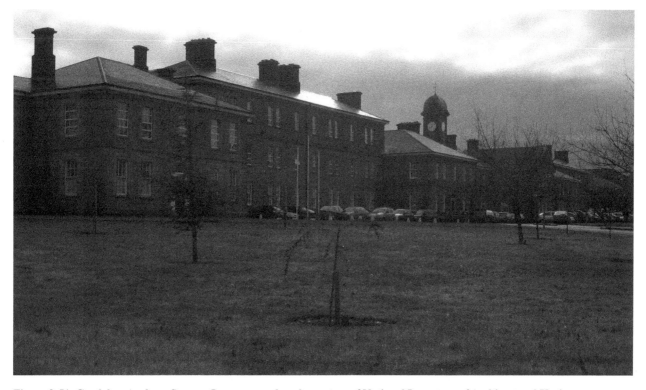

Figure 2-51. Castlebar Asylum. Source: Image reproduced courtesy of National Inventory of Architectural Heritage

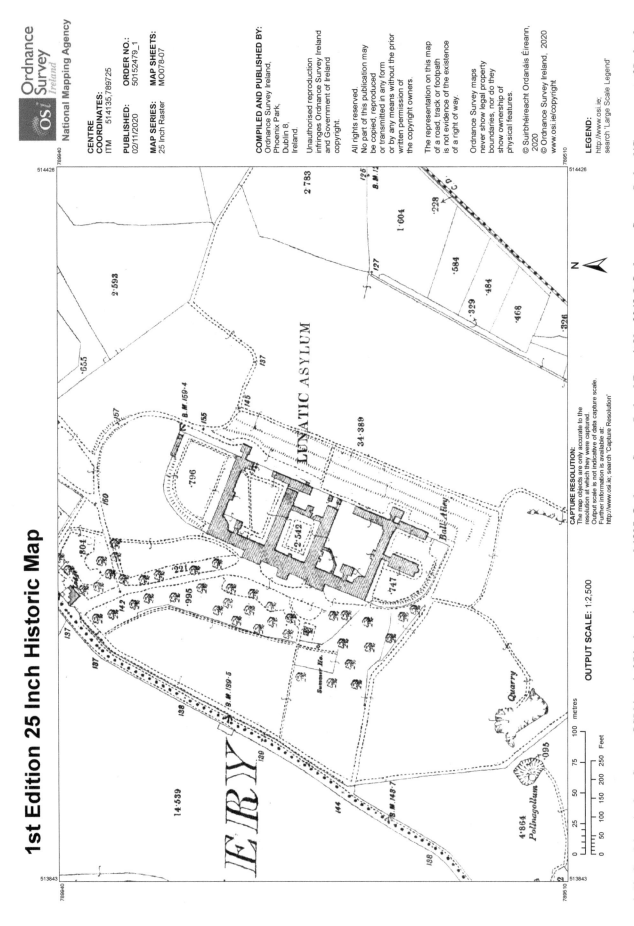

Figure 2-52. Castlebar Asylum. Source: OSI historic 25 inch series, surveyed 1895. Ordnance Survey Ireland Permit No. 9248 © Ordnance Survey Ireland/Government of Ireland.

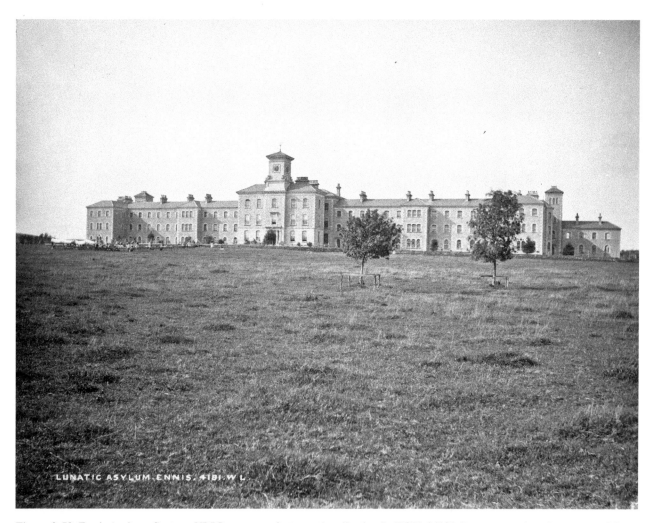

Figure 2-53. Ennis Asylum. Source: NLI Lawrence photograph collection L_ROY_04181. Image reproduced courtesy of the National Library of Ireland.

The extremely rapid industrialisation and consequent growth of Belfast saw the Antrim lunacy district divided into two, with Antrim patients accommodated at a new asylum opened in 1899 (although not fully completed until 1900), also built on the broad arrow plan (*ILC* 1901: xvi). A new general asylum was opened for the Dublin asylum district at Portrane in 1904. Both Antrim and Portrane adopted the pavilion system which was then prevalent in England, with blocks connected by corridors arranged in echelon, but favoured the broad arrow design with pavilions relatively widely spaced and distant from the central administration (as at Menston, Figure 2-19). The pavilion layout allowed for patient classification and prevented the spread of disease but prioritised control and containment.

The asylum at Purdysburn, for patients from Belfast District, was the last general lunatic asylum to be completed in Ireland, and replaced one of the very first asylums to be constructed. Construction at Purdysburn began in 1902, when four villas were built to designs by a local architectural firm (Graeme Watt & Tulloch). In 1909 construction began on the colony proper and hospital, admin, recreation hall, churches and further villas were added to the site, this phase reaching completion in 1913. The designer of this part of the asylum was G T

Hine, although working drawings and supervision of construction were carried out by a local firm, Graeme Watt & Tulloch.

2.3.3. Colony asylums in Ireland

From the 1860s a trend towards fragmentation of asylum sites is observable in Ireland, as elsewhere. Detached hospitals were commonly added to asylum sites (e.g. Armagh, Richmond, Clonmel) and this tendency appears to have accelerated from the 1890s. Detached hospitals were intended for the care of those suffering from 'bodily illness and requiring special care and watchfulness', and were built separately in order to benefit from the latest thinking in hospital design and construction (ILC 1892: 95). For instance, the detached hospital at Armagh, completed in 1897 had better heating than the main asylum and was built on higher ground to the north of the asylum site, where it benefitted from more efficient ventilation (ILC 1893: 90, Dictionary of Irish Architects).[8] Some asylums also erected smaller structures, sometimes

[8] This addition to Armagh asylum was the project of Dr William Graham who subsequently became the Medical Superintendent of Purdysburn (Quinn, 2011).

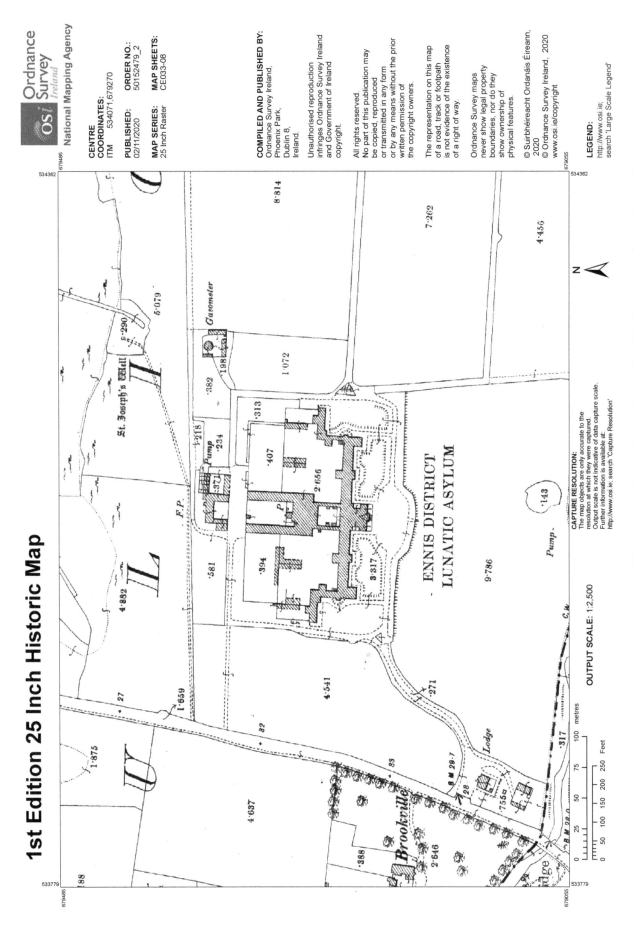

Figure 2-54. Ennis Asylum. Source: OSI historic 25 inch series, surveyed 1894. Ordnance Survey Ireland Permit No. 9248 © Ordnance Survey Ireland/Government of Ireland.

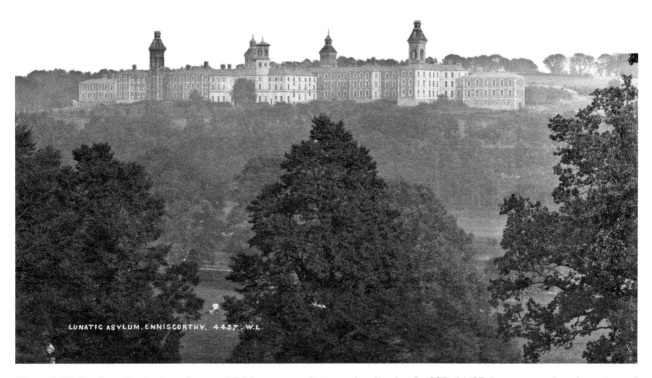

Figure 2-55. Enniscorthy Asylum. Source: NLI Lawrence photograph collection L_CSB_04437. Image reproduced courtesy of the National Library of Ireland.

of temporary materials, for patients suffering from infectious disease (e.g. Killarney) (ILC 1894: 206). The first asylum to provide detached accommodation for physically able patients appears to have been Monaghan, where villas (then referred to as 'blocks') were built as part of the design for the new asylum in 1869 (Figures 2-63, 2-64). It was stated that separate blocks allowed patients to be moved there who showed symptoms of improvement, allowing the different phases of disease to be 'more effectually dealt with than by the congregating of all classes of patients in one block'. The inspirations cited were Rouen, Prestwich and Chester, but this was the first asylum in Britain or Ireland to make such separate blocks part of the initial asylum design (*Irish Builder*, 1st June 1869). Subsequent to this, accommodation at existing asylums was often extended by the addition of separate blocks or pavilions, usually connected to the main asylum by means of corridors (e.g. Ballinasloe, Downpatrick) and some sites with pre-existing domestic dwellings available on the site used these for patients (e.g. Kilkenny, Portrane). However, Purdysburn was the only asylum in Ireland to use a full colony layout in the period before WWI. It was not until the decision was taken to build a villa colony at Purdysburn, that 'villas' so-called were occasionally added to other asylum sites around Ireland. For example, villas were built at Antrim, and Clonmel during the first decade of the twentieth century (Figure 2-66).

2.4. Scotland

Of the three asylum jurisdictions, (Ireland, England/ Wales and Scotland), the architecture of Scottish asylums is the most systematically and thoroughly recorded in the secondary literature. The unpublished thesis of Alison Darragh constitutes a gazetteer of all Scottish charitable and public asylums up to 1930, together with interpretation of their architectural development (Darragh, 2011). Harriet Richardson has also made important contributions to the history of Scottish hospitals, including asylums (Richardson, 1988; Richardson and MacInnes, 2010).

2.4.1. Institutional care of the insane prior to public asylums

Early institutional approaches to insanity in Scotland usually involved imprisonment, often at the local tollbooth, where the mentally ill were reputedly chained to the outer wall and abused by passers-by (Darragh 2011:8). The insane are known to have incarcerated and/or chained at tollbooths in Montrose, Perth, Aberdeen and Kilmaurs among other places. There were at this point few therapeutic treatments available, the insane being conceived as animal-like and insensitive with harsh treatment *de rigueur*, as elsewhere (Darragh 2011:11). With the establishment of infirmaries in the mid-eighteenth century, provision was sometimes made in hospitals for the mentally unwell but they were

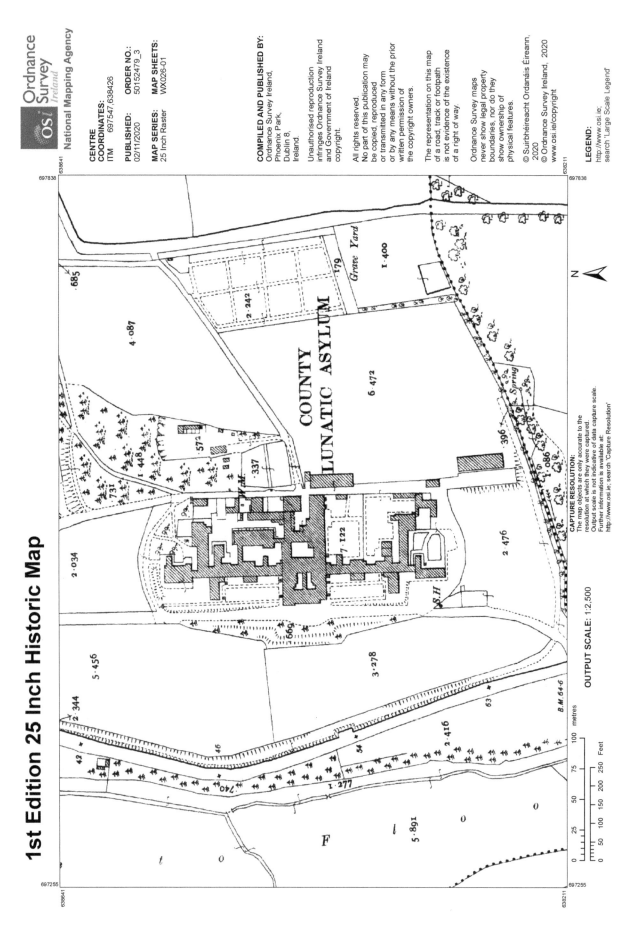

Figure 2-56. Enniscorthy Asylum. Source: OSI historic 25 inch series, surveyed 1903. Ordnance Survey Ireland Permit No. 9248 © Ordnance Survey Ireland/Government of Ireland.

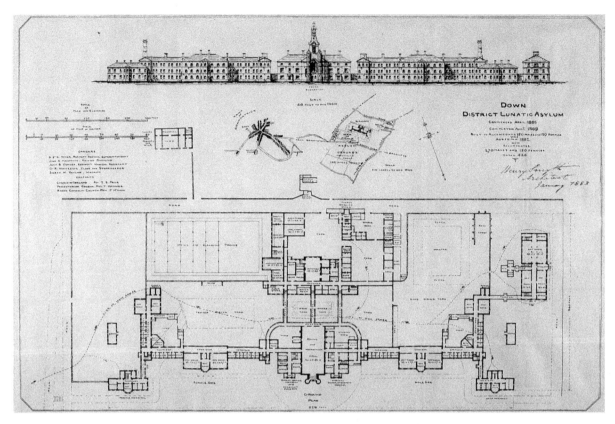

Figure 2-57. Down District Asylum, elevation and plan of asylum as extended in 1882 (built 1865-69). Source: reproduced with permission of Down County Museum.

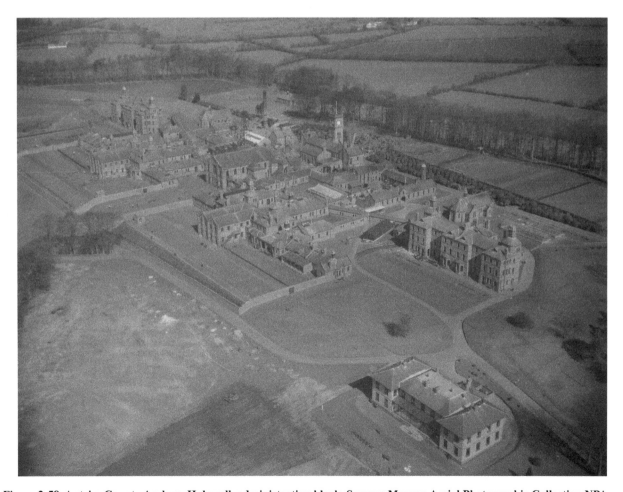

Figure 2-58. Antrim County Asylum, Holywell, administration block. Source: Morgan Aerial Photographic Collection NPA MOR1637. Image reproduced courtesy of the National Library of Ireland.

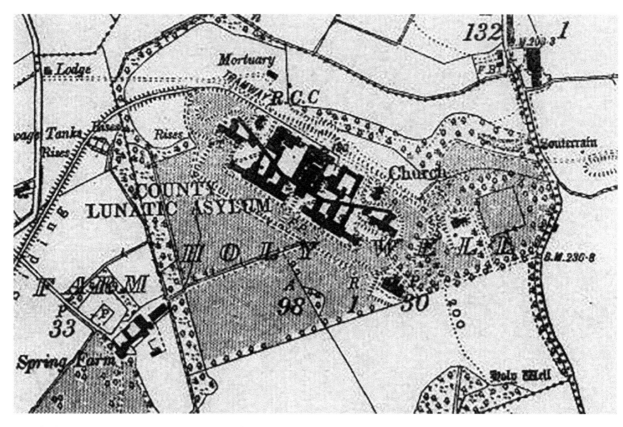

Figure 2-59. Antrim County Asylum, Holywell. Source: 6 inch to 1 mile county series edition 4, 1921.

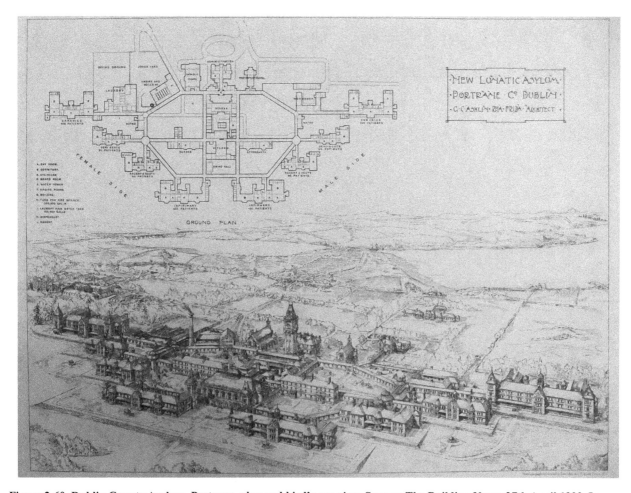

Figure 2-60. Dublin County Asylum, Portrane, plan and bird's eye view. Source: The Building News, 27th April 1900. Image reproduced courtesy of National Inventory of Architectural Heritage.

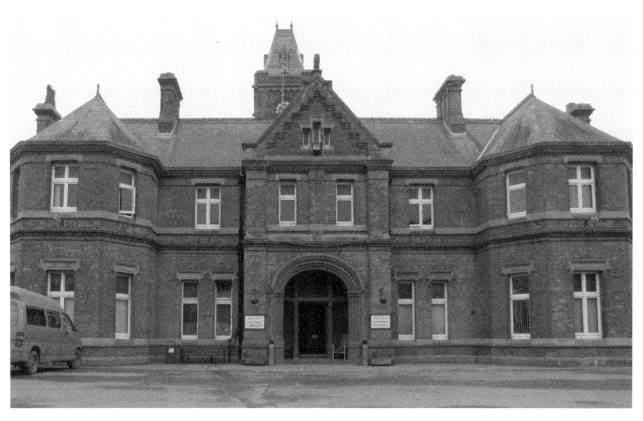

Figure 2-61. Dublin County Asylum, Portrane, entrance block. Source: Image reproduced courtesy of National Inventory of Architectural Heritage.

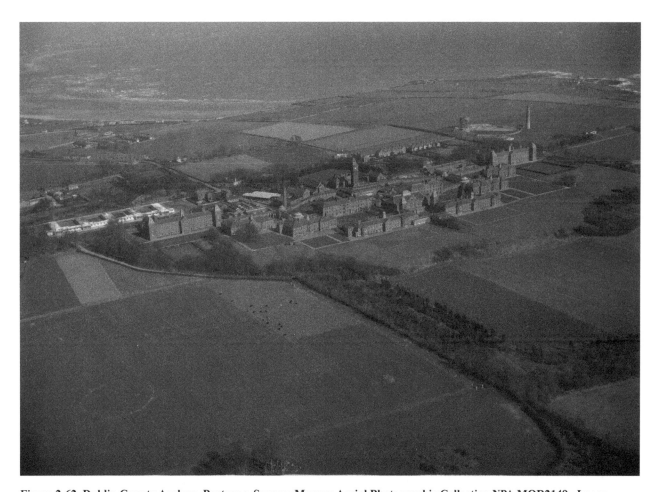

Figure 2-62. Dublin County Asylum, Portrane. Source: Morgan Aerial Photographic Collection NPA MOR2149. Image reproduced courtesy of the National Library of Ireland.

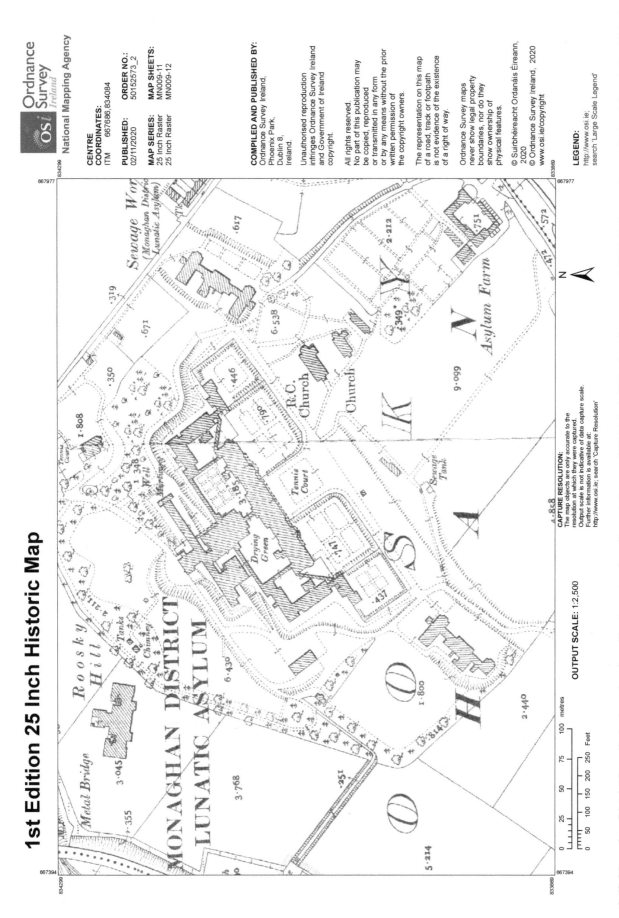

Figure 2-63. Monaghan District Lunatic Asylum showing villas to east and south-west. Source: OSI historic 25 inch series, surveyed 1907. Ordnance Survey Ireland Permit No. 9248 © Ordnance Survey Ireland/Government of Ireland.

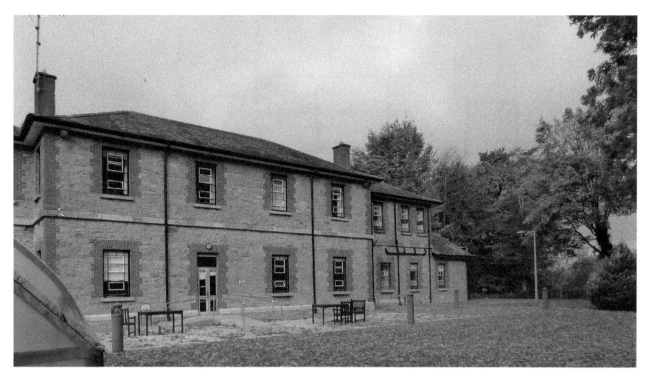

Figure 2-64. Monaghan District Lunatic Asylum villa (central section, wings demolished). Source: Author's photograph.

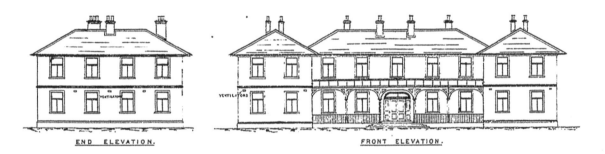

Figure 2-65. Antrim County Asylum, Holywell, villa elevations. Source: *Royal Commission on the Care and Control of the Feeble-minded. Minutes of Evidence relating to Scotland and Ireland on the original reference taken before the Royal Commission on the Care and Control of the Feeble-Minded with Appendices and Indexes. Volume III* **(1908). Image from ProQuest's House of Commons Parliamentary Papers. Permission provided by ProQuest LLC.**

generally considered a disruptive influence and were accommodated in separate wings or in a separate block (Glasgow, Aberdeen, Edinburgh, Dumfries Dundee and Inverness all had infirmaries with some accommodation for the insane). However, the type of accommodation provided was still of a carceral nature and often damp and dark (Darragh 2011: 15). Some charitable poorhouses also provided wards for the insane, such as that in Edinburgh, which was highly criticised by reformers as unsuitable due to its small size, unsuitable construction and local situation (Darragh 2011: 23).

The wealthier classes were able to avail of a network of private madhouses, but these did not necessarily provide superior accommodation, and were not subject to any kind of regulation. There was a considerable fear that these insitutions were capable of being exploited by those wishing to dispose of difficult relatives. The private madhouses were said to be overcrowded and the patients were restricted to an indoor life, or exercising within a small yard. Mechanical restraint was frequent and patients were observed sleeping 'together' on loose straw thrown into bed frames. Regulation came as a result of the *Act to Regulate madhouses in Scotland* in 1815 (55 Geo. III c.69), which required madhouses to obtain a licence and to submit to annual inspection from sheriffs and medical men (Darragh 2011:21).

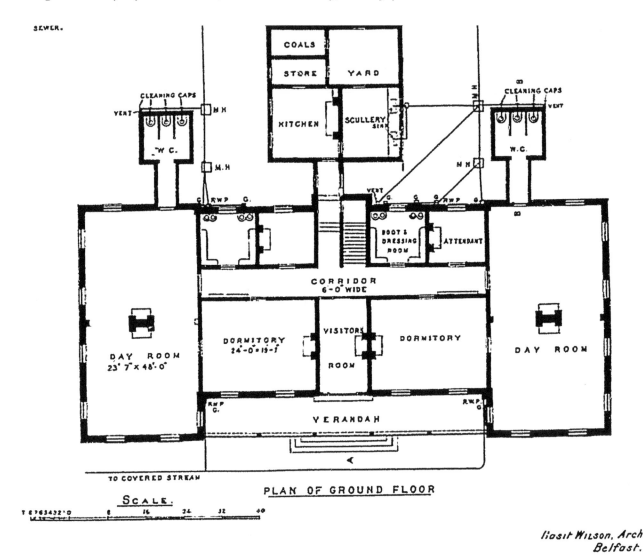

Figure 2-66. Antrim County Asylum, Holywell, villa ground plan. Source: *Royal Commission on the Care and Control of the Feeble-minded. Minutes of Evidence relating to Scotland and Ireland on the original reference taken before the Royal Commission on the Care and Control of the Feeble-Minded with Appendices and Indexes. Volume III* (1908). Image from ProQuest's House of Commons Parliamentary Papers. Permission provided by ProQuest LLC.

With the change to an enlightenment view of insanity, seven charitable asylums for the insane, accommodating both private and pauper patients and which were all to receive the royal charter, were established in Scotland in the late eighteenth and early nineteenth century. An unincorporated public asylum was built in Elgin in 1835 (as in some early English asylums, the building comprising ten cells was financed by subscription, but maintenance was provided by the poor rates), which accepted only pauper lunatics but the Royal Asylums accommodated both pauper and private patients. By 1818 the number of those identified as insane in Scotland can be estimated at c5,000, but of these only c750 were in any form of institution. The first asylum to be opened, in Montrose, was built by subscription and motivated by a desire to rid the town of the nuisance of the 'mad people being kept in prison in the middle of the street', to keep the insane in more humane conditions and to bring about a cure where possible. The early Royal asylums were small (for less than 150 patients), and the Aberdeen design may have been typical of the early style,

with a plain domestic building forming accommodation for the asylum keeper and attendants, forming one side of a quadrangle, the other three sides being divided into 16 single-storey cells for the patients (Darragh 2011: 55-58).

The design for Glasgow Royal Asylum by William Stark, was revolutionary, and provided a hitherto unknown level of comfort for insane patients (Darragh 2011:61). It was also very influential beyond Scotland, being the first hospital on a radial plan, and appearing to follow Bentham's panopticon approach (Figures 2-67, 2-68). The radial plan was adopted for the first phase of asylum building in Ireland and at two asylums in Devon and Cornwall, but later came to be seen as more suitable for prison design (Richardson & MacInnes 2010: 37-39). Dumfries and Perth, both by the same architect, William Burn, were heavily influenced by the design for Wakefield asylum and featured panoptic hubs, also a feature of Burn's design for the second Edinburgh Royal Asylum (Figures 2-69, 2-70). In architectural style, the Royal asylums were initially

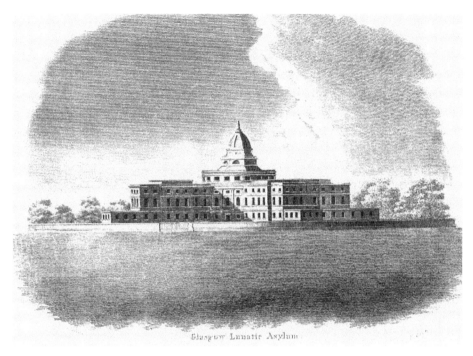

Figure 2-67. Glasgow Asylum, perspective view. Source: *Select Committee on provisions for better regulation of madhouses in England: Third report, minutes of evidence, appendix.* **Image from ProQuest's House of Commons Parliamentary Papers. Permission provided by ProQuest LLC.**

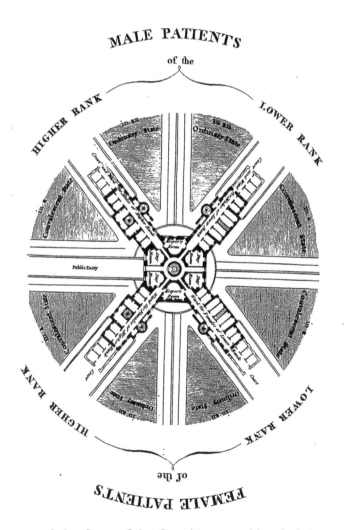

Figure 2-68. Glasgow Asylum, ground plan. Source: *Select Committee on provisions for better regulation of madhouses in England: Third report, minutes of evidence, appendix.* **Image from ProQuest's House of Commons Parliamentary Papers. Permission provided by ProQuest LLC.**

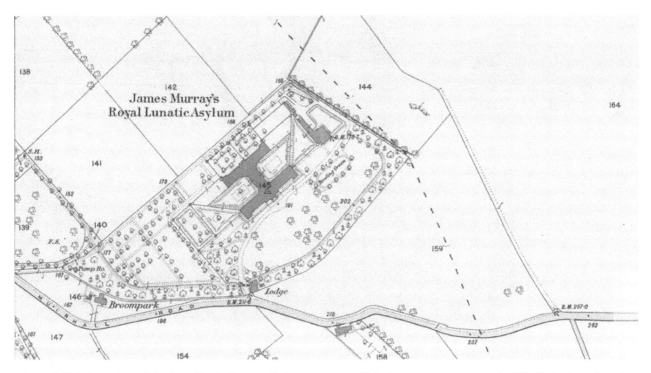

Figure 2-69. Murray Royal Asylum, Perth. Source: Ordnance Survey 25 inch to one mile, surveyed 1859-1860. Reproduced with the permission of the National Library of Scotland.

classical and sober but this changed with the construction of Gartnavel, the second Glasgow Royal Asylum (1843) in a Tudor Gothic style that was perceived as elaborate and palatial in character (Richardson and MacInnes, 2010: 41-42).

In addition to asylum accommodation, the insane were also accepted in Scotland's network of poorhouses, some of which had separate wards for these patients and Perth prison had a 'lunatic department'. Private accommodation for the insane was provided in 23

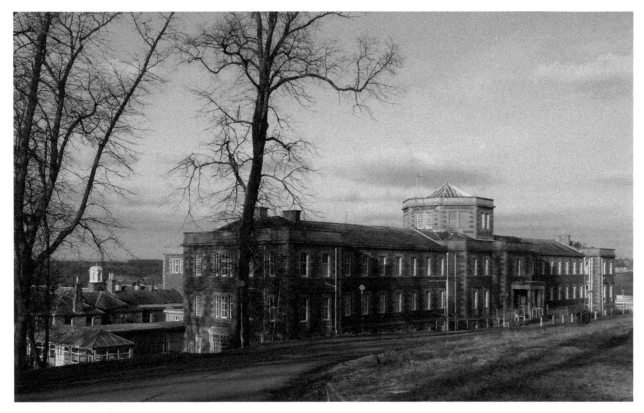

Figure 2-70. Murray Royal Asylum, Perth. Front elevation showing panoptic hub. Source: Rob Burke, Creative Commons Attribution Share-alike license 2.0 (CC BY-SA 2.0).

Table 4. Royal Asylums in Scotland with dates of opening and major additions.

Charitable (Royal) Asylums in Scotland (opening dates)	Plan Form	(middle phase of development)	(late phase of development))
Montrose (1)(1782)(obtained Royal Charter 1810)	Corridor	Montrose (2) (1857)	Separate Hospital Block (1888) Montrose (Carnegie House) (1895), Howden Villa (1901), North Esk Villa (1904)
Aberdeen (1)(1800)	Corridor		Aberdeen (Elmhill House) (1862), House of Daviot (1889) Separate hospital (1893)
Edinburgh (1)(1813)	Corridor	Edinburgh(2) (1837)	Edinburgh (Craighouse) (Bevan Villa) South Craig Villa) (1894)
Glasgow (1) (1814)	Radial	Glasgow (2) (1843)	Detached cottages for infectious diseases (1891)
Dundee (1) (1820)	Corridor	Dundee (2) (1880)	Dundee (Gowrie House) (1898)
Perth (James Murray's) (1827)	Panoptic Corridor		Two villas (1902)
Dumfries (Crichton Royal Institution) (1)(1839)	Panoptic Corridor	Dumfries (2) (1859)	Dumfries (3) (from 1898)(colony plan), male hospital block (1912)

licensed houses and 'idiot' children were provided for in two schools. In the early nineteenth century, unsuccessful attempts were made to establish public asylums, but by mid-century the charitable provision for the insane poor was overcrowded and pressure grew, stimulated by investigations made by the reformer Dorothea Dix, for a public system of asylums as had, by this time, been provided in Ireland, England and Wales (Darragh, 2011: 79-85).

2.4.2. Establishment of public asylum system

Following the passing of legislation in 1857 (Lunacy (Scotland) Act) (20 & 21 Vict. c.71), eighteen district asylums were built in Scotland in the period up to the First World War. Early asylums built in the 1860s were on a corridor plan and varied from a plain institutional gothic architectural style, to more elaborate styles such as the Jacobean of the Northern Counties Asylum (Figure 2-71,

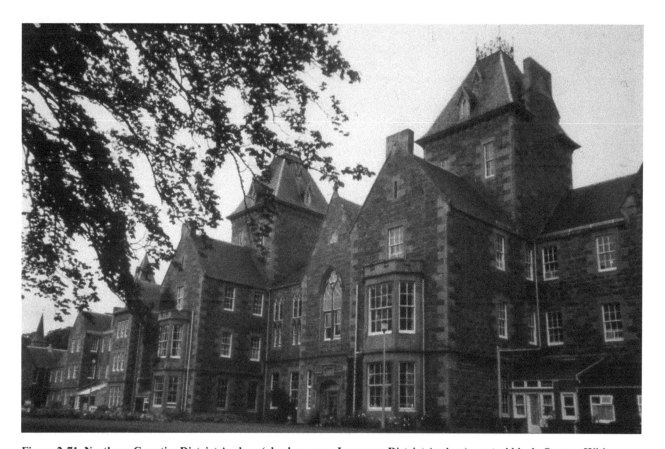

Figure 2-71. Northern Counties District Asylum (also known as Inverness District Asylum), central block. Source: With permission of Harriet Richardson, historic-hospitals.com.

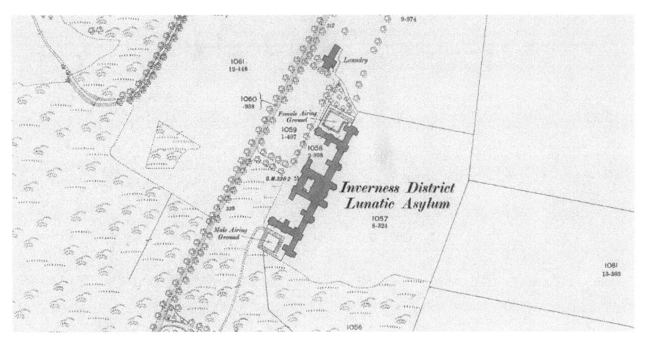

Figure 2-72. Northern Counties District Asylum (also known as Inverness District Asylum). Source: Ordnance Survey 25 inch to one mile, surveyed 1868. Reproduced with the permission of the National Library of Scotland.

2-72). Italianate styles were also used in the late 1860s and 1870s, and the plan form of asylums became more compact, perhaps reflecting the increasing provision of dayrooms and dormitories, as these replaced cells and galleries. After a gap of more than a decade, when no new asylums were built, construction of district asylums began anew in the mid 1890s with three relatively large examples constructed in the area surrounding Glasgow. These all used the pavilion plan which had become standard in

England at this period but only Lanark arranged pavilions in the English fashion, with a compact arrow layout that somewhat resembled Claybury (Figures 2-73, 2-74). The City of Glasgow and Govan district asylums used a layout which appears to have been unique to Scotland, consisting of pavilions arranged in a linear fashion, as 'wings' to each side of the administration buildings and a separate hospital on a corridor plan (Figure 2-75, 2-76). These two asylums effectively divided asylum accommodation into medical

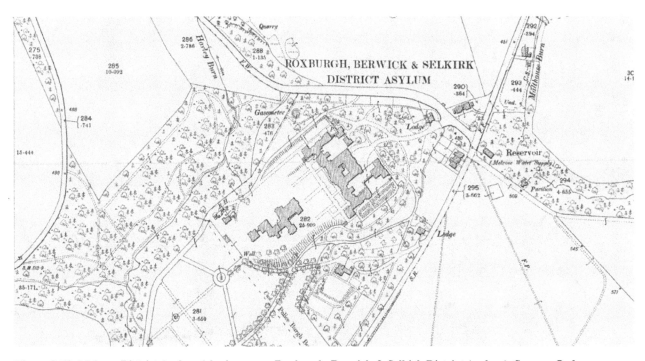

Figure 2-73. Melrose District Asylum (also known as Roxburgh, Berwick & Selkirk District Asylum). Source: Ordnance Survey 25 inch to one mile, surveyed 1897. Reproduced with the permission of the National Library of Scotland.

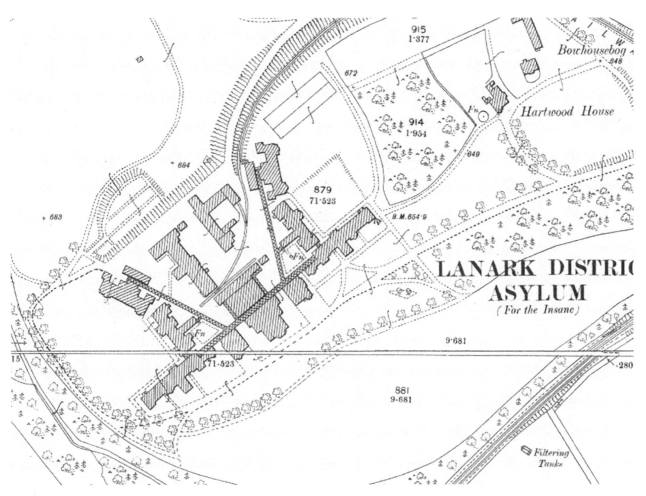

Figure 2-74. Lanark District Asylum. Source: Ordnance Survey 25 inch to one mile, revised 1896. Reproduced with the permission of the National Library of Scotland.

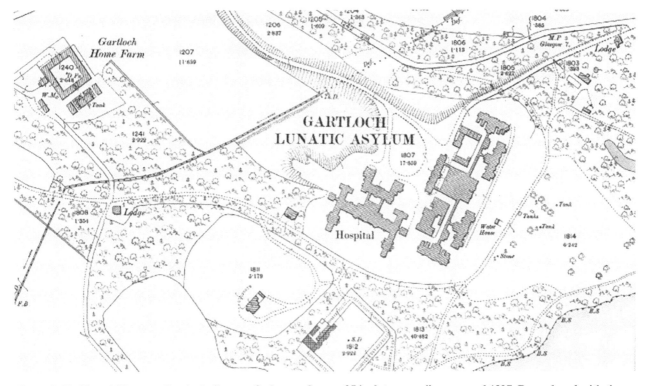

Figure 2-75. City of Glasgow, Gartloch. Source: Ordnance Survey 25 inch to one mile, surveyed 1897. Reproduced with the permission of the National Library of Scotland.

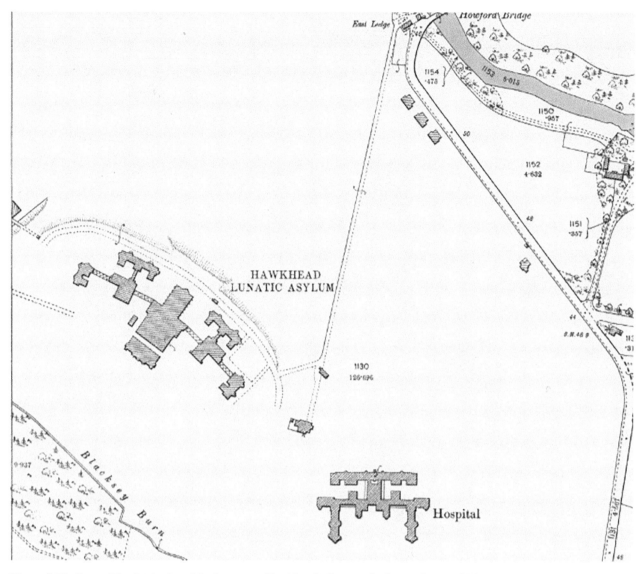

Figure 2-76. Govan District Asylum (also known as Hawkhead). Source: Ordnance Survey 25 inch to one mile, surveyed 1895. Reproduced with the permission of the National Library of Scotland.

and non-medical sections, thus providing more specialised treatment for those requiring it. As in other jurisdictions, the addition of separate hospital buildings to asylum sites became common from the late 1880s when a hospital was added to Montrose Royal. Hospitals were also added to Melrose, Ayrshire and Stirling District Asylums and Crichton Royal Institution, with hospital accommodation expanding to one half of the total provision in many asylums (Darragh, 2011:273).

There were several unique features to Scottish care for the insane poor in the second half of the nineteenth century. The first was 'boarding out', a system formally implemented by the Lunacy Act of 1857 whereby harmless, chronic patients (often those characterised as 'idiots' or 'imbeciles') were accommodated in the community. The system was regulated by the SLC who were charged with inspecting and maintaining standards. Patients were usually placed in cottages in farming or village communities with a suitable guardian, some communities

becoming accustomed to numbers of insane patients living among them. The numbers accommodated in this way grew from 1,804 in 1859 to 2,907 in 1908. Although Poor Law Unions in England sometimes supported the needy (including the insane) through out-relief, the system was not systematised in the same way as in Scotland, and Irish authorities resisted attempts to introduce boarding out (Bartlett and Wright, 1999: 7; Sturdy and Parry-Jones, 1999). The second feature was the removal of boundary and airing court walls in the second half of the nineteenth century due to the belief that patients' mental illness was exacerbated by close confinement with other patients. The walled airing courts also began to be seen as a type of 'mechanical restraint' which was increasingly seen as unacceptable within Scottish asylum discourse. Walls began to be removed at some asylums from the late 1860s, while others merely lowered them or replaced them with fences. External boundary walls or fences were also, according to the SLC, a rarity at Scottish district asylums, and these measures were thought to increase the patients' feeling of

Table 5. District Asylums constructed in Scotland under 1857 Act. (Two poor law asylums, Barony Parochial asylum (1875) and Greenock Poorhouse and Parochial Asylum (1879), have been omitted) (Source: Darragh, 2011).

Asylum Name	Opening Date	No of patients constructed for	Plan Form	Modifications
Argyll District Asylum	1863	275	Corridor	1881 – East House added. Villa added at unknown date.
Northern Counties District Asylum	1864	300	Corridor	1881 – additions, 1896-8 – hospital wards added to main building
Perth District Asylum	1864	202	Corridor	1894 – two villas added
Banff District Asylum	1865	90	Corridor	1880- separate block for chronic females, 1903 – villa for male patients
Fife and Kinross District Asylum	1866	200	Corridor	Further blocks added in 1869, 1879, 1892 and 1913
Haddington District Asylum	1866	90	Corridor	1908 – villas added for chronic working patients
Ayrshire District Asylum	1869	230	Corridor	1897, 1899 –villas added in grounds, 1904 – detached hospital
Stirling District Asylum	1869	220	Corridor	1893 – separate hospital added
Melrose District Asylum	1872	200	Corridor	1895-8 –hospital blocks added for males and females
Midlothian and Peebles District Asylum	1874	500	Corridor	
Paisley and Johnstone District Asylum	1876	100	Corridor	
Bothwell District Asylum	1881	180	Corridor	
Lanark District Asylum	1895	500	Pavilion	1904-7 – TB sanatorium
Govan District Asylum	1896	400	Pavilion with separate hospital	1908 – two pavilions added
City of Glasgow District Asylum	1897	382	Pavilion with separate hospital	1902 – farm and recreation hall added
Aberdeen District Asylum	1904	478	Colony	
Edinburgh District Asylum	1906	1000	Colony	
Renfrew District Asylum	1909	300	Colony	

liberty which would result in fewer escapes (Ross, 2014: 239-243). The open-door system derived from the same logic, doors were to be kept open during the daytime in all wards where this was practicable making asylums more reliant on the supervision of attendants to exercise control over patients (SLC Report 1881: xxxi-xxxv). It is unclear whether this system was widely practised in England and Wales, although Burdett claimed that 13 English County asylums were partly open and two idiot asylums fully open in 1891 (cited in Clarke, 1993:528).

2.4.3. Village/colony asylums in Scotland

As we have seen, after c1880, an earlier monolithic style of asylum construction, where all accommodation and services were contained within a single building, began to break down and a number of segregatory trends are observable, including the construction of separate asylum and hospital buildings (Darragh, 2011 257-273; Halliday, 2003: 295-305; Richardson, 1991; Ross, 2014: 283-305). The Royal (charitable) Asylums started to build or adapt separate houses in suburban areas for their private

patients (Aberdeen, Dundee, Edinburgh), usually on the scale of a hotel or large mansion house, and villas resembling middle-class dwelling houses were added to asylum sites at Banff, Dumfries, Perth, Montrose, Argyll, Ayrshire, and Haddington (Figures 2-77, 2-78). The 'village system' (as the colony asylum was often known in Scotland) constituted the fullest flowering of this trend, not only segregating patient accommodation, but actively dispersing it around a rural site. The only complete asylums to be built after 1900 in Scotland were built to this plan, which provided the majority of patient accommodation in bourgeois-style villas, laid out in the manner of a village or suburban settlement within a substantial rural acreage. The village layout was adopted for Crichton Royal Asylum's 'Third House' (commenced in 1898) and every one of the district asylums which were constructed in the period 1900-1914, namely, Kingseat (Aberdeen), Dykebar (Renfrew) and Bangour (Edinburgh) (Easterbrook, 1940). The village asylum in Scotland was directly inspired by the most influential German example of purpose-built colony for the insane, Alt Scherbitz, near Leipzig (Richardson, 1991). It was also the plan used for

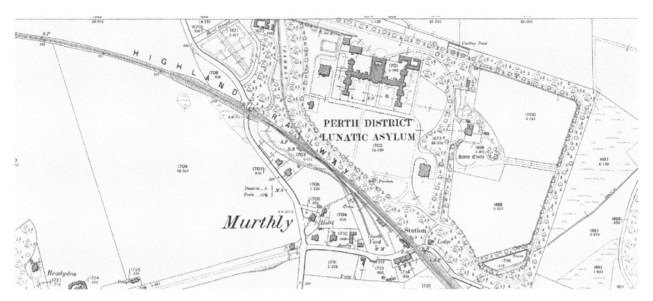

Figure 2-77. Perth District Asylum, villas shown to west and south. Source: Ordnance Survey 25 inch to one mile, surveyed 1895. Reproduced with the permission of the National Library of Scotland.

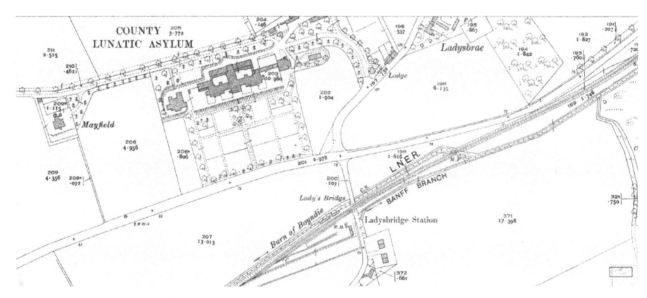

Figure 2-78. Banff District Asylum, villas shown to west. Source: Ordnance Survey 25 inch to one mile, revised 1928-9. Reproduced with the permission of the National Library of Scotland.

one of the largest asylums to be built in Scotland in the pre-war period, Bangour Village, which was twice as large as any hitherto built (although it did not reach full capacity for some time).

2.5. Germany

A number of selective surveys give a broad picture of the development of the asylum system in Germany. These include the work of Dieter Jetter (Jetter, 1971; Dieter Jetter, 1981) and N Müller (Müller, 1997) and the contextual work of Edward Shorter, Leslie Topp and Eric Engstrom (Shorter, 1997, 2007; Engstrom, 2003; Topp, Moran and Andrews, 2007).

2.5.1. Institutional care of the insane prior to public asylums

In the pre-asylum period in Germany, the raving insane were traditionally housed in cells or wooden cages, in the round towers of town walls, together with other ungovernable prisoners (Thompson & Goldin 1975: 59; Müller 1997: 187-189; Jetter 1971: 85-92). Early, more humane, attempts to care for or treat the insane were often based on monastic establishments or shrines, such as the shrine to St Dymphna at Gheel in Belgium. Gheel attracted many pilgrims from Germany and France and gradually led to the informal establishment of a colony of the insane, patients living with the villagers in their houses and the able assisting with domestic and farming work, which was gradually regulated and brought under state control (Jetter, 1981: 3-4). More systematic provision for the insane began with cells in the 'Burgerhospitaler' or public city hospitals, from the late medieval period. 'Landeshospitaler' were set up after the Reformation to divert monastic income towards education and the care of the poor and sick. Monastic separation of men and women continued, however, with separate institutions for each gender often widely separated. However, in these establishments the insane were often kept in chains. Highly influential for the establishment of the asylum system in Germany were developments in France which, under absolutist monarchy, brought forward a new type of 'Hôpital général'. The 'Hôpital de Bicêtre' for men and the 'Hôpital de la Salpetrière' for women contained from the outset large lunatic wards which became the cradle for the establishment of modern French psychiatry, with the work of Pinel (in particular his attempts to heal the chronically insane through 'traitement moral et philosophique' (psychological treatment)) and Esquirol becoming influential across Europe. The French model was followed in Germany on a smaller scale for the provision of the insane in such institutions as the *Zucht- und Tollhauser* (combined penitentiary and lunatic asylums (Dieter Jetter, 1981: 18-25).

Particularly notable is the segregation of the insane from other kinds of prisoner at the institution in Celle, one of the first *Zucht- und Tollhauser* (begun 1710) at a time where the insane and other prisoners were not clearly differentiated in other European institutions (Thompson & Goldin 1975: 62). The insane were housed in heated cells surrounding a courtyard that had cage-like lattice doors and privies in each cell with chained copper bowls for food, but wooden shutters instead of windows. In the first half of the nineteenth century, the German states generally combined accommodation for the insane with that for prisoners or the indigent poor and in the early nineteenth century the German physician and one of the first university teachers of psychiatry, Johann Christian Reil, wrote of his horror at the treatment of the insane in institutions. He commented,

> 'like criminals we lock these unfortunate creatures into mad-cages, into antiquated prisons, or put them next to the nesting holes of owls in desolate attics over the town gates or in the damp cellars of the jails, where the sympathetic gaze of a friend of mankind might never behold them; and we leave them there, gripped by chains, corrupting in their own filth' (quoted in Gold & Gold, 2015: 23).

2.5.2. Establishment of public asylum system

Early asylums in Germany were instituted as a result of agreements to compensate German princes after the Napoleonic wars which resulted in the secularisation of church property, including cloisters and castles which were then used to house insane patients. A number of new institutions were constructed from the 1830s including

Sachsenburg (1830), Illenau (1842), Nietleben (1844), Erlangen (1846) and Munich (1859) (Engstrom 1997: 17-18). Initially, separate institutions were constructed for curable (*heilanstalten* – healing institutions) and incurable (*pflegeanstalten* – nursing institutions) cases. By the mid-nineteenth century these two functions were often combined, for example, at Illenau (1842). This was an asylum of linear accommodation, organised by type of patient, curable/incurable, disturbed/quiet, with quieter patients also allocated accommodation according to social class. The church was architecturally at the centre of the building, rather than the doctors and administration, as was usually the case in an English asylum (Figure 2-79) (Thompson & Goldin, 1975: 62-7). Panoptic principles were adopted in only one German asylum, constructed in Erlangen in 1846, but this style was already considered outdated at the time (Figure 2-80) (Müller, 1997: 187). By mid-century there were 77 institutions for the insane in the German states, excluding Austria-Hungary, considerably more than in England at the same period, although one third of these were wards within larger hospitals. In the second half of the nineteenth century the proportion of patients being treated in private institutions also grew from three per cent to nearly 25 per cent, although this often reflected the duty of the state to care for patients within an overcrowded system. Before the German empire was established in 1871, German states administered their asylums in a variety of ways and, national legislation on the provision of asylums was never instituted in Germany, as it had been in other European states. The majority of institutions for the insane were situated in isolated rural locations which, as elsewhere, were said to be therapeutically beneficial (Engstrom 1997:18-19).

The institutions for 400 in Neustadt-Eberswalde (1865) and Dalldorf in Berlin for 1000 (1879) were inspired by the French system of agricultural colonies for the insane. This ultimately led to what was known in Germany as the 'pavillonsystem'[9] of separate dispersed villas for patients, as first practised at Alt Scherbitz. During the period 1876 to 1914, at least 26 examples of the 'pavillonsystem' were built in Germany, or opened as adjuncts to pre-existing asylums, earlier symmetrical layouts gradually giving way to layouts that were meandering and curvilinear. At these institutions the insane were encouraged to perform useful work, either agricultural or in workshops attached to the asylum, the belief being that lack of activity led to worsening of the symptoms of insanity and cognitive impairment (Müller, 1997: 188). City clinics for the acutely ill began to be opened from 1868, and institutional psychiatry and academic psychiatry began to draw apart, partly as a result of a dispute between major figures on either side (Dörries and Beddies, 2003: 158).

The clinics took a somatic view of the nature of mental illness as a disease of the brain and sought to treat it as a

---

[9] The terminology used in Germany differs from that used in England, where 'pavilions' usually refers to large blocks connected by corridors, rather than the villa or colony system.

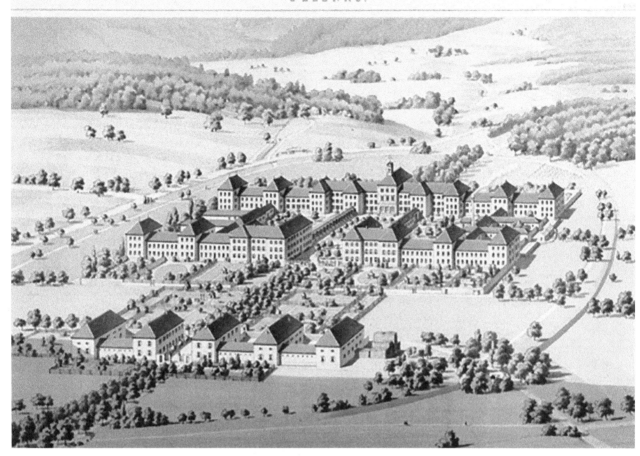

Figure 2-79. General view of the Illenau Sanatorium, 1865. Source: After a lithograph by J Vollweider and C Kiefer, Lithographic Institute L. Geissendörfer Carlsruhe.

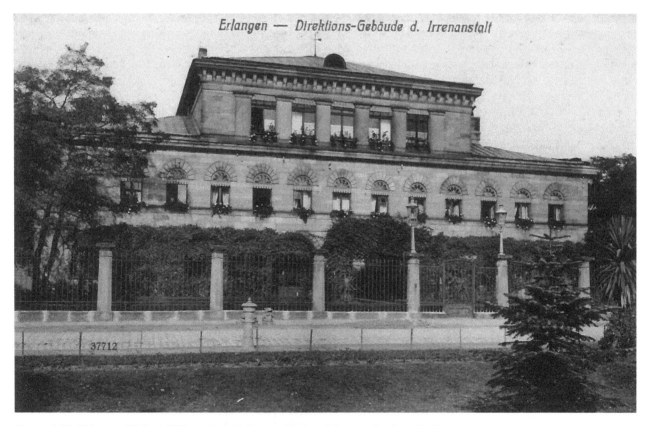

Figure 2-80. Erlangen Heil und Pflege Anstalt. Source: Postcard from author's collection.

Table 6. Colony asylums in Germany with year of opening (or year that pre-existing asylum opened colony accommodation) and number of patients. (Sources: Report of a Lancashire deputation, 1900; de.wikipedia.org; Burdett, Volume 1, 1891)

Asylum Location	Date of opening	Number of patients
Alt Scherbitz, Saxony	1876	450
Gabersee, Wasserburg	1883	?
Halle-Nietleben, Saxony	1887	400
Emmendingen, Freiburg	1889	1,000
Herzberge, Berlin (Figure 2-81)	1893	1,150
Untergöltzsch, Saxony	1893	600
Wuhlgarten, Berlin (Figure 2-82)	1893	1,000
Uchtspringe, Saxony (Figure 2-83)	1894	500
Zschadrass, Saxony	1895	500
Weilmünster, Wiesbaden	1897	1,000
Grafenburg, Rhine Province (Figure 2-84)	1899	800
Galkhausen, Rhine Province (Figure 2-85)	1900	800
Lüneburg, Lower Saxony	1901	800
Mecklenburg-Strelitz'sche, Domjuch	1902	130
Wiesloch, Nordbaden	1903	1,000
Weissenhof, Weinsberg (Figure 2-86)	1903	550
Warstein, Westphalia	1905	1,400
Eglfing/Haar, Munich	1905	1,250
Rheinhessen, Alzey	1908	400
Mainkofen, Deggendorf	1911	500
Herborn, Wiesbaden	1911	1,200
Warstein, Westphalia	1911	1,450
Bedburg-Hau, Westphalia	1912	3,000
Mühlhausen, Thuringia	1912	800
Stralsund, Pomerania	1912	400
Lübeck-Strecknitz, Schleswig-Holstein	1912	1,500
Reichenau, Baden-Württemberg	1913	910

physical illness in a setting forming part of a general or university hospital. As a result Germany was regarded as being at the forefront of psychiatry because of its emphasis on scientific research into the causes of mental illness (Beveridge, 1991: 380). Psychiatry and neurology formed a rich neuropsychiatric tradition in Germany and Austria which produced such prominent names as Griesinger, Wernicke, Krafft-Ebing, and Meynert (Renvoize, 1991: 71). In the early twentieth century, probably under the influence of treatments for TB, bed treatment in *Wachsaalen* or observation rooms began to be replaced by outdoor bed treatment, for which verandahs were often attached to the *Wachsaalen* and deck chairs and tents were purchased (Müller, 1997: 190). In Germany, as elsewhere, once a programme of construction of public lunatic asylums was undertaken, overcrowding of the system quickly followed and building of new asylums became necessary. Between 1877 and 1904 the number of asylums almost doubled

from 93 to 180 and numbers of patients almost tripled from 33,023 to 111,951 (Dörries and Beddies, 2003: 150).

2.5.3. *Colony asylums in Germany*

The Provincial Lunatic Asylum of Alt Scherbitz was founded near Leipzig in 1876, by Dr Johannes Moritz Koeppe and was taken over on his death in 1879 by his assistant Dr Albrecht Paetz, whose name is mostly clearly associated with the layout and regime (Sonntag, 1993: 26-30). By the 1890s, Alt Scherbitz had become 'a standard stop on asylum research trip itineraries' (Topp, 2007: 736). The immediate precursor was the *Ackerbaucolonien* or agricultural colonies for the insane that had been established in many places in Germany in the 1860s, following the example of Fitz-James in France, as annexes to 'closed' asylums. Alt Scherbitz represented a new departure, in that the amount of land was much extended, to about 1.5 acres per patient and all the patients were accommodated on a single site, with the vast majority (it was claimed 90 per cent) engaged in useful work, largely outdoors (Besser, 1881; Letchworth, 1889; Sonntag, 1993: 30).

Scottish asylum practice was also a significant inspiration for the regime at Alt Scherbitz and possibly also for its lay-out, part of the asylum being constructed after the Scottish Board of Lunacy reported on advances in patient liberty in 1881, as discussed below. Paetz lectured on the Scottish open-door system to the Annual Meeting of the Association of German Psychiatrists in 1886 and cites other pioneering Scottish developments, such as boarding out and the removal of walls and fences in his published work. Alt Scherbitz is described as the culmination of these ideas; a large agricultural colony combined with an asylum on the most modern principles of the free treatment of the insane which employs the open-door system '*nach schottischem Vorgange*' (after the Scottish precedent) for the first time in Germany and takes this system even further than it has been taken in Scotland through the construction of villas without connecting corridors (Paetz, 1893: 144; Sonntag, 1993: 29-30).

2.6. Development of the colony asylum in Europe

The earliest discernible attempt to marry agricultural work and family-style institutional provision for the poor was the 'farm school' system, inspired by Rousseau's ideas on education, originated by Pestalozzi in Switzerland in 1774 and carried forward by another prominent Swiss educator Fellenberg and his colleague Wehrli, in which children were engaged on simple agricultural tasks that were intended to make a meaningful contribution to their upkeep. By mid-century, schools with an agricultural component that sought to reform or protect pauper children were widespread across Germany, Switzerland, Holland, France and Belgium and were 'struggling into existence' in England (Fletcher, 1852: 4). The most celebrated examples of this trend were, Das Rauhe Haus, Hamburg (1837), and one of the imitators spawned by it, the reformatory colony of Mettray (1840), where juvenile inmates were dispersed

FIG. I. HERZBERGE ASYLUM.

GROUND PLAN.

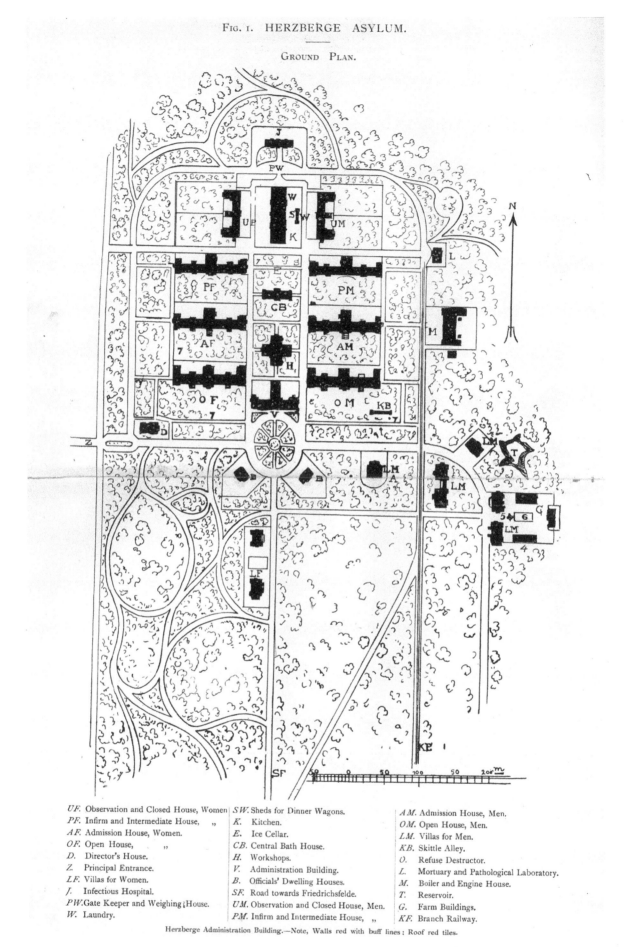

UF. Observation and Closed House, Women	*SW.* Sheds for Dinner Wagons.	*AM.* Admission House, Men.
PF. Infirm and Intermediate House, „	*K.* Kitchen.	*OM.* Open House, Men.
AF. Admission House, Women.	*E.* Ice Cellar.	*LM.* Villas for Men.
OF. Open House, „	*CB.* Central Bath House.	*KB.* Skittle Alley.
D. Director's House.	*H.* Workshops.	*O.* Refuse Destructor.
Z. Principal Entrance.	*V.* Administration Building.	*L.* Mortuary and Pathological Laboratory.
LF. Villas for Women.	*B.* Officials' Dwelling Houses.	*M.* Boiler and Engine House.
J. Infectious Hospital.	*SF.* Road towards Friedrichsfelde.	*T.* Reservoir.
PW. Gate Keeper and Weighing House.	*UM.* Observation and Closed House, Men.	*G.* Farm Buildings.
W. Laundry.	*PM.* Infirm and Intermediate House, „	*KF.* Branch Railway.

Herzberge Administration Building.—Note, Walls red with buff lines : Roof red tiles.

Figure 2-81. Herzberge Asylum, Berlin. Source: *Report of a deputation appointed to visit asylums on the continent with recommendations regarding the building of a new (sixth) Lancashire asylum* **(1900). Preston: Lancashire Asylums Board.**

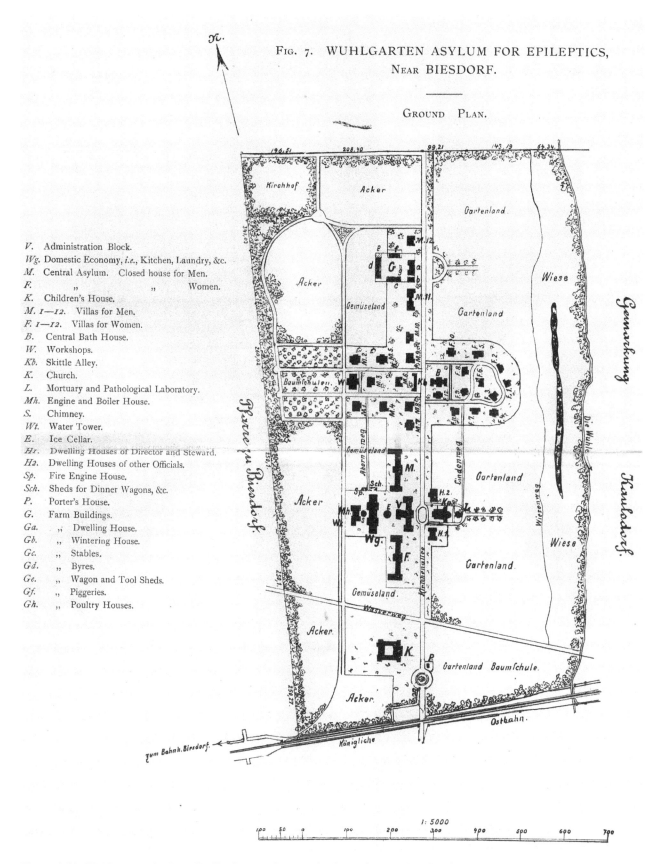

FIG. 7. WUHLGARTEN ASYLUM FOR EPILEPTICS, NEAR BIESDORF.

GROUND PLAN.

V.   Administration Block.
Wg. Domestic Economy, *i.e.*, Kitchen, Laundry, &c.
M.   Central Asylum.   Closed house for Men.
F.   „   „   Women.
K.   Children's House.
M. 1—12. Villas for Men.
F. 1—12. Villas for Women.
B.   Central Bath House.
W.   Workshops.
Kb. Skittle Alley.
K.   Church.
L.   Mortuary and Pathological Laboratory.
Mh. Engine and Boiler House.
S.   Chimney.
Wt. Water Tower.
E.   Ice Cellar.
H1. Dwelling Houses of Director and Steward.
H2. Dwelling Houses of other Officials.
Sp. Fire Engine House.
Sch. Sheds for Dinner Wagons, &c.
P.   Porter's House.
G.   Farm Buildings.
Ga.   „   Dwelling House.
Gb.   „   Wintering House.
Gc.   „   Stables.
Gd.   „   Byres.
Ge.   „   Wagon and Tool Sheds.
Gf.   „   Piggeries.
Gh.   „   Poultry Houses.

1: 5000

Figure 2-82. Wuhlgartern Asylum, Berlin. Source: *Report of a deputation appointed to visit asylums on the continent with recommendations regarding the building of a new (sixth) Lancashire asylum* **(1900). Preston: Lancashire Asylums Board.**

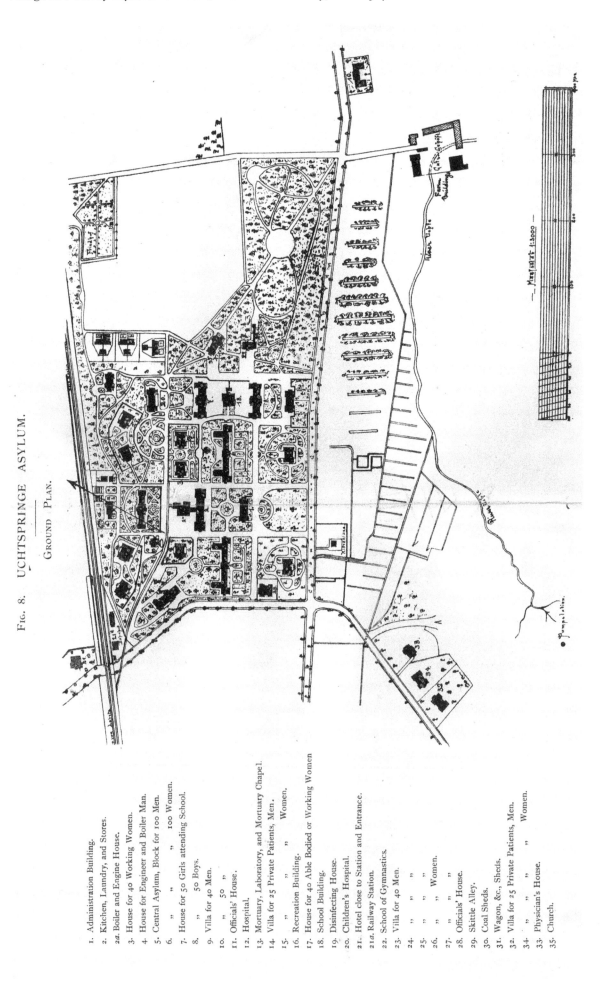

FIG. 8. UCHTSPRINGE ASYLUM.

GROUND PLAN.

1. Administration Building.
2. Kitchen, Laundry, and Stores.
2*a*. Boiler and Engine House.
3. House for 40 Working Women.
4. House for Engineer and Boiler Man.
5. Central Asylum, Block for 100 Men.
6. ,,   ,,   ,,   100 Women.
7. House for 50 Girls attending School.
8. ,,   ,,   50 Boys.
9. Villa for 40 Men.
10. ,,   50   ,,
11. Officials' House.
12. Hospital.
13. Mortuary, Laboratory, and Mortuary Chapel.
14. Villa for 25 Private Patients, Men.
15. ,,   ,,   ,,   Women.
16. Recreation Building.
17. House for 40 Able Bodied or Working Women
18. School Building.
19. Disinfecting House.
20. Children's Hospital.
21. Hotel close to Station and Entrance.
21*a*. Railway Station.
22. School of Gymnastics.
23. Villa for 40 Men.
24. ,,   ,,   ,,   ,,
25. ,,   ,,   ,,   ,,
26. ,,   ,,   Women.
27. ,,   ,,   ,,   ,,
28. Officials' House.
29. Skittle Alley.
30. Coal Sheds.
31. Wagon, &c., Sheds.
32. Villa for 25 Private Patients, Men.
33. Physician's House.
34. ,,   ,,   ,,   ,,   Women.
35. Church.

Figure 2-83. Uchtspringe Asylum, Rhine Province. Source: *Report of a deputation appointed to visit asylums on the continent with recommendations regarding the building of a new (sixth) Lancashire asylum (1900).* Preston: Lancashire Asylums Board.

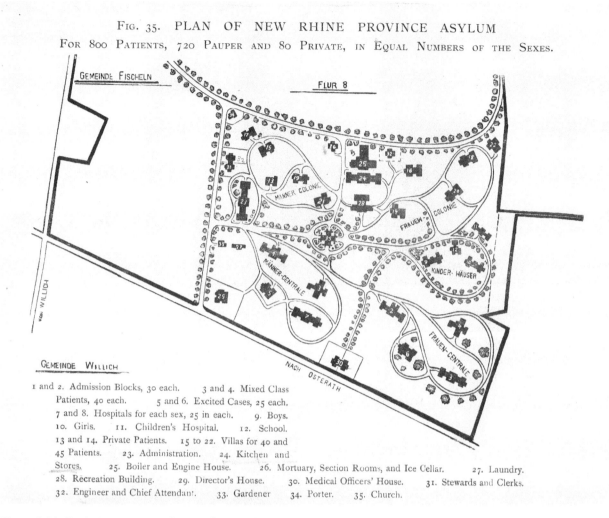

FIG. 35. PLAN OF NEW RHINE PROVINCE ASYLUM
For 800 Patients, 720 Pauper and 80 Private, in Equal Numbers of the Sexes.

1 and 2. Admission Blocks, 30 each. 3 and 4. Mixed Class Patients, 40 each. 5 and 6. Excited Cases, 25 each. 7 and 8. Hospitals for each sex, 25 in each. 9. Boys. 10. Girls. 11. Children's Hospital. 12. School. 13 and 14. Private Patients. 15 to 22. Villas for 40 and 45 Patients. 23. Administration. 24. Kitchen and Stores. 25. Boiler and Engine House. 26. Mortuary, Section Rooms, and Ice Cellar. 27. Laundry. 28. Recreation Building. 29. Director's House. 30. Medical Officers' House. 31. Stewards and Clerks. 32. Engineer and Chief Attendant. 33. Gardener 34. Porter. 35. Church.

Figure 2-84. Grafenburg Asylum, Saxony. Source: *Report of a deputation appointed to visit asylums on the continent with recommendations regarding the building of a new (sixth) Lancashire asylum* **(1900). Preston: Lancashire Asylums Board.**

into separate family-style 'houses' under paternalistic care and trained in agricultural work (Driver, 1990; Foucault, 1977: 293-296). These types of juvenile institution were a direct influence on the establishment of 'cottage homes' for pauper children in England from the 1870s, which sought to provide a village-like, 'natural' environment. Children were grouped into ersatz 'families' residing in detached houses often grouped around a chapel, school, infirmary and baths (Driver, 2004).

This pedagogical, reformatory trend was accompanied by a growing interest in the 'colonisation' of unemployed adults that may be traced initially to utopian reformers such as the socialist Robert Owen, also an educational reformer, who sent his own children to be educated by Fellenberg in Switzerland. Owen's 1817 scheme 'for the relief of the manufacturing and labouring poor' proposed 'villages of unity and mutual co-operation', to accommodate 1,200 people each (Owen, 1858). Owen claimed, it appears erroneously, that his scheme was the inspiration for the Dutch pauper colonies at Frederiksoord and Willemsoord which excited considerable interest throughout Europe following their establishment in 1818. Pauper families were housed in individual cottages on marginal land

and assisted to support themselves by farming. A flurry of pamphleteering exploring the possibility of 'home colonies' for the poor in Britain and Europe followed these developments and some fairly long-lived experiments took place, such as that of Owen's partner, William Allen, in Lindfield, Sussex (1825). Owen and two of his colleagues formed the 'Home Colonisation Society' in 1840 to raise funds for a farm known as 'Queenwood' in Hampshire, all these projects having the aim of making the poor self-supporting through working on the land, an occupation which was seen as 'morally superior' to manufacturing work (Harrison, 1969). In 1837, a French agricultural colony for the insane at Fitz-James, was established as an annexe to the main asylum at Clermont (Labitte, 1861). The same year Scottish alienist W A F Browne put forward his influential utopian asylum vision, advocating 'separate houses, in which the patients are distributed according to their dispositions and the features and stage of their disease', already by this time, a feature in a small number of private asylums in England and France. Browne further recommended that farms be attached to each establishment to provide agricultural work in the open air for patients (Browne, 1837: 185). It was also at about this time that interest was revived in the Belgian colony for the insane at Gheel following reforms by the Belgian authorities. At Gheel, patients were accommodated with local residents in a village community in pre-existing cottage dwellings, paralleling the Scottish practice of boarding-out (Andrews, 1998: 42-48). In the following decades the focus of attention shifted markedly from France, Belgium and the Netherlands to Germany. Established in 1867, a colony exclusively for epileptic patients at Bielefeld in north-west Germany inspired many imitators including the first therapeutic colony institutions in Britain (also exclusively for epileptics) including Bridge of Weir in Renfrewshire (1906). Bielefeld engendered an additional experiment, directed this time at the unemployed, the first German 'labour colony' which was established near to Beilefeld at Wilhelmsdorf in 1882 and led to the proposal for a 'farm colony' by William Booth in his influential work *In Darkest England and the way out* (Booth, 1890) (Figure 2-87). Many farm or labour colonies for the unemployed were established in Germany, Switzerland, Holland and Austria at this period and English copies were initiated at Hadleigh in Essex, and Midlocharwoods near Glasgow, among other places. Interest in the colony ideal as a means of organising the socially unproductive was relatively high from the 1890s and peaked in the period before the First World War. The colony asylum, as seen in Germany and replicated in Scotland and Ireland, was a bringing together of two ideals, that of the labour colony, in which the majority of asylum patients would be working on the land, and that of segregated domestic-style accommodation. The marrying of these two elements was a conscious one, as we can see from the comment of John Macpherson, Scottish Lunacy Commissioner that '[t]he village type of asylum ... combines the advantages of the home and of the labour colony' (Macpherson, 1905: 490). However, these two elements were not entailed by each other, and it would have been possible to build a traditional-style asylum or other institution in an agricultural setting where the majority of patients worked outdoors. However, in practice, the segregation of asylum accommodation into domestic-style villas and the provision of large areas of farmland to work on, usually occurred together in Europe, growing out of a European tradition, as has been discussed, and also out of an asylum tradition in the latter half of the nineteenth century of housing working patients in smaller-scale domestic-style accommodation. In the United States, the so-called segregate or cottage system, examples of which were constructed from the 1870s, does not appear to have made such a strong link between outdoor labour and domestic accommodation (Yanni, 2007: 79-84). At least initially, some of the 'cottages' on American sites were vast, housing more than 200 patients. It is therefore important to make a distinction between different kinds and styles of segregated asylum accommodation and agricultural sites for the insane. Terminology is another difficulty. Although the term 'colony asylum' has been used for ease throughout this study, no clear designation was made for this layout across national boundaries. In Germany, as we have seen the colony asylum was known as the 'pavillonsystem', in Ireland, it was called the 'villa colony', in Scotland, 'the village system', but the term 'segregate', 'cottage' or 'villa' system was also sometimes used. In this study, then, the term 'colony asylum' refers to an asylum inspired by Alt Scherbitz in Germany, in which the majority of patient accommodation is divided into domestic-style villas and these are situated within a rural landscape, usually in the style of a village or surburban settlement, the surrounding agricultural land providing an important source of health and employment for the patients.

2.7. Medical attitudes to insanity at the turn into the twentieth century

The two major approaches to mental illness in the nineteenth and twentieth centuries have been categorised as 'mentalist' or 'somaticist', that is, favouring either the mind or the body as the source of the symptoms that lead to a diagnosis of insanity (Gach, 2008: 689). In the first half of the nineteenth century the emphasis of therapeutic care for insanity was on 'moral treatment', based on the idea, following the philosopher John Locke, that madness was a fault in cognition, in which madmen put together 'wrong ideas ... and so make wrong propositions but argue and reason right from them' (Locke, 1824[1725]: 94; Skultans, 1979: 446-48). 'Moral'—in the sense of psychological or pertaining to thoughts and emotions—treatment, conceived of the insane as rational beings who needed to be encouraged to develop self-control through a system of rewards under the example and guidance of a benign 'Moral Governor' (Scull, 2015: 202-203). This was essentially a 'mentalist' approach which, as the century wore on, was increasingly challenged by an understanding of insanity as a disease of the nerves and brain, following the work of Wilhelm Griesinger at mid-century (Stone, 1998: 78). At first, the research of Griesinger and of Carl Wernicke, Theodore Meynert, and Paul Flechsig in Germany and Austria appeared to hold out hope that differences in brain structure would account for mental illness (Stone, 1998: 79-81). However, brain pathology did not reveal the brains of the insane to be structured any differently to those outside the asylums and researchers began to propose that insanity might be due to brain malfunction rather than anomalous structure, although the emphasis remained on somatic causes (Gold and Gold, 2015: 31). The second major development towards the end of the century, again in the German-speaking world, were the diagnostic categories developed by Emil Kraepelin, who, through observation of his patients over time, divided mental illness into two broad categories, 'manic-depressive psychosis' and 'dementia praecox' (later known as schizophrenia) (Scull, 2015: 263-265).

A third development was to have an influence far outside the world of asylums and psychiatry.[10] In 1857, Benedict-

---

[10] The discipline was known as 'mental science' at this period and the professionals concerned with its practice, 'alienists', reflecting the early dominance of the French in this field (*aliéniste*). The term 'psychiatrist' and the corresponding science of 'psychiatry' did not become widely accepted until after WW1, reflecting the dominance of the German-speaking world prior to the war.

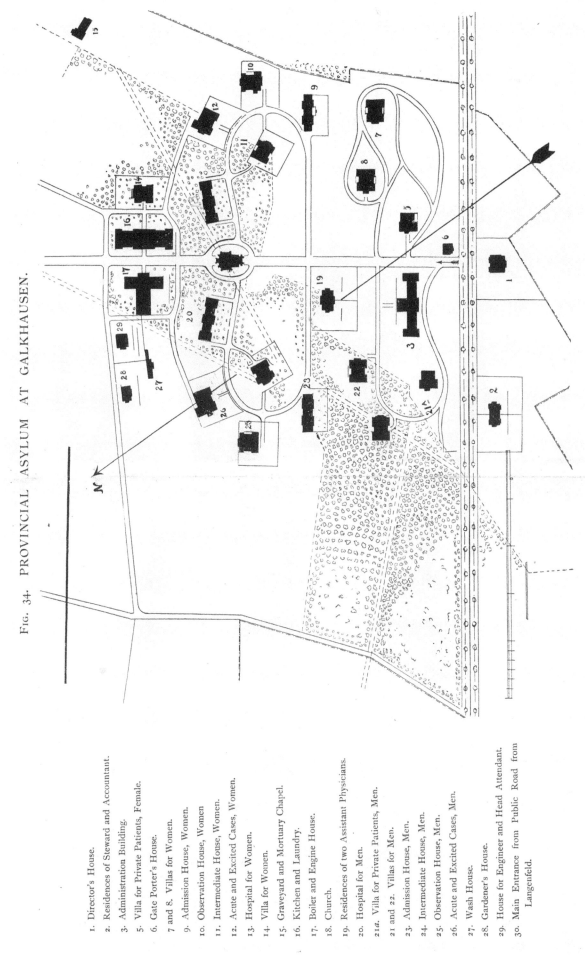

FIG. 34. PROVINCIAL ASYLUM AT GALKHAUSEN.

1. Director's House.
2. Residences of Steward and Accountant.
3. Administration Building.
5. Villa for Private Patients, Female.
6. Gate Porter's House.
7 and 8. Villas for Women.
9. Admission House, Women.
10. Observation House, Women.
11. Intermediate House, Women.
12. Acute and Excited Cases, Women.
13. Hospital for Women.
14. Villa for Women.
15. Graveyard and Mortuary Chapel.
16. Kitchen and Laundry.
17. Boiler and Engine House.
18. Church.
19. Residences of two Assistant Physicians.
20. Hospital for Men.
21a. Villa for Private Patients, Men.
21 and 22. Villas for Men.
23. Admission House, Men.
24. Intermediate House, Men.
25. Observation House, Men.
26. Acute and Excited Cases, Men.
27. Wash House.
28. Gardener's House.
29. House for Engineer and Head Attendant.
30. Main Entrance from Public Road from Langenfeld.

Figure 2-85. Galkhausen Asylum, Rhine Province. Source: *Report of a deputation appointed to visit asylums on the continent with recommendations regarding the building of a new (sixth) Lancashire asylum* (1900). **Preston: Lancashire Asylums Board.**

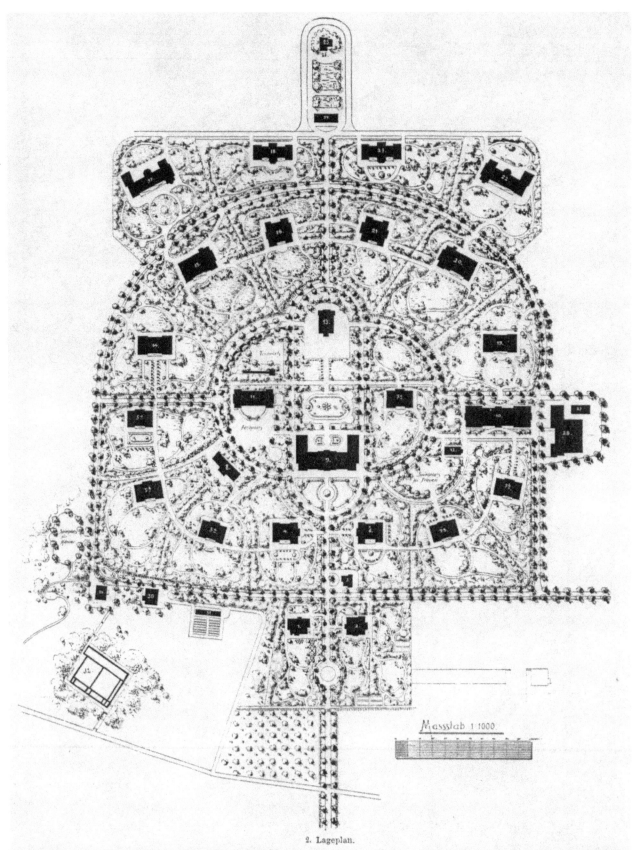

2. Lageplan.

1. Wohnhaus des Directors. 2. Wohnh. d. Oberarztes und Verwalters. 3. Portierhaus. 4. Offener Pavillon I. u. II. Cl. für Männer. 5, a, b, c. Offene Pavillons III. Cl. für Männer. 6. Offener Pavillon I. u. II. Cl. für Frauen. 7. a, b, c. Offene Pavillons III. Cl. für Frauen. 8. Werkstätte. 9. Verwaltungsgebäude. 10. Wirthschaftsgebäude. 11. Gesellschaftshaus. 12. Eishaus. 13. Betsaal. 14. Haus für halbruhige Männer. 15. Aufn.- u Ueberw.-Haus III. Cl. für Männer. 16. Aufn.- u. Ueberw.-Haus I. u. II. Cl. für Männer. 17. Ueberw.-Haus für unruhige Männer. 18. Lazareth für körperl. kranke Männer. 19. Haus für halbruhige Frauen. 20. Aufn.- u. Ueberw.-Haus III. Cl. für Frauen. 21. Aufn.- u. Ueberw.-Haus I. u. II. Cl. für Frauen. 22. Ueberw.-Haus für unruhige Frauen. 23. Lazareth für körperl. kranke Frauen. 24. Desinfections- u. Trockenhaus. 25. Sectionshaus mit Leichenhalle. 26. Kegelbahn. 27. Kohlenschuppen. 28. Kessel- u. Maschinenhaus. 29. Metzgerei. 30. Bäckerei. 31. Gewächshaus. 32. Kläranlage.

Figure 2-86. Weissenhof Asylum, Weinsburg (1903). Source: The Weinsberg Clinc at Weissenhof by Chief Medical Officer Dr. Dietz (1903). Stuttgart: K. Hofbuchdruckerei zu Gutenberg, Carl Grüninger (Klett und Hartman).

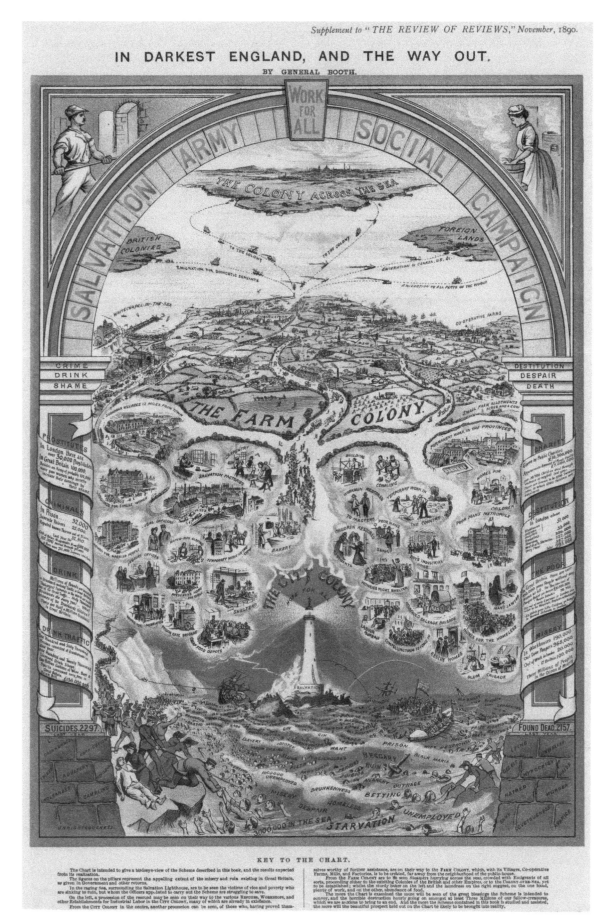

Figure 2-87. William Booth proposed colonies, both at home and abroad, as a solution to the 'problem of the unemployed'. 'Lunatic asylums', 'madmen' and 'idiotcy' [sic], float in the stormy sea at the bottom of the image, and numbers and cost of pauper lunatics are given on the right pillar. Source: Booth, W. (1890) *In Darkest England and the Way Out.* London: Bradley T Batsford. Reproduced courtesy of Cornell University – PJ Mode Collection of Persuasive Cartography.

Augustin Morel attempted to account for the incessant increase in Europe of GPI, epilepsy, suicide and crime by developing the by then widely-held belief that insanity was hereditary. He felt that his patients exemplified an accumulation of generations of faulty characteristics, a 'pathological momentum' that he called degeneration. According to Morel, degenerate characteristics could initially be acquired through alcoholism or slum living conditions and be transmitted to succeeding generations, becoming worse with each generation (Shorter, 1997:94-95). Morel believed, however, that the social causes of degeneration such as poverty and vice could be corrected and arrest the decline of the generations (Stone, 1998: 97). Degenerationist thinking became the motive force behind the eugenicist movement amid fears of irreversible racial decline and the belief that degenerate 'stock' should not be permitted to reproduce. Degenerationist ideas were also widely held in the psychiatric profession and by some of their most influential members such as Henry Maudsley, who recommended examining patients for the outward marks of 'inward and invisible peculiarity of cerebral organization' (quoted in Shorter, 1997: 97).

In attempting to clarify the ideas about madness that informed the development of the colony asylum in Scotland and Ireland, it has been necessary to rely more fully on the medical superintendent of Purdysburn than his colleagues in Scotland. This is because, not only was Graham the only medical superintendent to have pushed for the establishment of a colony asylum (all the others were appointed after the decision was made), he has also left by far the most detailed legacy in terms of his opinions on the causes and treatment of insanity. However all the medical superintendents discussed here, William Graham (Purdysburn), John Keay (Bangour Village), Charles Angus and Hugh De Maine Alexander (Kingseat) and Robert Dunmore Hotchkis (Dykebar) received much, if not all, of their medical training in Scotland and can be assumed to have been influenced by the broad climate of psychiatric thought prevailing in Scotland.

We know, for example, that the medical superintendents mentioned above largely concurred with the understanding that mental illness ultimately had physical causes and that a predisposition to mental illness was hereditary but that the tendency could remain dormant. A multitude of factors, including toxins and environment, could cause a hereditary weakness to be expressed in the form of mental illness, giving external factors a large role to play in the development of insanity (Kingseat Annual Report, 1910; Bangour Village Annual Report, 1908; Dykebar Annual Report, 1910, 1911; BDLA Annual Report 1898, 1899, 1903; Graham, 1901: 695).

William Graham elaborated on these themes in his Annual Reports. Graham was not alone in believing that the relentless increase in the numbers of insane came from the ranks of the poor, rather than the better-off classes. He stated that mental illness 'increases as we descend the scale of culture', and suggests that reproduction of the 'unfit'

should not be sanctioned, demonstrating his adherence to degenerationist ideas (BDLA Annual Reports, 1902, 1905). Graham believed that the bulk of mental derangement was due to neglect or violation of 'fundamental hygienic laws', because the poor lived in unhealthy surroundings and behaved in ways which were detrimental to health (BDLA Annual Report, 1900). He believed that among the poorer classes there had been an ongoing process of degeneration in those whose food and environment were defective, producing the 'thin, stunted, anaemic figures that populate the lower quarters of our great cities' (BDLA Annual Report, 1901). The increase in numbers of the insane was due to the emigration and lower reproduction of the middle classes, leaving those classes who did not have 'healthful existence' within their reach and were reduced to 'starvation, disease, stunted development and moral degradation' (BDLA Annual Report 1903). Graham found that the majority of the patients (70 per cent who entered the asylum were dirty and unkempt, 'their bodies the happy hunting-ground of a myriad parasites' (BDLA Annual Report 1901). The connection between the mental and the physical was such that an illness which appeared in one generation as a physical weakness or disease, could reappear in another as an insane predisposition. Graham contended, therefore, that when the guardians of public health addressed themselves to physical diseases such as tuberculosis, they were also addressing themselves to 'ills of the mind' (BDLA Annual Report 1910). He saw fatigue and depression as most common 'in our great cities' and held that 'half the existing insanity could be banished or contracted to inconsiderable limits, were the hygienic conditions in the home, the school and the factory what they ought to be' (BDLA Annual Report, 1905, 1902). He suggested that 'the over-crowded tenement houses should be replaced by buildings in which proper hygiene and pure air would enable men and women to live decently' making explicit a link between a healthy environment and morality (BDLA Annual Report 1905). Important causes of insanity were diet, drink and the 'very air we breathe', 'the unhygienic conditions of life' and 'defective morals and lack of self-control' (BDLA Annual Report 1901, 1911). Vice of any kind, including abuse of alcohol, involved a 'profuse waste of vitality' or a 'leakage of nervous energy' which 'must end sooner or later in mental and physical bankruptcy' (BDLA Annual Report 1905, 1912). Graham seems to claim a two-way relationship between mental weakness and unhealthy practices and poor environments. Alcoholism, for example, could be a cause of bodily changes that could be inherited or alternatively it could be the result of degeneracy producing a 'weakness of brain and nerve which leads to a want of self-control' (BDLA Annual Report, 1903).

Graham proposed education in the 'predisposing and exciting causes' of madness and also the 'rules and principles of a preventive kind' and suggested that children should be trained in hygienic principles with all schools providing a gymnasium and a swimming-bath so that the body could be developed to a state of efficiency and beauty (BDLA Annual Report 1902). Good hygiene included the 'beneficial and invigorating effect of judicious exercise in the open air' which had the additional benefit of allowing the deleterious products of respiration to be removed from buildings by natural ventilation (Annual Report 1901). Utilitarian work in which the patient was brought into contact with 'reality' was seen to be the best kind of therapy and contact with nature gave steadiness, poise and balance, the soil being 'a permanent source of recreative energy'. (BDLA Annual Report 1908). Work in the open air was the ideal employment for the mentally disturbed because Nature represented 'solidarity, reality, order and cohesion', expressing the higher rationality that he wished his patients to aspire to (BDLA Annual Report 1911). Fresh air, exercise and salubrious surroundings was one of the most effective ways to benefit 'the diseased brain' (BDLA Annual Report 1898). Graham asserted that the villa colony system brought the patient into the 'healthy currents of normal social life', the inherently sane and healthful practices of bourgeois living lifting the patients above the unhealthy lifestyles of the poor. Good treatment in an asylum produced patients who improved more rapidly and were cured more quickly but also who were more tractable, amiable and mild, took more interest in their surroundings, were more cheerful and showed greater zest for life (BDLA Annual Report 1898, 1899). The following chapter will provide detailed biographies of the sites and buildings in this study, including the circumstances of their construction and treatments used, where known.

3

Study Sites: Scotland

In the following two chapters, starting in this chapter with the three Scottish sites, a short biography of each site is given, setting out the processes and ideologies informing the decision to build a new asylum and the timeline of its construction, including the relative contributions of architects, medical personnel and administrators. These chapters also contain a short description of selected buildings on each site, particularly those that provided accommodation for patients, and elaborate on the regime and the views of madness and its cure held by the first medical superintendents.

3.1. Aberdeen District Lunatic Asylum (Kingseat)

3.1.1. Introduction

Provision for the insane poor in Aberdeen began with the founding of the Aberdeen Royal Infirmary in 1742, a small hospital of 40 beds, which reserved some rooms on the lower floor as 'Bedlam cells'. In 1800 the charitable Aberdeen Lunatic Asylum was opened for 15-20 patients with gradual extensions bringing numbers up to 600 by 1880, necessitating the building of a branch asylum at Daviot ('The First British Village Asylum', 1906). The main asylum, by this time designated 'Royal', was rebuilt and reopened in 1896, and the city authorities paid for pauper patients to be accommodated there and in the local poorhouses, the nearest district asylum being situated in Banff. Aberdeen district was also said to be an early pioneer of the 'boarding out' system, which commenced in the parish of St Nicholas in 1865 (Macgibbon & Ross, 1887). However, by 1904 the numbers of patients provided for was small, being 7.6 per cent in the Aberdeen City Lunacy District as opposed to 18.7 per cent in Scotland as a whole (*Aberdeen Free Press*, 24th October 1904). Chronic patients tended to be accommodated in poorhouses rather than being boarded out (Kingseat Annual Report 1911).

Following an 1898 enquiry into the increase of lunacy in the north east of Scotland by the Scottish Lunacy Commissioners (SLC), a decision was taken to create a separate District Lunacy Board for Aberdeen and this was duly carried out the same year (Darragh, 2011: 123). The ACDLB was identical with the city parish council of Aberdeen and its members were drawn from the untitled middle classes, living for the most part at street addresses in Aberdeen (ACDLB Minutes 8th November 1901). In May 1899, a sites and buildings committee of 15 members was appointed to find a suitable site for a new asylum (*Aberdeen Journal*, 16th September 1901).

3.1.2. Construction of asylum

In November 1899, two estates were purchased outside Aberdeen, Rainnieshill and Kingseat, amounting to 1700 acres in total (Rainnieshill was later sold, the Asylum Board having acquired the water rights, leaving an estate of c400 acres) and Alexander Marshall Mackenzie was appointed architect for the new asylum buildings (*Aberdeen Journal,* 8th November 1899; 23rd November 1899; 25th April 1900)

In December of 1899, a deputation, consisting of the chair, two members and the clerk of the ACDLB together with A Marshall Mackenzie, the architect, visited Alt Scherbitz. The visit to view the 'segregated system' at Alt Scherbitz, followed the recommendation of the Lunacy Commissioners (St Anne and Ville Juif, Paris and Herzberge, Berlin were also on the itinerary) (*Aberdeen Journal*, 13th December 1899). In March 1900, the same deputation (one of the members was replaced) set off to visit asylums in Scotland and England including Perth, Rainhill, West Riding, Claybury and Cane Hill and in June, a delegation (without the architect) visited the asylum at Larbert,[1] which was considered to be 'partially segregated' (*Aberdeen Journal*, 16th March 1900; 4th June 1900). The ACDLB concluded that the 'advantages of the segregate type of asylum appeared so manifest' that Alt Scherbitz was chosen as the model to be followed 'with the modifications rendered necessary by climate and other local conditions' (*Aberdeen Journal*, 4th June, 1900).

The SLC visited the proposed site on 15th March and were said to be 'highly pleased', pronouncing it suitable for the building of an asylum. Marshall Mackenzie's drawings had been prepared by August 1900, but there was some initial criticism of these on the grounds that there was a 'large amount of useless and expensive ornamentation', although this was denied by Mackenzie and the drawings were exhibited at the Royal Scottish Academy in 1902 (*Aberdeen Journal,* 15th August, 1900; 1st September 1900). The asylum was described initially as 'segregated' in design, later the term 'colony' was used, moving finally to 'village', in conformity with the term used for Bangour Village, Edinburgh. Twenty-seven buildings occupied a site of 30 acres and the remainder of the 400 acre site was to be used for farming, gardening and for a recreation ground, the site being described as sloping 'pleasantly to the south' and having a 'background of

---

[1] The main asylum at Larbert was opened in 1869 and a separate hospital was added to the site in 1893, dividing the patient accommodation into two (Darragh, 2011: 142)

rising ground, well wooded' (in order to provide shelter). The asylum was to be built for 550 patients with the possibility of expansion to 700 (*Aberdeen Journal,* 5th December 1900).

A mason was appointed in January 1901, who was to use stone quarried on the site, and the ceremony of cutting the turf took place on the 12th of that month. A member of the ACDLB described the asylum at the turf-cutting ceremony as 'the first buildings of the kind in Britain and he had no doubt that the Continental people would get a few 'tips' after the asylum was erected'. (*Aberdeen Journal,* 14th January 1901). In February, it was noted that Belfast and Edinburgh were following Aberdeen's example by building new asylums on the colony model (*Aberdeen Journal,* 19th February 1901).

A ceremony, costing £100, took place on 14th September 1901 to lay the foundation stone (the foundation stone is at the north-west corner of the hospital building). A considerable furore erupted over this expense and, perhaps as a consequence, the official opening when patients were finally admitted in May 1904 was extremely low key. Quarrying and road-making, trenching and laying-out of the grounds, formation of the vegetable garden and work on the farm was all carried out by patients saving over £400 in labour (Kingseat Annual Report, 1905).

In 1902 there was some evidence of attempts to cut costs. The glass used was to be 26 oz thirds 'free from specks, waves or other defects' rather than 26 oz seconds and three coats of varnish over oil stain were deemed adequate instead of four for the woodwork. The woodwork of the steward's house was to be stained and varnished, not painted which would have required more maintenance (ACDLB Minutes 21st April 1902).

In February 1902 the SLC reminded the ACDLB of a number of points relating to the fitting and furnishing of the asylum including that 'there should be nothing special about the windows which are not in ordinary dwellings. Upholstered chairs and sofas should have a vacant space between back and seat, so as to prevent concealment of articles. Crockery should be of good ordinary stoneware. Dining tables should be numerous and small' (ACDLB Minutes 11th February, 1902).

The asylum was opened for public inspection on 30th April, 2nd and 3rd May 1904, invitation cards being issued for the purpose (ACDLB, 12th April 1904). A thorough inspection of the asylum by the SLC took place on 11th May and it was pronounced complete, and 'of admirable and economical construction'. It was said that the patients,

'were provided with suitable and comfortable furniture, that the arrangements for heating, lighting and generally for carrying on the work of the Asylum were efficient; that the arrangements for a water supply, for the extinction of fire, and for the disposal of sewage were satisfactory; and that the Asylum was

provided with a suitable and adequate staff' (ACDLB 19th June, 1904).

The official opening took place on 16th May 1904, (although some of the asylum buildings remained unoccupied until 1906) when patients were brought from the Aberdeen Royal Lunatic Asylum and from the two city poorhouses. The opening of the asylum was reported in the *British Medical Journal* in 1904 describing the asylum 'on the detached villa system' as 'splendidly situated on rising ground … about twelve miles from the city' with the furnishing and equipment said to be 'of the most modern description' (ACDLB 10th April 1906, *British Medical Journal,* 21st May 1904). However, the wider reaction to the asylum appears to have been muted and it was not until 1905 that the asylum was mentioned as the 'first village asylum opened in Great Britain' in the course of a lecture by John Macpherson given at the Royal College of Physicians, Edinburgh, which was subsequently reported in the *JMS*. Macpherson commented that,

'The village type of asylum has not only greatly facilitated our methods of dealing with the insane, but it has permitted us to see how in the future the problems of undertaking the suitable disposition of the accumulating masses of the insane for whom asylum treatment is absolutely necessary are to be solved. It combines the advantages of the home and of the labour colony. It has taught us how to cheapen the construction of asylums while rendering them more efficient and more adaptable to their purpose; and above all, it has shown us that the hard lot of the insane can be made a little brighter and happier than under the old, more expensive, and more cumbersome method of erecting palatial prison-like buildings' (*JMS* 50 (1905): 471-490*)*.

The *BMJ* gave a glowing report of the asylum in 1906 and concluded that it had been considerably cheaper to build than other Scottish asylums at £253 per bed, as opposed to Glasgow (£466), Lanark (£348) and Govan (£461). The cost of maintaining patients at Kingseat was estimated at £25 per head per annum, while boarding out cost £19, but many patients were not suitable for boarding out (the BMJ cites the 'danger of offences against females') and so the extra cost was justifiable ('The First British Village Asylum', 1906).

The final cost of the asylum was £130,468 including £11,260 for furnishings (ACDLB Minutes, 10th July 1906). It was said that the aim in the construction and management of the asylum was 'economy without sacrifice of efficiency', signifying that any measures that were seen to be excessive in terms of decoration or comfort had to be justified against the understanding that they were therapeutic for this 'deserving' category of poor (*British Medical Journal,* 24th November 1906).

Shortly after the opening a journalist visiting the asylum described the buildings as 'cheerful and homelike…

without architectural pretensions' and as having 'a simple beauty in harmony with their surroundings and with the purpose for which they are intended'. It was noted that the asylum is 'far from the smoke and din of the city' and that Aberdeen paid for 'the cleanliness of its stone-paved streets by the nerve-shattering noise of its traffic' (*British Medical Journal*, 24th November 1906). However, he criticised Kingseat on the grounds of its overly sumptuous accommodation,

'...the "home" which is made for its inmates is perhaps a trifle luxurious. The patients with the stigmata of degeneracy writ large upon them and their cheap "slops" [shoddy manufactured clothing][2] hanging in ungainly folds about their awkward limbs, produced a curious effect of incongruity with the suburban aestheticism of their environment' *(British Medical Journal*, 24th November 1906).

The *BMJ* concluded that,

'The asylum is as free as it is possible for an institution to be from the prison-like appearance and depressing environment which in popular conception are inseparable from a madhouse. There is no evidence of restraint of any kind, though everywhere discipline, gentle but firm makes itself felt ... It is recognized by the Aberdeen municipal authorities that insanity cannot be cured by bricks and mortar, even in the most massive doses. We earnestly commend their method to the notice and imitation of certain public bodies in England, which appear to think that the solution of the lunacy problem is to be found in covering as much ground as possible with palatial buildings. In this, as in other things, their motto would seem to be *Ad majorem Concilii gloriam.* In the Kingseat asylum the foremost consideration has been the greatest good of the sufferers for whose relief it is intended' *(British Medical Journal*, 24th November 1906).

Farm buildings were added to the site in 1911 and a new hospital block was added in 1914-16. Further villas and attendants' accommodation were constructed in the 1920s (Darragh, 2011: 16-17).

The hospital was closed on 28th July 1999 and the site has since been converted into housing. Of the original buildings, most still survive and the exteriors, at least, have been retained. The administration building and original hospital building are derelict and in a poor state, while the laundry, kitchens, workshops and two of the original villas have been demolished. Eight of the original villas survive and are now houses or flats and the recreation hall is currently being converted. The original layout, while somewhat eroded by housing developments on the outskirts of the estate, remains largely legible.

---

[2] Patients did not wear a uniform but were supplied with clothing by the asylum from a standard range of sizes and it is likely, therefore, that much of this was ill-fitting.

3.1.3. *Treatments*

It was said in 1906 that approximately 30 per cent of the patients at Aberdeen (i.e. c140) were of the harmless 'fatuous' category, i.e. cognitively impaired. A British journalist visiting the asylum thought that the patients manifested 'the Scottish character' and were 'quiet, decent bodies'. There were 86 admissions in 1907 of whom 27 were actively suicidal and eight had homicidal tendencies. Fourteen patients had general paralysis of the insane which was 'attracting a large amount of attention just now on account of the increase of the malady in the large towns' (Kingseat Annual Report 1907).

Patients are described in their notes in terms of the ways in which their behaviour falls short of social norms e.g. Noisy, cannot feed himself, destructive of clothing, suspicious, abusive, excitable, no self-control, impulsive, uncleanly, delusional, sullen, takes no interest, weak-willed, alcoholic, emotional, mischievous, spiteful. Descriptions are usually measured but occasionally can be quite intemperate—'dirty little monkey sticks her head up the chimney', 'her manner is that of a spoiled child', 'filthy-minded low type, always making disgusting remarks and has no sense of propriety' 'sings and dances in a grotesque manner' (GA GRHB8/1/1-2 Kingseat patient case notes, vols 1 and 2, 1904). Instances are recorded of patients breaking furniture, light fitments and windows and tearing clothes.

Patient notes from the year 1904 suggest that diagnosis fell into four main categories: dementia (senile, chronic, secondary, incipient), mania (chronic, delusional, intermittent, acute, recurrent, alcoholic), melancholia (senile) and imbecile/idiot (moral) with occasional diagnoses of GPI, 'folie circulaire' (now known as bipolar disorder) and epilepsy or eleptiform insanity. Pregnant patients were always discharged before they gave birth but the reasons for this are unclear (GA GRHB8/1/1-2 Kingseat patient case notes, vols 1 and 2, 1904).

The lack of verandahs for open air bed treatment at Kingseat was lamented a few years after the opening and it was stated that a sanatorium (for TB) would not be necessary if there was adequate verandah accommodation for the patients to be out in all weathers (Kingseat Annual Report 1908). Although many buildings had verandahs, some on three sides, these simply consisted of a roof and timber supports and were not suitable for patients who were unwell.

All patients were treated in bed on admission until the acute mental symptoms had subsided. Patient case notes state that in most cases the 'ordinary treatment' was given which consisted of rest in bed followed by open-air exercise and/or light manual labour and nourishing food (GA GRHB8/1/1-2 Kingseat patient case notes, volumes 1 and 2, 1904). Close observation took place for about a month and patients then went to an open or a closed villa. In the closed villas, billiards was available as a reward to patients who did not become 'excited'. Patients in the open or 'parole' villas were free to wander around the grounds. The *BMJ* concluded that,

'The principle on which the asylum is conducted is that the true treatment of insanity is by plenty of good food, fresh air, suitable occupation varied with amusement, and such medical ministrations as may be needed in individual cases' (*British Medical Journal* 24th November 1906).

Games were to be regarded as a means of treatment 'as the interest taken in them is often beneficial mentally' and they 'soften the suspicions' of patients towards their fellow men (Kingseat Annual Report 1911). Cricket, reading, solo whist, billiard and bagatelle were recreations and asylum entertainments took place on Wednesday of each week. In 1904 the asylum purchased much of the entertainment equipment including billiard tables, bagatelle tables, seven cottage (upright) pianos, one grand piano for the recreation hall, one organ, a gramophone and 36 records, an optical lantern and the use of 50 slides per week (ACDLB Minutes 12th April 1904). Summer entertainments included cricket, a 'strawberry treat' during the season and dancing on the green to the strains of a bagpipe. A bowling green and tennis and croquet lawns were laid (Kingseat Annual Report 1905). Entertainments during the winter consisted of a fortnightly dance, alternating with magic lantern and gramophone (a Columbia gramophone and a number of records were donated to the asylum in 1905), concerts and drama. Cinematograph was added to the entertainments in 1906 (Kingseat Annual Reports 1905, 1906, 1913). The medical superintendent asked for several years for a curling pond because at other asylums 'the patients play it with great zest and it provides amusement and outdoor exercise at a monotonous time of year'. This request was granted in 1914 (Kingseat Annual Report, 1914). Being a good sportsman was approved of. It was noted that a male patient 'takes a hack on the shins at football very philosophically and always "plays the game"' (GA GRHB8/1/1-2 Kingseat patient case notes, volumes 1 and 2, 1904). The *BMJ* records that the nurses played out of doors with the female patients but it was 'sad to note that the women did not take much active part in the sports, looking on with apathetic indifference at the efforts of the nurses to amuse them' (*British Medical Journal*, 24th November 1906).

Dr Angus requested that electric baths be provided at the hospital, one in each of the male and female sections. Electric baths were used for the treatment of adolescent melancholia, stupor and delusional insanity and combined hydrotherapy with electric treatment consisting of an earthenware or wooden bath with metal plates each end connected to an electric current. The electrification of a patient was thought to bring about 'improved colour, greater activity, increased appetite and...sounder sleep' (Hide, 2014:140; *JMS* 47 (1901):245-50). Sometimes 'stimulant treatment' was advocated for melancholic patients, which could consist of diluted whiskey, the external application of hot water bottles and doses of phosphoric acid or strychnine. Some patients who refused to eat were tube fed, and those who were noisy at night or annoyed other patients were moved to single rooms. Others were given a 'hypnotic' usually paraldehyde, sometimes veronal. Bromide was given for epilepsy—the first anti-epileptic to be widely used from the 1860s. General Paralysis of the Insane (GPI) was treated by inoculation with tuberculin or sodium nucleniate to produce a febrile reaction. Nourishing diet could consist of eggs and milk for infirm/senile patients (GA GRHB8/1/1-2 Kingseat patient case notes, volumes 1 and 2, 1904).

Thomas Clouston of Edinburgh Royal Asylum calculated that the recovery rate for Scottish asylums was equal to the recovery rate of ordinary hospitals by the early years of the twentieth century (Kingseat Annual Report 1907). The admission rate here and across Scotland was felt to be falling by 1907 and it was 'probable that the burden which lunacy entails upon the country had reached its limit' (Kingseat Annual Report 1907). In 1910 recoveries were 44.6 per cent, the highest yet recorded. Those patients who had a greater chance of recovery were the melancholics and those who had had an episode of mania or melancholia after a drinking or opium binge, in which case the hospital could dry them out, or as the result of a shock or lifestage such as perinatal. Some cases of recurrent mania were in and out of the hospital but even those who had recovered were often kept at Kingseat for weeks or months until discharge. Some violent patients who had attempted murder on their relatives were admitted, but at least one was reported to the procurator fiscal as he was 'too dangerous a patient for the wards of an ordinary asylum' suggesting he was taken to an institution for criminal lunatics (GA GRHB8/1/1-2 Kingseat patient case notes, vols 1 and 2, 1904).

3.1.4. Escapes, restraint and injuries

The Annual Reports contend that restraint was kept to a minimum and mention restraint only in the context of the most violent patients. Patients were examined for marks and bruises on entering and any new marks or bruises had to be accounted for to the SLC if they were to ask during their inspection visits. The asylum was run on the principle of the 'open door' except for two of the villas and there were no boundary walls around the asylum, yet Annual Reports record few escapes, accidents or injuries in the early years.

In 1906 there was one escape that was discharged after 28 days having not been brought back, and four other escapes were brought back (Kingseat Annual Report 1906). In 1909 the *BMJ* reminded its readers that there were no walls around the asylum (there had been two escapes that year, both of which had been brought back within a day) and the medical superintendent stated that the idea of not being shut in had in itself 'a restraining influence on the patients' (*BMJ*, 20th May 1909). He put the lack of escapes at Kingseat down to the restraining effect on the patients of the 'idea of not being shut in' and asserted that the term 'escape' was merely 'a statutory expression' (Kingseat Annual Report 1908). The medical superintendent stated that Alt Scherbitz had by contrast to Kingseat, high fences and palings round some of the closed villas.

A patient died in 1906 after rupture of the intestine following a struggle with an attendant (no blame attached to staff, however). In 1907 one man was restrained eight times because he was 'violently excited and harboured dangerous antipathies towards some of the attendants' and a patient was injured by catching her hand in the roller of an ironing machine in the laundry. The same year, one attendant was requested to resign 'for being unable to account in a satisfactory manner for an injury sustained by a patient while under his charge'. In 1909 there were four cases of seclusion in cases of epileptic excitement and violence. A patient broke a window and jumped through it, breaking his leg, a fractured rib was sustained during a struggle with attendants, following which an attendant was dismissed, and a patient slipped on the floor and broke his leg. In 1910 a female patient jumped through a window and sustained injuries and in 1912 a woman patient drowned herself in a horse trough. There were eight escapes this year, five due to patients breaking their parole. In 1913 three patients escaped by breaking windows and two men who were not recovered were removed from the register. Two patients were struck by the shot of hunters shooting rabbits in a nearby field (Kingseat Annual Reports, 1908-1914).

Patients could be visited on Wednesdays and Saturdays, and on public holidays from 2pm to 5 pm, by not more than two friends at a time. Relatives were required to see doctors on their first visit to get information about the patient and were enjoined to be cheerful and not refer to anything that 'might cause the patient to be discontented'. The patient was to be treated as though they were suffering from bodily illness. They could not be given knives, money, matches or alcohol and visitors were not to post letters given to them by the patient but they could bring fruit, tobacco, snuff, sweets or cakes, newspapers and books. These were given to the attendant who would give them to the patient. The asylum authorities could refuse permission to visit (ACDLB Minutes 11th June 1907).

3.1.5. Staffing

The asylum was staffed by a medical superintendent and an assistant medical officer, a matron and two assistant matrons (one for day and one for night), and a house steward. The Matron and Assistant Matrons were trained hospital nurses. The day staff consisted of 26 nurses and eight attendants, a ratio of around one to eight patients, while on night duty were seven nurses and three attendants, giving a proportion of one to 29. The majority of the staff were women, and female nurses were intentionally employed on male wards, with eight nurses on day and two on night duty in the male division. Two male wards in the hospital were staffed by nurses day and night and a male villa was supervised by two nurses, while an attendant and

his wife supervised another male villa. Once appointed, Dr Angus was keen to introduce female nurses as soon as possible, with the support of a Lunacy Commissioner,

> 'I am strongly of opinion that for both economy and efficiency female nurses should be employed for male as well as for female patients, wherever practicable – in fact, as far as possible like the staffing of a general hospital. My experience is that, when the right type of nurse is got, she is more sympathetic and kindly, her nursing is more efficient, and even irritable male patients are more amenable to her influence than to the influence of a male attendant. By this method we would not only have greater efficiency in nursing, but a saving would be effected on the wages bill' (ACDLB Minutes 29th July 1903).

Married male attendants were thought to represent an increase in quality and stability of staff so suitable accommodation should be provided for them. Staff cottages were needed so that staff could be near the asylum in case of emergency (Kingseat Annual Report 1906). Accommodation for married staff was therefore built, in 1907, to designs by D & J R McMillan (Kingseat Annual Report 1907).

3.1.6. Site

The *British Medical Journal* reported on the asylum's opening that it was at an elevation of 439 feet above sea level, 'the air is pure and bracing and around stretches a wide landscape bounded by mountains' (*British Medical Journal*, 21st May 1904) (Figure 3.1).

Kingseat was planted with trees during the construction process with the aim of creating 'a beautifully wooded village' (*British Medical Journal*, 21st May 1904). In

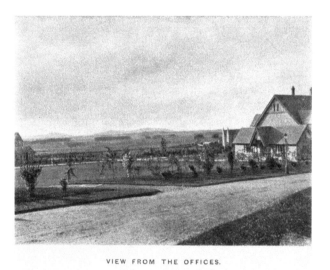

VIEW FROM THE OFFICES.

Figure 3-1. Kingseat Asylum: view from the administration block approximately westwards. Source: Kingseat Annual Report 1906, GRHB8/6/1. Courtesy of NHS Grampian Archives.

1908, a line of firs was planted from the mortuary to the football ground and along the south boundary (these trees are still present) and a cinder path was constructed through the woods to allow patients to walk at a distance from the asylum (Figure 3-2).

The asylum's elevation above sea level was an important therapeutic factor. Patients were said to enjoy to the full the quiet country life and the pure, bracing air of Kingseat (Kingseat Annual Report 1905). The asylum was well wooded and protected on the east, gently sloping to the south west and 'commands an extensive view of mountain scenery'. Also the lack of boundary walls meant there was 'absolutely no feeling of restraint or limitation of movements' (Kingseat Annual Report 1904-5). The patients in closed wards walked around the circular roads of the asylum for their exercise until a mile long path was made in the woods up to Beauty Hill (Kingseat Annual Report 1913). Dr Angus was instructed to erect notice boards and to employ a policeman on Sundays when necessary to warn the public from trespassing on the Asylum grounds, suggesting that the danger of public trespass was seen as more pressing than the danger of the patients escaping (ACDLB Minutes, 25th September

1903). It was reported in 1914 that new exercise paths were a success and allowed privacy when the grounds of the institution were open on visiting days (Kingseat Annual Report 1914). Several items were purchased for the outdoor use of patients, namely; forty garden seats from Messrs Edwards and Rae at ten shillings and nine pence each, 130 straw hats for patients at one shilling each and 60 garden hats at four and a half pence each (ACDLB Minutes, 14th June 1904).

Parole involved the patient giving their word that they would not go beyond the precincts of the asylum. In 1908, it was reported that this had not been broken more than six times in four years (Kingseat Annual Report 1907). Men were said to be more reliable in not breaking their parole than women. The comparative isolation of the hospital allowed parole to be granted to larger numbers of patients and it was found that,

> 'patients who are irritable, discontented and lazy when confined, become more contented and begin to work on their own initiative on being allowed greater liberty... Parole is the most valuable asset of the villa type of asylum and renders patients contented, hard working and loyal and friendly towards others.'(Kingseat Annual Report 1913).

Farmwork was seen as providing 'the very best form of tonic for the convalescent cases prior to their discharge' and by 1913 the farm was supplying all the needs of the asylum (Kingseat Annual Report 1913). Farm work was held to be a,

> '...natural, healthy and sane interest which tends to promote recovery or at all events contentment and easy management. Work on the grounds must however be less valuable as a curative agent, as being less varied and mentally stimulating than farm work'.

It was felt undesirable for the patients to do work which merely employed them, as was common in prisons or workhouses, rather than work which was useful (Kingseat Annual Report 1909). By 1907, 250 of the patients were working usefully, of the men: 79 on the land, 13 as clerks/tradesmen/messengers and 60 in household work. Thirty-four of the women were employed in the kitchen, laundry and admin block, 36 at sewing/knitting, and 28 in ordinary household work. All patients that were able to work were expected to do so, and a newspaper report of 1904 stated that the value of outdoor work 'in promoting health of body and mind' was fully recognised at Kingseat. Work consisted of polishing the floor 'till you can see your face in it' and dusting 'imaginary specks off the leaves of the hot-house grown plants'. Work on the farm and on the grounds was encouraged but no patient was compelled to do this (*Aberdeen Free Press*, 24th October 1904). In 1902 the board complained to the architect that there was too much machinery in the laundry which 'limited the means of useful occupation for the female patients'. However, the architect countered that the machinery could be a fall back

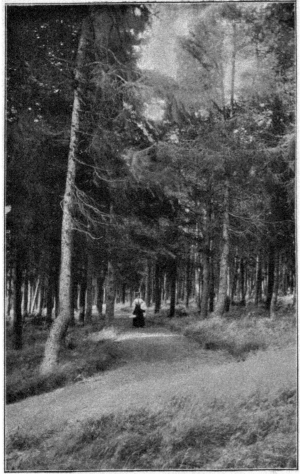

The Benefit of Parole.

Figure 3-2. Kingseat Asylum: view of patient walking in the grounds. Source: Kingseat Annual Report 1911 GRHB8/6/1. Courtesy of NHS Grampian Archives.

if suitable patients were not available (ACDLB Minutes, 14th January 1902). There is some evidence to suggest that labour was seen as somewhat less important for women than it was for men. For example, in 1905 it was recorded that, while 129 men were working of the 370 patients, only 76 women were industrially employed (*British Medical Journal*, 24th November 1906). Women were also much less likely to be employed outdoors. Patients were not compelled to work or do activities but their refusal to participate was noted with displeasure. 'Not much of a worker', 'does not do a stroke of work' appears in patient case notes (GA GRHB8/1/1-2 Kingseat patient case notes, volumes 1 and 2, 1904).

3.1.7. Layout

The layout of Kingseat follows very closely the idealised garden city layout put forward by Ebenezer Howard in his 1898 publication 'Tomorrow: a practical path to real reform' (Figures 3-3, 3-4). Subsequent domestic settlements built on garden city lines in Britain e.g. Letchworth and Welwyn Garden City did not use Howard's layout, so Kingseat is perhaps the only example of a self-contained settlement built according to Howard's original plan, on a miniature scale (Howard's original garden city was to cover 1,000 acres with a population of 32,000) (Howard 1898: 14, 22). A contemporary newspaper article reprinted a 'prize essay' describing Kingseat as a,

'picturesque little village on the fine slope of Beauty Hill … No high wall, in fact, no fence of any kind, surrounds Kingseat, its outward appearance with its finely laid out grounds, bowling greens, cricket and football pitches &c being more like a modern garden city' (GA GRHB8/6/2 Scrapbook of newspaper cuttings) (Figure 3-5, 3-6).

3.1.8. Selected buildings

Gate Lodges

The asylum is entered from the main road through a gatescreen—there are three of these (a further gatescreen opened into the Medical Superintendent's house), accompanied by lodges, to the north of the site. This is a departure from the German model, Alt Scherbitz, which consciously dispensed with gatescreens and lodges. The gatescreens provide a barrier between the asylum and the public road which appears to have been, at least partly, motivated by a desire to keep the public out and thus protect the privacy of patients and staff. The splitting of the entrance into three, along a relatively short stretch of road appears excessive, but each entrance conducts the visitor onto a different part of the site. The 'gardener's lodge' to the west of the site conducts the visitor to the administration building or the hospital, while the

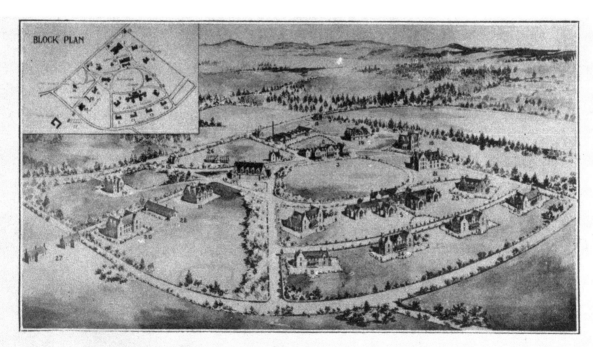

KINGSEAT ASYLUM—FOR THE ABERDEEN CITY DISTRICT LUNACY BOARD.

1. Laundry and Power House
2. Kitchen and Store.
3. Administrative Block.
4. Recreation Hall.
5. Hospital.
    (for 116 Patients).
8. Closed Villa
    (for 32 Male Patients).
9. Observation Villa
    (for 39 Male Patients).
10. Colony Villa
    (for 42 Female Patients).
11. Colony Villa
    (for 32 Male Patients).
13. Closed Villa
    (for 36 Female Patients).
14. Medical Superintendent's House.
15. Gardener's Lodge.
16. Steward's House.
17. Engineer's Lodge.
18. Mortuary.
19. Colony Villa
    (for 32 Female Patients).
20. Colony Villa
    (for 42 Male Patients).
21. Nurses' Home.
23. Observation Villa
    (for 39 Female Patients).
24. Closed Villa
    (for 36 Male Patients).
25. Closed Villa
    (for 32 Female Patients).
26. Greenhouses.
27. Labourers' Cottages.
28. Workshops.

Figure 3-3 Kingseat Asylum: perspective drawing and plan. Source: Kingseat Annual Report, 1905) GRHB8/6/1. Courtesy of NHS Grampian Archives.

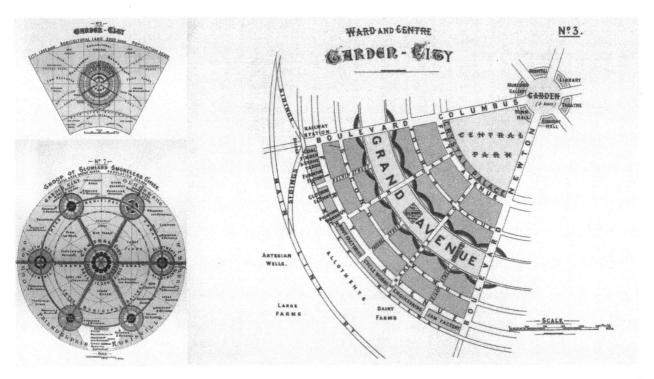

Figure 3-4. Ebenezer Howard's garden city diagrams. Top left: Garden City. Bottom left: Group of Cities. Right: Section of Garden City. Source: Howard, Ebenezer (1898) *Tomorrow: a peaceful path to real reform.*

engineer's lodge provides easy access to the laundry, boiler houses and kitchens. The mortuary has a separate entrance on the edge of the estate, most likely because it was thus made easier to remove bodies and conduct funerals without distressing the remainder of the asylum population.

Administrative Block

The administrative block uses the traditional institutional style of central pediment with matching pediments to either side and renders it more informal and domestic in scale (Figure 3-7). Gables replace pediments and matching large

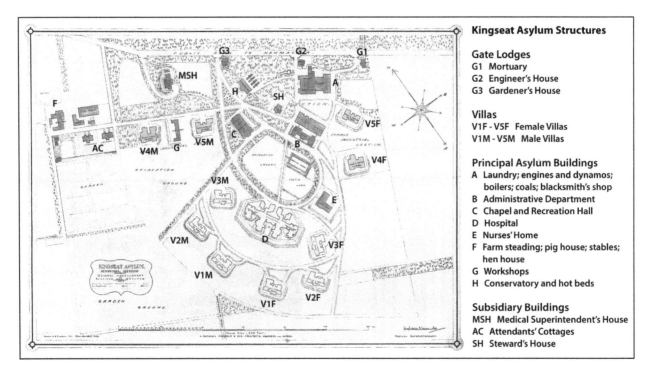

Figure 3-5. Kingseat Asylum layout. Source: Annotated architect's drawing dated 1906, reproduced in Jenkins & Marr (1997) *Kingseat Village Proposals.*

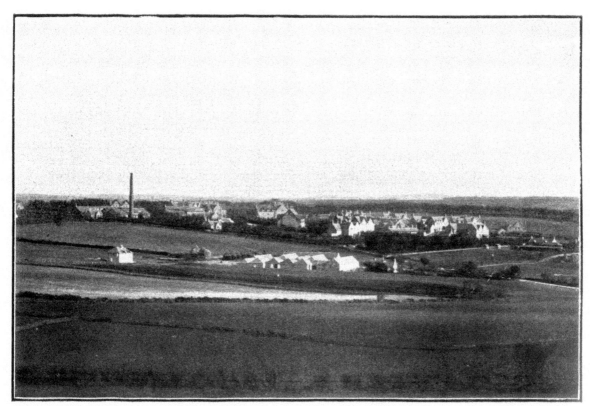

General View--Kingseat Mental Hospital.

Figure 3-6. Kingseat Asylum: general view showing absence of walls and rural situation. Source: Kingseat Annual Report, 1912, GRHB8/6/1. Courtesy of NHS Grampian Archives.

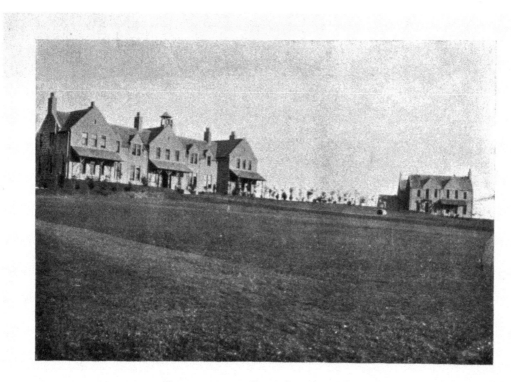

THE ADMINISTRATIVE BLOCK.

Figure 3-7. Kingseat Asylum: administration block. Source: Kingseat Annual Report 1906, GRHB8/6/1. Courtesy of NHS Grampian Archives.

and small wallhead dormers add variation to the roofline in the intervening bays. The windows are significantly larger on the ground floor than on the upper floor. The entrance bay is marked by a circular opening at attic level replicating the 'oculus' often found on institutional buildings, although some photographs suggest that this was formerly fitted with a clock. On the roofline of the central gable is a bellcote composed of shaped wooden supports and a leaded pyramidal roof with finial. The bell was fitted for 'the purposes of summoning the inmates to worship and meals' (*British Medical Journal*, 24th November 1906). Although only one verandah remains, an original photograph shows that tiled, wooden verandahs sheltered the ground floor windows of all three forward facing gables. The admin block contained accommodation for attendants on the upper floor.

Hospital

The hospital building consisted of a central two storey section with reception areas for patients and single storey side wings catering for depressed and excited cases (corresponding to the old categories of manic and melancholic) with sick wards to the rear. Isolation wards, connected by an open verandah to the main building, accommodated four patients on each side (*British Medical Journal*, 24th November 1906) (Figures 3-8, 3-9). The main frontage was approximately 285 feet in width including the side wings and the hospital was divided centrally along gender lines with males to the west and females to the east

.The WC facilities were deliberately isolated from the rest of the hospital by their position on the edges of wards, which allowed for two sets of windows opposite each other and therefore allowed the rooms to be cross-ventilated. Separate WC and lavatory arrangements had to be made for female attendants in the male wards of the hospital. A number of single rooms are provided—five in each ward for excited cases, and four in the sick wards (with a further single room accessible from the corridor outside the sick ward) and a 'strong room' and a 'padded room' accessible from the corridor outside the depressed ward. Pocock brothers (a London specialist supplier to asylums) were paid £197 for the padded rooms (ACDLB Minutes 12th July 1904). The male padded room was subsequently moved to the corridor where it could be more efficiently ventilated and where other patients would not be disturbed (ACDLB Minutes, 8th October 1907).

All the wards have at least one bay window at the end, in the excited ward, these face south east (female), north west (male) and south west and in the sick ward, south west. The isolation wards and the reception areas for patients (which also contain a charge nurses' sitting room with a bay window) face north east, suggesting less privileged accommodation because it was occupied by fewer numbers and those passing through to the main wards. A window in the front ward to the east of hospital was subsequently made into a French window to give access to grounds and to the coal store lying immediately behind it and to the front west ward (ACDLB Minutes 24th November 1903).

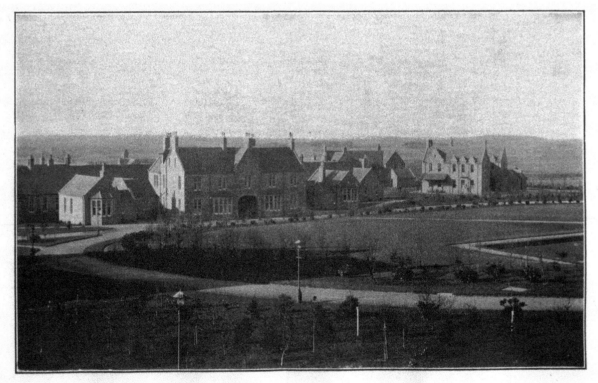

MENTAL HOSPITAL.   Nos. 2 and 3 Male Closed Villas.

Figure 3-8. Kingseat Asylum: hospital building. Source: Kingseat Annual Report 1909, GRHB8/6/1. Courtesy of NHS Grampian Archives.

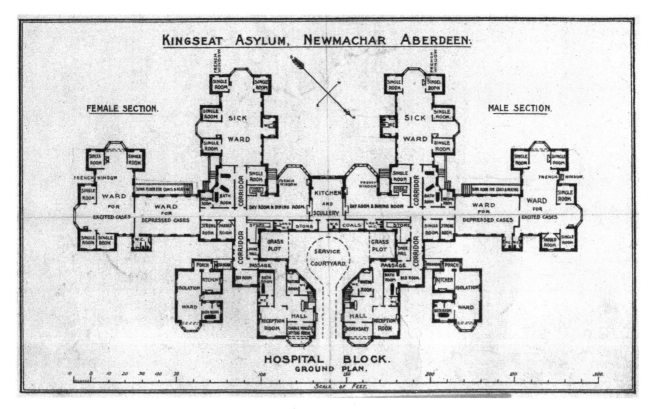

Figure 3-9. Kingseat Asylum: plan of hospital. Source: Kingseat Annual Report 1905, GRHB8/6/1. Courtesy of NHS Grampian Archives.

The reception area for patients comprised a waiting room, reception room and bathroom suggesting that patients were examined and bathed before they went onto the wards. The hospital had four further baths on each side, three for patients in the excited, depressed and sick wards and one for the isolation ward. The *BMJ* reported that the bath fittings were 'excellent; a bath can be filled to the depth of 9 inches in 30 seconds, and emptied in about the same time' (*British Medical Journal*, 24th November 1906). No plan has survived for the upper floor of the central block, but it is known to have contained accommodation for nurses and doctors during the day, consisting of parlour/sitting room and bathrooms ('The New Asylum at Kingseat', 1901).

The depressed/excited wards were fitted with curtain poles and hung with curtains, which may have been used to regulate the amount of stimulating light reaching patients (Figure 3-10). Net curtains appear also to have been fitted in order to filter out glare at the bay windows. The bedsteads are identical to those in the villas, wooden with low ends and backs and lacking ligature points. A conscious decision was taken that the hospital bedsteads were to be of pitch pine rather than iron (ACDLB Minutes, 24th November 1903). Plants and flowers are a strong feature of the room with plants on bentwood stands at intervals along the length of the ward and beside the bay window. Numerous pictures hang from the walls and also a smaller hanging item, probably a medical chart for each patient. Ventilation grilles are shown in the ceiling, the hospital being ventilated, initially, by the Plenum system, making it one of the first institutional buildings to use this

very early air-conditioning (controlling both humidity and heat) system (Kingseat Annual Report, 1907).

Villas

Dr Angus considered that 'the idea of a home is the foundation of the colony system of Asylum' and that the departure from domestic life in a traditional asylum was not conducive to comfort and happiness (Kingseat Annual Report 1904-5). Life in the villas was intended to be as homelike as possible and this is explicitly connected with some villas being under female supervision and all the doors being open during the day, the patients being allowed to go in and out at will. However, the hospital ward for excited male patients and the closed villas for epileptics and mental cases requiring special supervision were staffed by male attendants. Dr Angus was commended for 'assimilating as completely as possible the nursing arrangements of an asylum to those of a general hospital'. The dayrooms and dormitories were approvingly described by the Commissioners as 'bright and comfortable in aspect and well ventilated' (Kingseat Annual Report 1907). The stock of plants in the greenhouses was able to 'liberally and punctually' supply the institution with flowers all the year round' and dayrooms were supplied with objects 'calculated to interest the inmates' including newspapers, periodicals and indoor games (Kingseat Annual Report 1906).

There were five villas for males and five for females divided into two sections, 'industrial' or 'colony' and

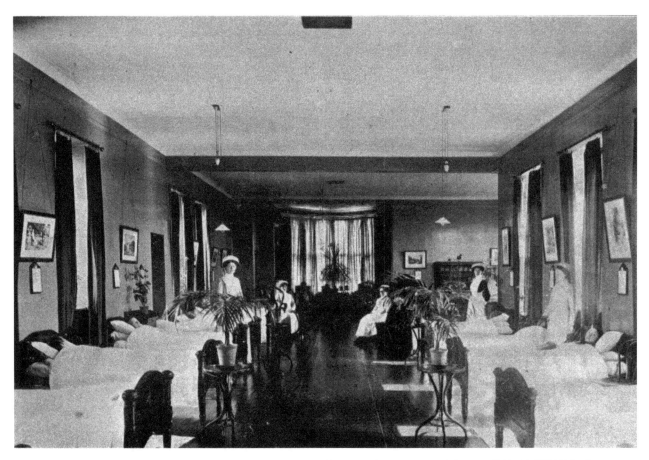

Figure 3-10. Kingseat Asylum: female depressed/excited ward. Source: Kingseat Annual Report 1911, GRHB8/6/1. Courtesy of NHS Grampian Archives.

'medical'. Two of the three villas in the medical section were 'closed', i.e. doors were locked during the day, all villas being locked during the night and the third villa was an 'observation villa'. The three medical villas were situated within easy reach of the hospital building, with male villas grouped to the west and female villas to the east. The 'closed' male and female villas were situated close to each other, while the 'observation' villas (number three) were either side of the hospital and less accessible to each other. The female industrial villas were situated near the laundry and kitchens where many of the females would have worked. The male industrial villas were likewise situated near the farm and workshops, the traditional male places of work. There was a clear spatial division between industrial and medical sections and between male and female open villas. The architect wanted to build all the villas (two on each side) in the industrial colony in the 'old English' or 'woodwork' style with projecting eaves and gables as he thought it looked 'exceedingly well'. However, this idea was rejected by the Board on the grounds of expense and ultimately only one villa on each side was built in 'old English style' (ACDLB Minutes 14th January 1902, 27th January 1902).

Halliday suggests that the accommodation at Kingseat constitutes a 'ladder of progress' with the patients moving from the reception wards in the hospital to the closed villas, open villas and eventual discharge (Halliday

2003: 305-310). However, this seems simplistic, as many patients who were treated in the hospital never entered the villas and it is likely that those who did were usually seen as 'chronic' or long-term patients who were either unlikely to recover or whose residence was likely to be lengthy. Halliday's assertion about the categorisation of patients into 'violent' and 'quiet', 'dirty' and 'clean', 'curable' and 'incurable', while congruent with some descriptions of the asylum, should be examined next to the most detailed list of how patients were categorised, which is found in the Annual Report for 1906. This report suggests that patients were categorised along three main lines once they had been through an initial period of observation. Cases of an acute or physically ill nature remained in the hospital together with those who were on the way to recovery. All other patients, largely consisting of incurable and chronic cases were transferred to the different villas and these were categorised according to their capacity for work and the type of work they could do, and additionally according to the amount of supervision they required. Therefore, the categorisation was less in terms of their condition, but in terms of their significance for the operation of the asylum—could they contribute their labour to the running of the asylum and how much supervision would they need to do so? Only villa four admitted long-term convalescent patients who presumably were expected to improve and leave the asylum. These relatively healthy patients were, however, probably critical to the smooth running of the asylum and would have contributed much needed labour power.

Villa One

Villa one (male) housed patients who were supervised by four attendants. The male patients in this villa were epileptics and 'impulsive cases' i.e. those who were categorised as 'untrustworthy in consequence of restless habits, or delusions likely to render them troublesome or offensive, or of a tendency to run away, or commit offences'. This villa was locked during the day and had constant supervision day and night (Kingseat Annual Report, 1906; 'The New Asylum at Kingseat', 1901). At least one primary source suggests that the patients in this villa were expected to work, despite their condition ('The New Asylum at Kingseat', 1901). Villa one (female) for 42 patients did not come into use for some time.

Villa Two

Villa two (male) was a closed villa of 36 beds for incurable cases who worked but required observation (although less so than those in villa one). The villa was supervised by three attendants and continuously at night. Villa two (female) had 33 beds and 3 nurses and was used for epileptics and impulsive cases (Kingseat Annual Report, 1906).

Villa Three

Villa three (male) was an observation villa with 42 beds and three attendants. It was for incurable patients who required less observation than those in villa two and was supervised at night by patrol. The female equivalent observation villa had the same number of beds but four nurses supervising and was for 'quiet epileptics and incurable cases who work, but require observation'. The female villa was supervised continuously at night (Kingseat Annual Report, 1906).

Villa Four

Villa four(female) had 46 beds and was for patients engaged in dressmaking, millinery and the repair of clothing. They were supervised by a 'sewing nurse' and two regular nurses. The sewing villa was said to be for convalescent cases and was patrolled by night supervision. Villa four (male) was for farm and garden workers, convalescent and chronic patients who were supervised by one attendant and one nurse (Kingseat Annual Report, 1906).

Villa Five

Villa five (male) (Figure 3-11) was originally designated for tradesmen and skilled artisans and could house 32 patients who were supervised by two nurses. Villa five (female) housed 34 patients, supervised by two nurses and was the dwelling for kitchen and laundry workers. It was an open or 'parole' villa and the cases who lived here were 'chronic' and worked on the grounds and in the workshops. Supervision at night was by night patrol rather than by staff who lived in the villas (Kingseat Annual Report, 1906).

3.1.9. Medical superintendents at Kingseat and their views on insanity

Charles Angus, a graduate of Aberdeen University, was appointed Medical Superintendent at Kingseat in March 1903 (ACDLB Minutes, 1st April 1903). Although he had been working as a medical superintendent of the Aberdeen Royal Infirmary and not at an asylum, he had previously had ten years experience at Aberdeen Royal Asylum. He had continued to make a

'...special study of mental derangement and its treatment in all its bearings and to make a special study also of asylum construction and administration and... he had visited and made himself familiar with the construction and working of the asylum at Alt Scherbitz in Germany' (*Aberdeen Journal*, 19th March 1903).

He was the candidate for the position to have visited Alt Scherbitz and the trip may have been influential in his appointment. Angus died prematurely in 1906 and was succeeded by Dr Hugh de Maine Alexander who remained in post until 1933 (GA GRHB8/6/8 Kingseat Hospital commemorative booklet).

Dr Angus was described as a 'doctor, farmer, gardener and general engineer all rolled into one' (*Aberdeen Free Press*, 24th October 1904). He was initially much concerned with the furnishings of the new asylum and in a letter to the ACDLB in 1903 he called furnishings a 'very heavy and important undertaking and one that requires most careful consideration'. He noted that,

'...with our most recent and improved methods of housing and treatment, the type of furnishing has undergone a corresponding change. The heavy furniture has given place to a lighter and more comfortable furnishing. The old form or bench, where formerly there were seated five or six patients, frail in body and irritable in temper, presumably resting, where the one was constantly leaning up against the other, and thus increasing their irritability and excitement, has given place to light arm-chairs, where each patient is comfortable and isolated, and where he remains contented, resting both body and mind, and thus tending to hasten his speedy recovery' (ACDLB Minutes, 29th July 1903).

Dr Angus and his assistants were praised by the Commissioners during the construction of the asylum because,

'there were many matters to be determined, arising out of the novelty of the type of the Asylum, in which they had nothing to guide them but their own judgement and initiative, for there was no precedent to appeal to' (Kingseat Annual Report 1905).

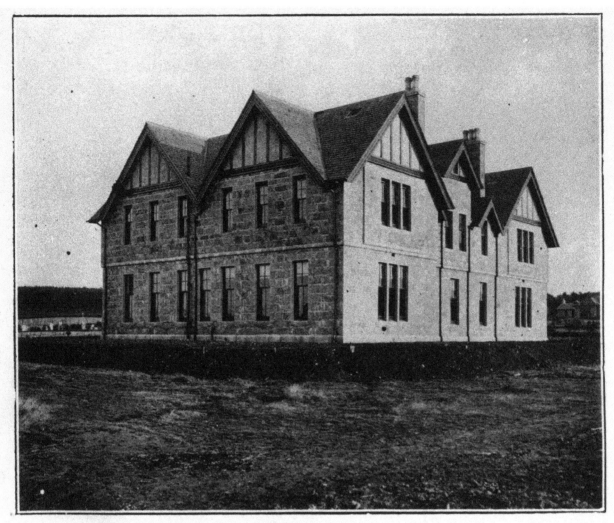

MALE COLONY VILLA.

Figure 3-11. Kingseat Asylum: male colony villa 5. Source: Kingseat Annual Report, 1905 GRHB8/6/1. Courtesy of NHS Grampian Archives.

Dr Angus summarised the advantages of the 'new village system',

'…it looks less like an institution, it allows of the patients being more easily classified and grouped; it tends to diminish the effects of any noise or excitement among the chronic patients by localising the disturbance; it minimises the risk of fire. On the other hand, it requires a larger staff and it is perhaps less easy to supervise'.

Angus found that the hospital was preferred to the villas by curable patients because there was more going on there and companions were more easily found (Kingseat Annual Report 1907).

The promotion of individuality was seen as the key aspect of the 'colony system'. Dr Angus wrote,

'Individuality is prone to be lost in a crowd and with the loss of individuality goes loss of initiative and mental energy. Appeals to the personal initiative are more successfully made to patients living in small communities, with attendants coming intimately and constantly in contact with them. It has also been proved that when patients are living in small, selected groups, there is an absence of that noisy excitement which is so disturbing and injurious to those who are recovering from their mental ailments. Patients with special characteristics of mental disease such as epileptics, paralytics, and those of faulty habits, are separated from those whose habits and taste in their personal tidiness are unimpaired' (Kingseat Annual Report 1905).

Angus's successor Dr Alexander commented on the hereditary nature of mental illness,

'We all admit the importance of heredity, but its ill effects do not equally embrace all forms of mental disease. Insanity is mainly produced by the action of morbid external causes, various physical affections and diseases, infections and toxins etc. In those in whom a hereditary predisposition is strongly present, unsuitable education, occupation or environment play their part' (Kingseat Annual Report 1910).

He also showed the influence of eugenic thinking in stating that 'weak-minded, morally facile and immorally vicious women' should be permanently segregated because they produced children who were chargeable to the rates and 'mothers transmit insanity and epilepsy with much greater frequency than do fathers' (Kingseat Annual Report, 1911). A good many of the admissions were suffering from the 'insanities associated with infection and exhaustion'. Causes of insanity are listed as 'syphilis, uraemia, Huntington's chorea' as well as alcoholism. Persons with mania and melancholia exhibited physical characteristics such as being run down and having bad teeth (Kingseat Annual Report, 1909). Loss of 'self-control' was often seen as the crisis precipitating admission to the asylum but it was felt that many patients had been ill for months preceding this and the 'legal nature' of admission papers was preventing patients from receiving earlier treatment. The medical superintendent stated that,

> 'Hereditary predisposition is the chief predisposing factor in the causation of insanity but its effect might be more or less neutralised if the principles of mental and physical hygiene were attended to throughout the life of the individual so predisposed' (Kingseat Annual Report, 1907).

The connection between syphilis and general paralysis was noted in 1912 when ocular signs of dementia had also been discovered (Kingseat Annual Report 1912). Physical disorders were seen to be at the root of most mental conditions (Kingseat Annual Report, 1910). However, a newspaper article complained that too much money was being spent on the insane without a full understanding of the causes of insanity,

> 'Of what avail our Kingseat inmates playing themselves back to reason by means of billiards or bowls or piano music, if the incoming stream of lunatics continues as great as the outgoing?'

The article expressed concern that little progress had been made in understanding insanity compared with other branches of medicine, but summarised the current view which was that lunacy was due to brain disease or changes of structures in the brain and that 'whatever tends to impair the general health may under certain circumstances produce insanity'. Criticism was made of asylum superintendents who were 'more concerned with pigs than prognosis' and did not carry out original research or pathological study (*Aberdeen Free Press*, 29th April 1906).

3.2. Edinburgh District Lunatic Asylum (Bangour Village)

3.2.1. Introduction

Early provision for the insane in Edinburgh consisted of the City Bedlam built in 1678 and about a dozen cells attached to the Royal Infirmary. In 1746 the earlier Bedlam was replaced by a larger building containing 21 cells with

64 inmates, both private and pauper. A Royal asylum was opened at Morningside in 1813 but this catered initially only for wealthier patients until an agreement with the city authorities in 1844 opened it up to the insane poor. With the gradual growth in numbers of the insane, increasing reliance was placed on boarding out, accommodation of chronic patients in the poorhouses and removing Edinburgh patients to other district asylums around the country. However, the pressure of numbers eventually becoming too great, Edinburgh was constituted a Lunacy District in 1897 (*JMS* 57 (1911): 408-411; EDLB Minutes, 18th February 1901).

John Sibbald, a Commissioner in Lunacy for Scotland, was a strong advocate for the 'village' system,[3] as practised at Alt Scherbitz, publishing a pamphlet to this effect in 1897, which was circulated among the members of the newly-appointed Edinburgh District Lunacy Board (Sibbald, 1897). The same year, a deputation of the Board made a visit to 'certain asylums in France, Germany and England', namely: St Anne and Ville Juif, Paris; Dalldorf, Herzberge and Wuhlgarten, Berlin and Alt Scherbitz, Leipzig (*Report of Edinburgh Deputation*, 1897).

The deputation of five members of the Board (a separate deputation visited some English asylums, namely Claybury, Canehill and Menston) concluded that,

> '...there can be no question of the excellence of the Alt Scherbitz system of dealing with the insane. None of us is an expert in lunacy, but it does not require the eye of an expert to note the many advantages possessed by the segregating system. The separate dwellings, the home-like surroundings, the freedom from restraint, the substitution of gardens for airing yards, bedrooms for dormitories, sitting rooms for halls, and roads for corridors, cannot fail to have a soothing and beneficial effect on the patients requiring treatment in an asylum.'

They found Alt Scherbitz to be 'altogether different from anything the deputation ever saw before...the most striking feature of the place is the *absence of the appearance of an institution*' (italics in original). The asylum is particularly praised for 'having none of that dead uniformity of design which produces monotony...Monotonous uniformity has been avoided, whether it be in the design of the villas or the pattern of the teacups.' The EDLB recognised that Alt Scherbitz was the 'logical development of the open-door system' which had originated in Scotland (*Report of Edinburgh Deputation*, 1897).

3.2.2. Construction of asylum

The estate of Bangour, about 15 miles from Edinburgh and comprising 950 acres, was purchased in 1897. A competition to design the asylum was held in 1898, in consultation with Sir John Sibbald, specifying that

---

[3] 'Village' was the term most often used in Edinburgh for the system that was elsewhere often known as 'colony' or 'segregate'.

the design be 'framed on the principle of segregation' practised at Alt Scherbitz, and the contract was awarded to Hippolyte J Blanc of Edinburgh. The architect undertook visits to asylums in Germany, France, England and Scotland, and had many of the features of Alt Scherbitz in mind when he designed the asylum (Blanc, 1908; EDLB Minutes, 17th June 1901). Sir John Sibbald was secured as medical adviser to the new District Board of Lunacy after this visit (*JMS* 57 (1911):408-411).[4] The Chairman of the EDLB stated in 1901 that,

> 'A great change has taken place in medical ideas as to treatment of the insane. They are no longer shut up within confined barracks, condemned to seclusion and surrounded by high stone walls. The new theory—and it is a humane one—is that their daily life should be made as near as possible to what it is when living absolutely free of restraint—in fact living a natural life, relieved of worry and anxiety, living in a bracing district of country in thoroughly sanitary dwellings, with adequate food supplies, and ample recreation ground for exercise and amusement' (EDLB Minutes 1901).

Preparation of the site began in 1898 but no building work commenced for several years. From the outset, the proposed cost of the asylum caused consternation among ratepayers and hence difficulties for the EDLB. They fell back on both their statutory and moral obligation to provide for the insane. The 'one outstanding feature of the age in which we live is the desire to alleviate suffering in every form'. The opinion was expressed by board members that there was no compulsion to provide hospitals for the sick but there was an imperative to provide asylums for the insane because a greater duty existed to provide treatment and cure for insanity which was the worst misfortune and hardest to cure (EDLB Minutes, 18th February 1901).

By 1901, large sums had been spent on the construction of a private railway to bring building stone to the site, and on roads and other preparation work. The Commissioners of Lunacy (Sibbald having retired by this stage to take up his post as adviser to the EDLB) commented on 'unnecessary costliness in matters of detail', specifying window mullions, crow-stepped gables, string courses, mouldings and balustrades. They stated that these features were 'out of place in the buildings of a village asylum erected for poor people, and they will add nothing to their efficiency as a means of caring for or curing the insane' (*British Architect*, 27th December 1901).

Blanc was asked on several occasions to redraw the plans with the aim of reducing costs and eventually, George T Hine, the foremost asylum architect of the era, was invited to comment on the cost of the plans and whether or not it was justified. He expressed admiration for Blanc's designs calling them 'an ornament to the country and a landmark in the history of asylum building'. Hine advised on some

minor modifications to cut costs such as modifying the interior treatments (*British Architect* 12th September 1902).

The undue delay in deciding on the asylum design led to the decision to erect barrack-like structures of iron and wood on the site which were begun in 1902. The first patients were accepted into these 'villas' in 1904 and they ultimately became the 'industrial' housing for men when the asylum was completed. The villas were rebuilt at a later period in brick and are still present on the site today. Although they were originally built of less durable materials, they were not intended to be temporary, and indeed have stood the test of time. However, they were not part of Hippolyte J Blanc's original plan for the asylum (which can be seen at Figure 3-12).

The asylum's opening on 3rd October 1906 was given extensive coverage in both the architectural and medical press. *The Builder* of November 10th 1906 reported that the asylum was composed of detached buildings distributed 'without formality or attempt at regularity' (Figure 3-14). They termed the new layout, the 'villa or segregate system' whose main feature was the 'avoidance of everything suggestive of restraint such as enclosing yards'. The buildings were small and were 'treated with such variety of form and environment as to destroy all appearance of official residence'. The buildings were of 'simple, natural design' and interest was imparted by a variety of external treatments, in 'exposed stone, harling, tiled and green slated roofs'. Simple variations in form were able to give a 'fair architectural effect'. It was thought to be the first complete example of the 'segregate system' (but in fact Aberdeen was earlier) (*The Builder*, 10th November 1906).

The asylum could accommodate 750 patients, although offices and admin buildings were built to meet the needs of 1,000, so that future expansion could be accommodated. The recreation hall was still to be built at this period and the hospital was still under construction (*BMJ*, 13th October 1906) (Figure 3-13). The final cost was c£300,000 and the former Prime Minister, Lord Rosebery, who performed the opening ceremony, made a speech reported in local and national newspapers which was highly critical of the expense of asylums such as Bangour and the wastefulness of spending money on those who could not be cured (*The Lancet,* 27th October 1906).

The architect of Bangour Village, Hippolyte J Blanc, addressed the Royal Institute of British Architects in 1908, emphasising the main therapeutic features of the village asylum and Bangour in particular, freedom, and greater facility for the classification of patients. There were no gates, walls, fences or lodges at the approach to the asylum, or walls or fences around the buildings, and it therefore gave an impression of startling openness when compared with the typical asylum layout. The vast majority of the patients, including those suffering from acute mania or serious depressive illnesses, were housed in villas of between 35 and 50 individuals, modelled on domestic houses and forming a settlement that was intended to

---

[4] Sibbald retired as a Lunacy Commissioner in 1899 and advised the EDLB until his resignation in 1904 (*BMJ*, 6th May 1905)

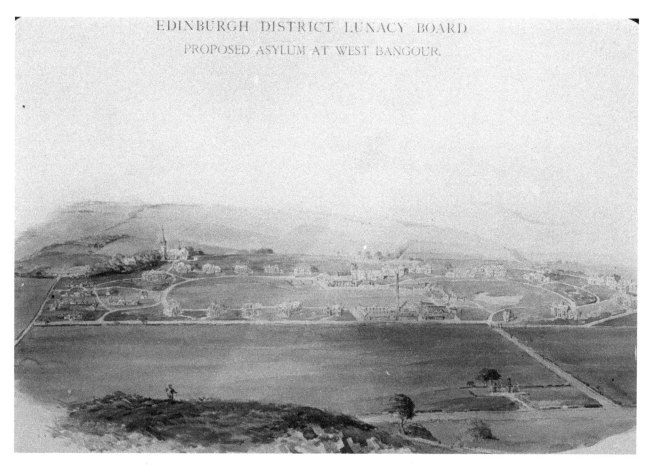

Figure 3-12. Bangour Village Asylum: original design, bird's eye view. The asylum as built was much modified. Source: Image LHB44/26/5. Courtesy of Lothian Health Services Archive.

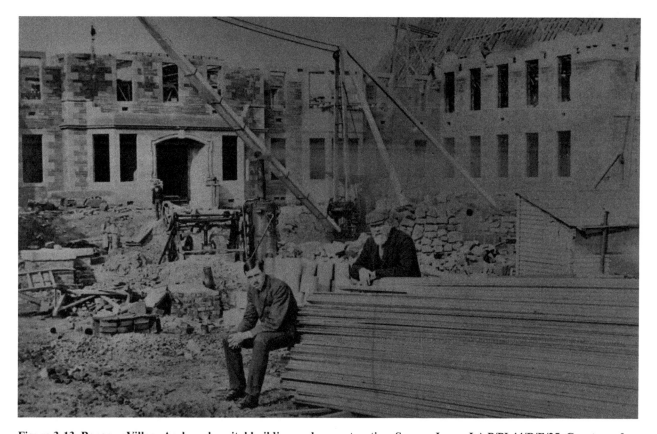

Figure 3-13. Bangour Village Asylum: hospital building under construction. Source: Image LA P/PL44/B/E/25. Courtesy of Lothian Health Service Archive.

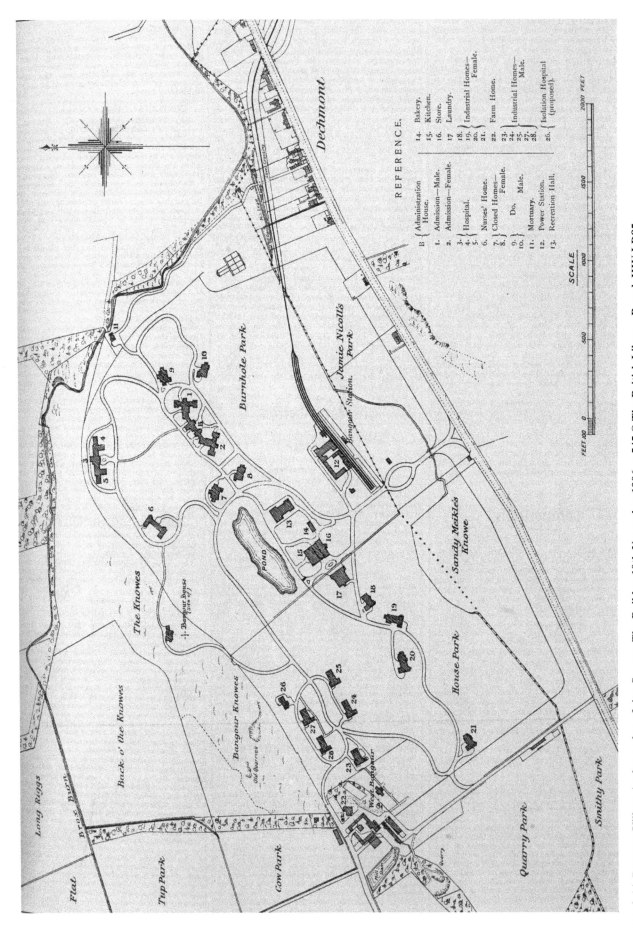

REFERENCE.

B { Administration House.
1. Admission—Male.
2. Admission—Female.
3. } Hospital.
4. }
5. Nurses' Home.
6. } Closed Homes—Female.
7. }
8. } Do. Male.
9. }
10. }
11. Mortuary.
12. Power Station.
13. Recreation Hall.
14. Bakery.
15. Kitchen.
16. Store.
17. Laundry.
18. }
19. } Industrial Homes—Female.
20. }
21. }
22. Farm Home.
23. }
24. } Industrial Homes—Male.
25. }
27. }
28. }
26. } Isolation Hospital (proposed).

SCALE

FEET 100   0   500   1000   1500   2000 FEET

Figure 3-14. Bangour Village Asylum: plan of site. Source: The Builder, 10th November 1906, p.545 © The British Library Board, HIU.LD85.

112

resemble 'an ordinary village' or 'an ordinary city suburb'. For the patients, the home-like appearance 'must be less depressing than are the more or less formidable large pavilion buildings' (Blanc, 1908).

In the ensuing discussion on Blanc's paper, George T Hine, the foremost asylum architect of his day, commended Blanc on being one of the first to design an asylum on the colony system and admitted that England was moving 'at a less rapid pace' having only experimented with erecting a few detached villas in the grounds of traditional asylums. But he thought that not enough was known about the working of the villa system in practice and warned that 'in a few years the promoters of this scheme in Edinburgh might probably think they had gone a little too far' (quoted in Blanc, 1908). Hine's architectural colleagues were much more forceful in their condemnation, foreseeing difficulties with supervising and administering the village asylum, and criticising the sanitary arrangements. Doubts were raised about the capacity of the insane to appreciate the greater integration of the village layout with its beautiful surroundings and it was suggested that the supposed advantage of less institutional feeling was chimerical. The village asylum was vilified as a 'backward' step and one critic went so far as to position the Scottish Lunacy Commissioners as subalterns, claiming they were 'less intelligent' than those in England for having passed such a scheme (Blanc, 1908).

By 1911, Edinburgh, with a population of 355,000, has 1,200 persons identified as insane and unable to pay for treatment. Of these, 745 were resident in Bangour, over 300 were boarded out in private dwellings, 105 remained at the Royal Asylum and the remainder were at other asylums or homes for 'imbeciles' (Bangour Village Annual Report, 1911). Patients at Bangour Village cost £27 per annum covering the cost of food, clothing, salaries and wages and not including the cost of buildings or their upkeep (Halliday 2003: 166).

During the First World War, patients were transferred to other centres and Bangour became a war hospital from 1915 until 1922 (Hendrie & Macleod, 1991). A church was added to the site as a war memorial and opened in 1930. Various additions were made to the site over time, notably a large addition to the nurses' home in 1931 (Darragh, 2011: 60). The hospital was closed in 2004 and the site remained empty and derelict for some years before being purchased for redevelopment as a housing estate.

3.2.3. Staffing

The ratio of nursing staff to patients in the Medical Section, was one to eight by day, and by night, one to 22. In the industrial section, the ratio was one to 14 by day and one to 154 by night making the overall staffing ratio— one to 11 by day, and one to 46 by night. There were 23 unmarried attendants at the asylum in 1908 who had bedrooms in the men's industrial homes with no common sitting room or recreation room and they were inclined to

wander into the local villages when off duty and get into trouble. It was thought a separate attendants' home should be built for them. There was concern about pensions and retaining staff because the work was said to be 'repugnant' (Bangour Village Annual Report 1908). Asylum staff were advised to get out of the asylum on their days off (Hendrie & Macleod, 1991).

Providing a separate residence for nurses was seen as a good way of attracting high quality staff, i.e. kindly, well-educated and refined. They were to be given 'civilised conditions of life' and be out of the sphere of work during the time of their recreation in a residence where they could see and help one another and compare notes and at the same time live the life of 'honest and cultured' human beings. The work was trying and difficult and if it were to be done under humane and civilised conditions they had to have a reasonable number of nurses and give them reasonable time for self-improvement and recreation. Female staff were preferred where possible as they were thought to give 'improved nursing' (Bangour Village Annual Report 1907).

It was thought that better quality staff were attracted by providing quarters for married couples, so cottages were to be built at Dechmont Village and Bangour farmsteading (Bangour Village Annual Report 1909). However, Sibbald wanted cottages for attendants to be placed far away from patient accommodation because the wives and families of staff could undermine the discipline of the institution (EDLB Minutes, 28th November 1900).

3.2.4. Site and layout

Bangour Village Asylum was 14 miles from Edinburgh, and 960 acres in extent including about 200 acres of woodlands. The land was from 500 to 700 feet above sea-level on sloping ground with a southern exposure (LHB44/6 Edinburgh War Hospital pamphlet) (Figure 3-15). The Board aimed to provide three quarters of an acre per patient, in excess of the regulations of the SLC, which stipulated half an acre (EDLB Minutes, 18th February 1901). In 1908, 40 per cent of the men were working on the land, while female patients were working in the laundry and kitchens and 80 were engaged at sewing and knitting (Bangour Village Annual Report 1908).

The site was divided into two parts, the medical section in the eastern part of the site, with hospital, admission wards and villas for all patients requiring special treatment or medical supervision and the 'industrial' section comprising villas for patients with 'chronic' mental illness and convalescents. There was no gate lodge at the entrance to the site and the asylum presented no centralised building embodying the institution, the administration building being a two-storey structure of an unimposing character and relatively distant from the entrance. The hospital was likewise removed to the back of the site. The asylum itself, therefore, 'disappears', as in the Alt Scherbitz model. There was no surrounding wall to the asylum and villa

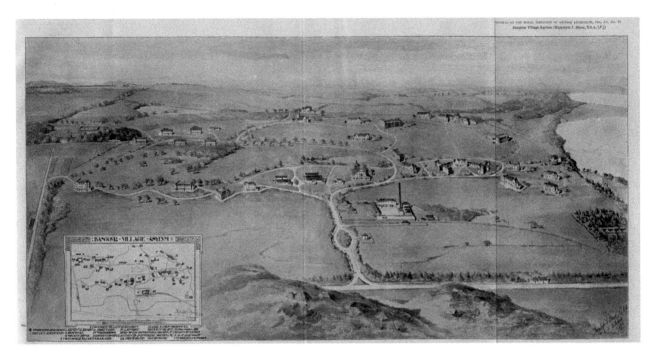

Figure 3-15. Bangour Village Asylum: perspective view. Although largely as built, some buildings are depicted (four additional villas, for example) that were never constructed. Source: Blanc, H J (1908) *Bangour Village Asylum*, **RIBA Journal XV (10), pp.309-26. Special Collections, Queen's University Belfast.**

gardens were for the most part, unfenced, a few having the kind of low fence that would be typical of the garden of a suburban dwelling. The buildings were laid out in an informal style mimicking an unplanned development that had grown up organically. Curving roadways connected the buildings in a series of continuous irregular loops nearly four miles long in total which replaced the lengthy linear or hemispherical corridors of a pavilion layout.

The 'village' was placed near the lower border of the Bangour estate, on ground sloping to the south, near the Edinburgh/Glasgow road. The medical section accommodated 346 patients, a number which it was envisaged, could be increased,

> '...by building more villas or an infirmary for senile cases. The roads, drains, water-pipes and electric cables have been laid in such a way that additional buildings can be erected at any time with a minimum of inconvenience and cost'.

Water was supplied by gravitation from a reservoir, rather than using a water tower. The reservoir was constructed on the estate at a height of 700 feet above sea-level, with a capacity of 16 million gallons, the asylum using 56,000 gallons a day (Bangour Village Annual Report 1908). It was well stocked with trout and a boat house was added so that medical staff could use the reservoir for recreation on their days off (Hendrie & Macleod, 1991).

3.2.5. Selected buildings

The buildings, which were of 'freestone, from various quarries in Scotland' showed a variation in building forms and orientations, which was intended to 'destroy all appearance of official residence' and interest was imparted by 'variety of external treatment in exposed stone, harling, tiled and green slated roofs' (Blanc 1908). Some villas were replicas or near-replicas of each other, e.g. acute villas for males and females are on the same plan, as are observation villas and the four women's industrial villas are of only two different types, but each villa is orientated slightly differently and the villas are positioned irregularly around the site, deriving variety from their aspect and environment. Villa dayroom windows, for the most part, look out onto the rural site rather than other asylum buildings. The asylum was bounded on two sides by public roads and 'such a road passes through the farm-steading and close to houses occupied by patients', the discursive highlighting of this accessibility emphasising the openness of the site (Keay, 1911). The villas also ranged in size so that more difficult patients were accommodated in smaller numbers for closer supervision. The acute villas were the smallest, having 32 patients, observation villas housed 40 and the villas for chronic patients were largest at 46-50. The absence of corridors, walls and fences meant that patients leaving the villas and moving between buildings walked out into the open grounds. Potential escapes or difficulties in managing patients outdoors had to be addressed either by vesting more trust in the patients or by increasing attendant supervision, rather than depending on the built environment.

Other buildings comprised an administration block with admission wings, a hospital, a nurses' home for 88 nurses, a farm, recreation hall, bakery, kitchen, power station, mortuary, store and laundry. Emphasis is continually placed in EDLB Minutes on the efforts made to save money.

Cheap finishes were used, e.g. internal linings on walls of dayrooms were of yellow pine rather than hardwood. 'As regards the exterior of the buildings there is little that can be called simply decorative', and there was no decorative finishing on the interiors except inside the Board Room. 'Quiet and reposeful' colours were used such as greens and blues, 'as the influence of red on nervous patients is well known to be pronouncedly irritating' (*British Architect* 5th October 1906). The furnaces burned coke so that smoke could be avoided. Ventilation was by opening doors and windows and was assisted by air inlets placed behind the radiators.

Gate Lodges

Bangour Village is the only asylum of the three Scottish institutions considered here that dispensed with entrance gates and gate lodges, in an emulation of Alt Scherbitz.

Administration House (Figures 3-16, 3-17)

The Administration House contained a board room and dispensary and quarters for three assistant physicians, as well as a billiard room for staff recreation. Admission wards for male and female patients were in wings to either side of the central block and accommodated 46 patients of each sex. The patients were examined and observed here for several days before being passed to the appropriate ward. A doctor's room with photographic studio with glass roof and sides, bathroom and single rooms were grouped round a vestibule at the visitors' entrance on each side,

partitioned off from the occupied wards 'so that nothing tending to depress may be observed by anyone coming for first treatment' (Blanc 1908). The Administration Block is unassuming and domestic in architectural character, a quality which was unusual in institutional building and came in for some criticism when the asylum opened. The *British Architect* commented that,

'the administration block [is] generally the most commanding portion structurally of public institutions, but [was] in this case constructed by the board in one of its fits of parsimony, and look[s] pretty much as if it were trying to sink out of sight in offended dignity' (*British Architect*, 5th October 1906).

The admission wards were originally conceived as separate blocks but, at the request of Sibbald, the design was changed to incorporate the blocks into the administration building (EDLB Minutes 1905). A verandah was added along the length of each admission wing at the recommendation of the Lunacy Commissioners in 1908 (Bangour Village Annual Report 1908). The verandahs in front of the admission wards were occupied in 1909 and were seen as giving rest in bed in the open air to many patients. For those who remained in the wards, they provided 'increased space, better air, and peace and quietness' (Bangour Village Annual Report 1908). Open-air treatment was found of benefit in cases of a 'more chronic nature associated with a reduced condition of bodily health'. Enlargement and improvement of verandahs was carried out in 1910 so they could be used all year round and night and day. The

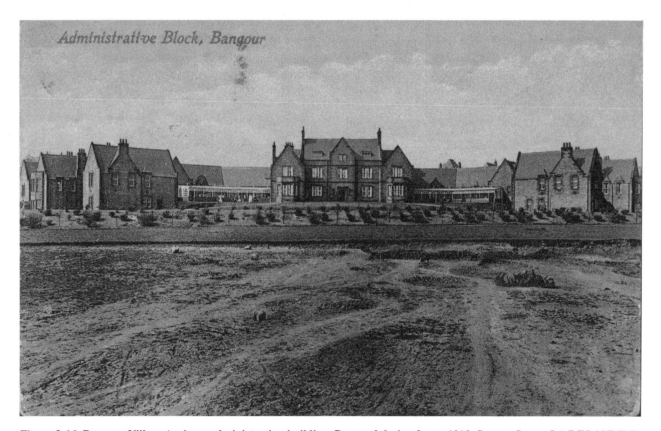

Figure 3-16. Bangour Village Asylum: administration building. Postcard dating from c1910. Source: Image LA P/PL44/B/E/7. Courtesy of Lothian Health Service Archive.

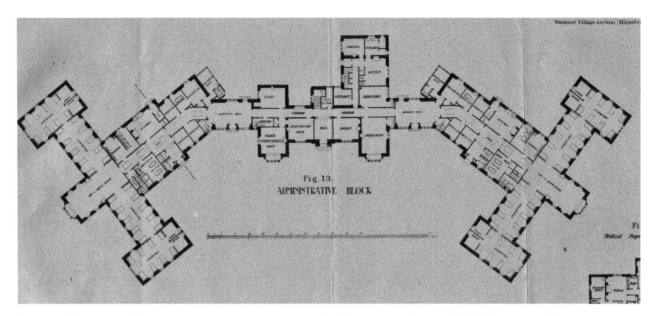

Figure 3-17. Bangour Village Asylum: plan of administration building. Source: Blanc, H J (1908) *Bangour Village Asylum*, RIBA Journal XV (10), pp.309-26. Special Collections, Queen's University Belfast.

verandahs were increased in width and fitted with roller shutters for protection during wet and stormy weather, the open-air treatment being thought to be of 'great benefit in many cases of mental disorder as in other diseases' (Bangour Village Annual Report 1909).

Hospital (Figures 3-18, 3-19)

The hospital of 90 beds was for those requiring medical care and nursing due to bodily illness. The hospital was completed on 30th June 1908, well after the official opening of the asylum in 1906. It was described in the Annual Report of 1909 as occupying a 'fine, commanding site', overlooking the medical section, sheltered on the north side by ground rising behind it and open to the south (Bangour Village Annual Report 1909). There were three wards on each side, two on the ground floor and one on the first floor (one of 12 and two of 14 beds) as well as four side rooms on each side, accommodating 45 of each sex. Patients were each allowed an area of 100 to 110 superficial feet, much more than the 60 superficial feet allowed for each patient in the industrial homes. A hoist

near the centre of the building could lift a patient in bed to the first floor (Blanc 1908).

Also part of the facilities were, an operation room, a laboratory for clinical and pathological work, a lecture room for training nursing staff and an electrical department. Attached to the wards were covered and protected verandahs and sun-rooms in which 'the open air treatment of disease can be conveniently carried out' (Bangour Village Annual Report 1909). More verandahs were added to the hospital c1911 (Bangour Village Annual Report 1911). The open wards of the hospital were praised in 1910, 'one may walk from one end of the hospital at Bangour to another, through male and female divisions, without requiring a key or a nurse to show the way' (*JMS* 56 (1910): 626).

Villas

The villas were all built to a similar plan with variations as to detail, layout and number of storeys. Each villa had a central flat-roofed section to the main building which

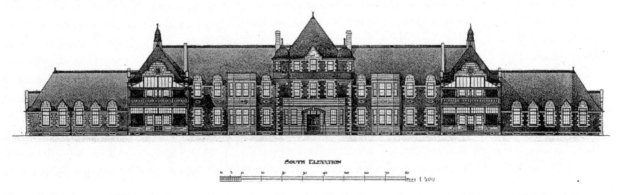

Figure 3-18. Bangour Village Asylum: south elevation of hospital block. Source: Academy Architecture 1906. Special Collections, Queen's University Belfast.

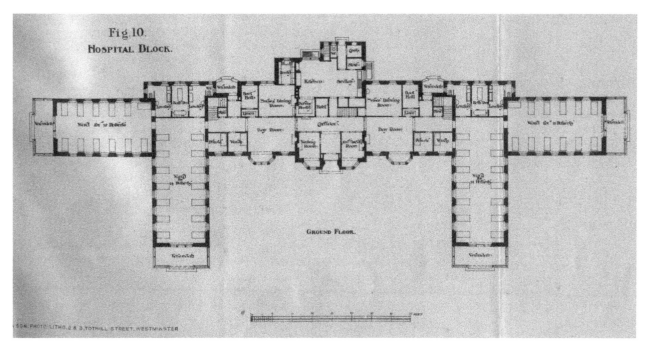

Figure 3-19. Bangour Village Asylum: plan of hospital block. Source: Blanc, H J (1908) *Bangour Village Asylum*, **RIBA Journal XV (10), pp.309-26. Special Collections, Queen's University Belfast.**

was not visible from ground level, and single-storey flat-roofed projections containing WCs and a boot hall, which were covered with 'asphalte'. Eaves did not overhang but terminated at an eaves course of dressing stone. Each also had an emergency stair tower, joined to the main building on one side and separately roofed, which was surmounted by a cupola and finial with a ventilator. The original plans suggest that flues within the walls led up to the ventilator, while fireplaces provided flue ventilation on the other side of the building.

Each villa 'is provided with electrical appliances for ventilation by fans, wherever special ventilation is considered essential, such as in the boot-rooms and lavatories' (Blanc 1908). In dayrooms and dormitories, ventilation was provided by the windows and by fresh-air inlets in the window recesses at floor level 'under key control of the attendants'. This allowed for incoming air to be warmed by radiators in the winter. Vitiated air was to exit through grated openings in the wall near the ceilings and taken through glazed brick flues into an outlet shaft and ventilator in the roof containing an electric fan (*British Architect*, 5th August 1898). The kitchens in each villa were used for dealing with special diets and for washing up, but the majority of food was brought from the central kitchen. Each villa featured two staircases for easy evacuation of patients in case of emergency (Blanc 1908).

WCs in all the villas were the 'white glazed pedestal wash-down'. This was of a special design with rounded corners on the cistern. 'No chain nor connecting rod is visible, the flush being produced by a gentle pressure of the finger upon a pin concealed within a slotted tube attached to the wall. There are no knobs or projections of any kind to which patients of suicidal tendency can attach

a hold.' The divisions between WCs were of Sicilian marble, one and a quarter inches thick, with a 20 inch gap beneath them and rising four feet six inches from the floor. This was presumably so that patients could be observed through the gap if necessary. The floors of the bathrooms were laid with terrazzo 'rounded at the angles of the floor and walls', to assist cleaning. The architect emphasised the measures taken to ensure ventilation of the WCs 'Cross-ventilation is provided by windows. The water-closet wing is in height a single story only, no occupied buildings being built over it. Each, in addition to cross-windows, has an extract shaft carried up in the main gable, with electric fan for ventilation' (Blanc 1908). The wash-hand basins were installed without traps and spilled 'directly into a continuous open gutter formed in the terrazzo floor'.[5] This arrangement would have had the advantage that objects could not easily be inserted into the sinks and block them. A special bathhouse had been proposed for the patients at one point but this was thought to pose a risk to health to patients walking to and from the bathhouse in inclement weather. The baths in each villa were separated by low screen and had 'semi-enclosed dressing boxes'. The baths were specially designed to be lower than usual with a five inch broad flat edge for the patient to sit on while being dried and with a 'shallow cavetto on the underside to prevent the patient securing a hold'. The windows were also specially designed with a mechanism that automatically opened the top sash when the lower sash was raised. There was no visible mechanism 'for patients to tamper with' and the system encouraged the natural circulation of air. 'Baffle boards' were placed in the open gap in

---

[5] At Blanc's RIBA presentation, this arrangement was criticised by another architect as unsanitary (Blanc 1908: 325).

wards containing bedridden patients to diffuse the air current (*British Architect*, 5th August 1898).

Closed Villas (Numbering of the villas below conforms to the plan of the site at Figure 3-14)

Closed villas, male and female, were for patients requiring continuous or special supervision due to their mental symptoms and were completed during 1907. They were designed with window restraints and other fitments so that patients could not injure themselves (Hendrie & Macleod, 1991). The villas were of two sizes (acute and observation), accommodating 32 and 40 patients and were close to the administration house and the admission wards (Figures 3-21, 3-22). Each 'closed' villa had on the ground floor a dining room, two dayrooms, bath-room, lavatory, boot and cloak rooms, nurses' dining room, kitchen and scullery. On the first floor was the patients' sleeping accommodation consisting of dormitories in which the space for beds was broken up by low wooden screens, about four and a half feet in height, 'so as to afford a simultaneous open view for nurses' and allow the patients to be observed easily (Blanc 1908). The dormitories were different sizes in order to provide 'variety'. There were also some single rooms and a parlour and bedroom for the charge nurse (other nurses slept in the Nurses' Home). The accommodation for patients in these villas was similar to that in the industrial homes except that the number of rooms was greater and they were of smaller size so that there were fewer patients in any one room. The furnishings of the closed villas were similar to those in other parts of the institution but the dining tables only seated four. Small tables facilitated the classification of patients at meals and the special supervision of those who required it (Bangour Village Annual Report 1907). The single rooms were about ten feet square, containing one bed and all had double doors. Two of the villas (seven and nine) had four single rooms, the other two (eight and ten) each had six, one of which was a padded room (the only padded rooms in the asylum) (Bangour Village Annual Report 1908; Blanc, 1908). It was proposed, likely by Sibbald, that extension of night nursing to all patients would decrease the need for single rooms, which were used for locking patients up at night to reduce the need for supervision. Single rooms were used for the sick, restless, suicidal and excited/noisy but in the opinion of Sibbald, 'it should be recognised that to lock such patients into single rooms at night is, from a medical or scientific point of view, no advance upon the methods of treatment followed in the last century' (EDLB Minutes, 28th November 1900).

VILLA NINE – OBSERVATION (MALE)

It had been intended that this villa would be used for males requiring observation, but the asylum had been built with less accommodation for women than for men, even though it transpired on opening, that there were more female patients, so villa nine was converted for use as a hospital for senile and infirm women (Figure 3-23). 'Being able to make such alterations so easily was one of the

advantages of the segregate system', reported the medical superintendent after this change (Bangour Village Annual Report 1908).

VILLA TEN – ACUTE (MALE)

Villa ten was built as a 'closed' or 'acute' villa for males, intended to accommodate 33 patients and was begun in June 1905 and completed in 1907 (Figure 3-24). The acute villa was said to 'supply the minimum accommodation according to the requirements of the Act and is compressed in a simple and economical form' (EDLB Minutes, 18th December 1901).

The villa is situated towards the east of the site, overlooking the recreation field. It is also very close to the administration block and admission wards, so that patients could be easily transferred once admitted. The building is orientated with its long axis west to east, its main elevation and front doorway facing southwards. The building material is Scottish sandstone of a cream to pink/orange hue. The stone has a roughly stugged finish and the ashlar blocks are laid in discontinuous, random courses. Dressing stones are of Locharbriggs sandstone which is used for quoins, window surrounds, plinth course, eaves course and other decorative highlights. In scale, the building resembles a large domestic villa and the domestic idiom is emphasised by the two forward-facing gables on the front elevation and the decorative features such as the wallhead dormers on the upper floor which are surmounted with circular-headed gablets finished with cornices and pointed finials.

The main entrance to the villa is within a single–storey projection at the east of the building forming a porch and its position within a re-entrant angle means that it is concealed from view when the building is approached from most directions. The path to the house leads to the nurses' entrance at the rear which is accorded less emphasis in terms of decorative treatment and size. The main doorway is emphasised with Locharbriggs sandstone dressings which form an elliptical-headed arch and moulded architrave. A second entrance on the south elevation, originally fitted with double-leafed doors, leads to and from a dayroom and can be considered an informal entrance and exit for patients to the verandah (no longer present). A contemporary photograph of villa eight (the identical villa on the female side) (Figure 3-22) shows the verandah which appears to be composed of a lean-to glass roof supported by cast-iron pillars. The gable at the west of the elevation projects slightly (six inches) from the façade, emphasising the feature (an oriel was originally planned for this elevation but the projection of the gable was said to be sufficient to create the effect of an oriel. Double 'air inlets' are fitted just below the plinth course under every window to ventilate the space between foundation and floor.

Windows are six over six sliding sashes to all openings. The ground floor windows on the south elevation are mullioned and each double window is in two, three-foot wide (0.9m) sections and is seven feet (2.13m) in height. To the right of

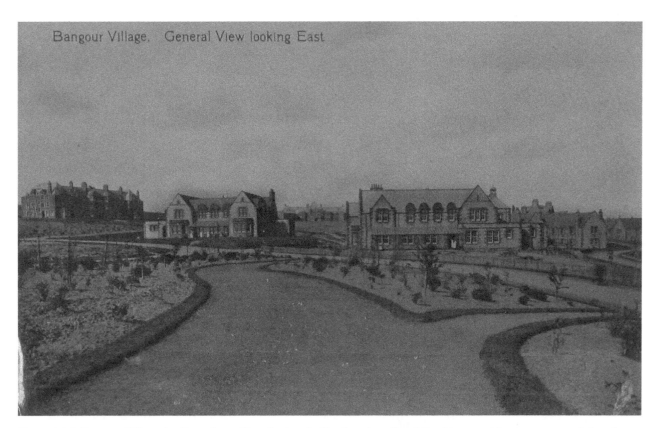

Figure 3-20. Bangour Village Asylum: view of female closed villas (numbers 7 and 8) with nurses' home to extreme left and part of administration block visible to extreme right. Source: Image LA P/PL44/B/E/2. Courtesy of Lothian Health Services Archive).

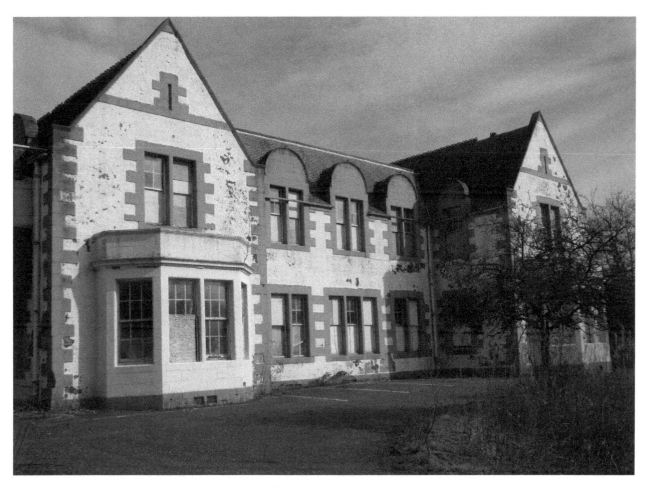

Figure 3-21. Bangour Village Asylum: observation villa (female). Source: Author's photograph.

119

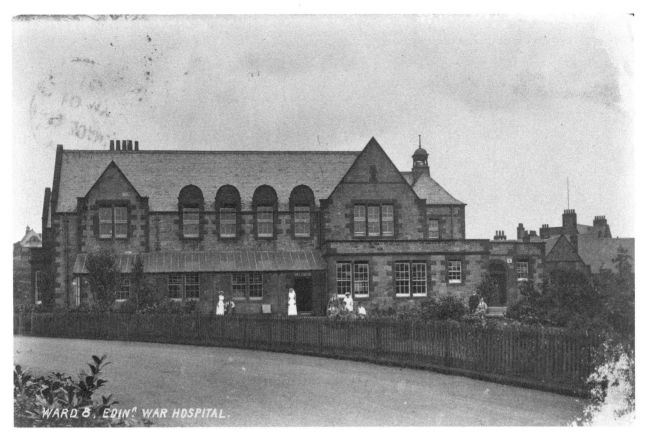

Figure 3-22. Bangour Village Asylum: acute villa (female) (image dates from c.1915 when the asylum was in use as a war hospital). Source: Image LA P/PL44/B/E/6. Courtesy of Lothian Health Services Archive.

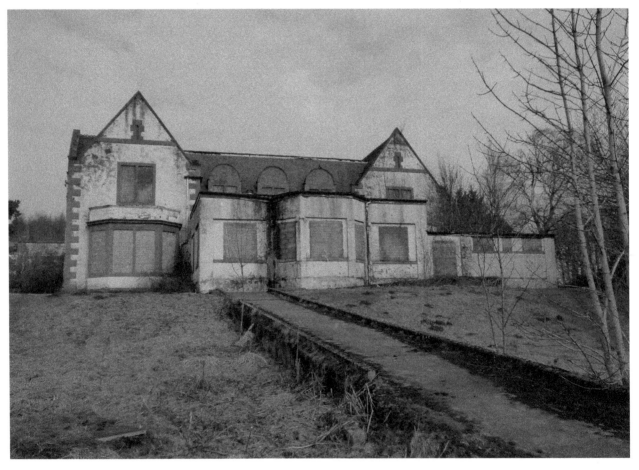

Figure 3-23. Bangour Village Asylum: observation villa (male) Source: Author's photograph.

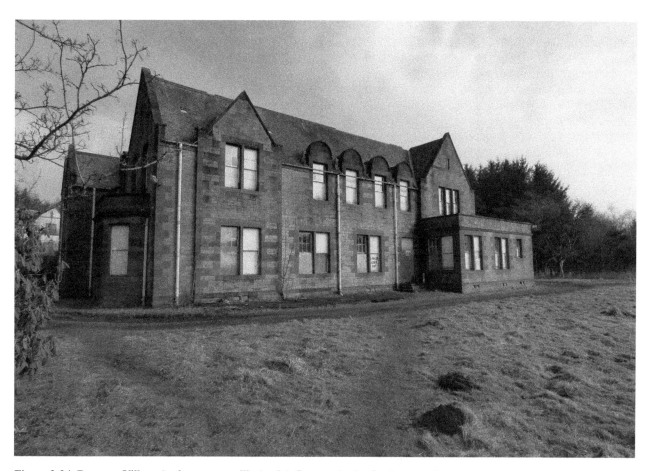

Figure 3-24. Bangour Village Asylum: acute villa (male). Source: Author's photograph.

the single storey projection is a window of dimensions two feet, nine inches by four feet, six inches (0.84m x 1.37m). This window lit one of the villa's single rooms, which would have been used for the confinement of agitated or disruptive patients. The contemporary photograph at Figure three suggests that the window was of normal appearance externally, but the original plan (Figure four) shows that internal shutters were fitted in order to exclude light or prevent breakage/escape. Windows on the upper floor are smaller than those on the lower floor, two feet six inches wide (0.76m) on the gables, while the wallhead dormers are three feet, three inches wide (one metre). The roofing slates are Coniston, having a greenish tinge and hand-worked irregularities, while the ridge tiles are of red clay.

The north elevation is effectively the back of the house, but is in fact the elevation most visitors, staff and patients would have initially approached from the main path. The soil pipes leading to the sewers are on this elevation, as are the chimneys. Architecturally it is less formal than the main elevation, with a greater variety of forms and greater asymmetricality.

Ground floor windows on this elevation are for the most part smaller than on the main elevation, being in the main two feet six inches wide. The lavatory is lit by two windows, a mullioned window in two sections and a single window, all six feet in height, while the bathroom is lit by two similar mullioned windows. Two very small windows of two feet by three feet light a storeroom and the WC within the 'stair tower' (the stair tower expressed the presence of the stairs within, but the staircase is, in fact, contained within the main body of the building). The only window approaching the dimensions of those on the south-facing elevation is that lighting the nurses' sitting room which is three feet, six inches by seven feet and is within a re-entrant angle, facing eastwards, where it would only have received early morning sun. The windows on the first floor gable are two feet, nine inches wide, slightly wider than those below, but are single windows only rather than bipartite mullions. These light single rooms and air inlets are let into the walls of these rooms, presumably so that ventilation could be provided even when the windows were closed due to any disruptive behaviour of the patient within. Both these windows were fitted with internal shutters.

The wing to the right, which is structurally almost completely isolated from the rest of the building, contains three single rooms and one padded room on the upper floor, the only padded rooms in the asylum being situated in the male and female acute villas. Two single rooms are situated on the eastern facing portion of this wing and are fitted with windows two feet, nine inches in width and with air inlets below. They would also have been fitted with internal shutters. A gable on this elevation allows for greater headroom for the patients within. The roof ridge of this wing is spanned by a plain rectangular chimney with five flues, one coming from the kitchen range, another from the fireplace in the nurses' sitting room. The other flues may have been connected to the basement boiler or may have been attached to ventilation grilles within the patient accommodation. A single air inlet on the north facing elevation ventilates a 'glazed brick duct' of irregular shape that extends along one wall of the padded room. The purpose of this is unclear, but may have facilitated the removal of bodily fluids from the room.

As in the industrial homes the internal spaces of villa 10 are arranged to replicate those of a domestic dwelling, with living spaces on the ground floor and sleeping accommodation on the upper floor (Figure 3-25). However, the ground floor rooms share with the industrial villas the same characteristic of rooms opening into each other, rather than off a central hallway, as would be more common in a domestic house. The rooms are smaller than those in the industrial villas and are all of a rectangular

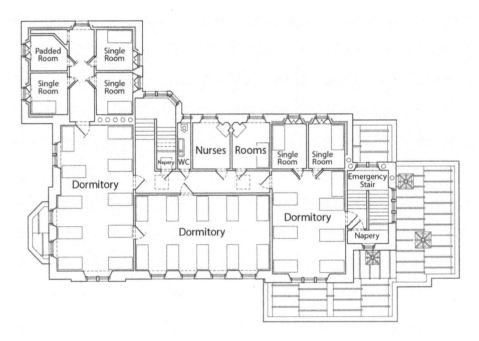

First Foor

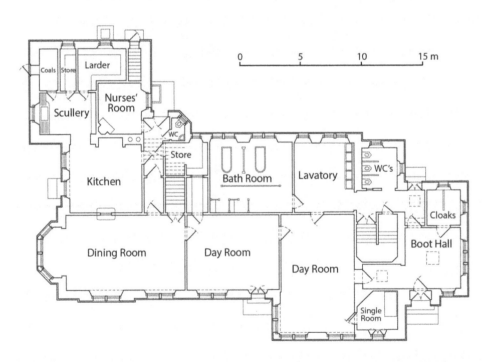

Ground Floor

Figure 3-25. Bangour Village Asylum: plan of villa 10, ground floor and first floor. Source: Redrawn by L Mulqueeny of Queen's University Belfast after original plans, NRS RHP49150 National Records of Scotland.

shape that is easily surveilled from any position in the room. The 'best' rooms in the house, those that are largest and have a south-facing orientation, for greater exposure to light, are reserved for patient use. The dining room is endowed with a large west-facing, canted bay window that would have created a light-filled space during the evening meal and also allows for a measure of cross-ventilation, when windows to west and south are opened. The middle dayroom is lit and ventilated from only one direction, but the dayroom to the right also achieves a measure of cross-ventilation and evening sunlight by dint of projecting a few feet forward of the main elevation. However, this room also has a 'single room' opening off it, which would have been used to seclude patients who were exhibiting disruptive behaviour. This room can only be entered from the dayroom and is effectively isolated from the rest of the villa by being surrounded by thick walls in a single-storey section of the building. The cloakroom, boot hall and WCs are also included in this single storey section, all these rooms being thus isolated and achieving a measure of cross-ventilation with windows on two (adjacent) elevations. The bathroom and lavatory are not cross-ventilated and are incorporated in the main section of the building, suggesting that they were not seen as potential sources of disease. The nurses' sitting room is at the back of the building, with an east-facing window, where it would only have received early morning light. It is therefore in a secondary position in regard to the spatial hierarchy of the building. The nurses' WC is located conveniently near to their sitting room and is not cross ventilated. The staircase to the upper floor leads directly out of the dining room, rather than being accessed from a hallway, again to give the staff greater control over the movements of residents.

The upper floor again situates the patient accommodation in the best rooms, with two dormitories for ten patients and one for seven at the south-facing front of the building. The eastern elevation is entirely obscured by the emergency stair tower which is isolated from the rest of the building, which suggests that early morning sunlight was not seen as an important requirement. The left-hand dormitory, however, does have a lengthy western elevation and would have received light in the evenings. The dormitories all open off a central corridor, making nurse access to individual rooms during the night easier, but generally reflects the static position of patients during sleeping hours. Sitting rooms for nurses on night supervision are at the back of the building and are north facing, in a similar position to the adjacent single rooms for patients that would have been used for disciplinary control. However, the single rooms differ from the nurses' sitting rooms in the consideration that has been given to ventilation, with air access inlets in the walls and electric fans in the ceilings. The single WC on this floor suggests that chamber pots may have been used in addition. The majority of single rooms and the only padded room are contained in a virtually self-contained annexe at the rear of the building. Accessed from a corridor, opening off the dormitory on the left, two of the rooms are lit from the west and two from the east, but are likely to have been among the darker rooms in the

house for the majority of the day, perhaps because of the fears of manic patients being over-stimulated by light.

Industrial Homes (Female)

Industrial homes for women occupied the lower portion of the grounds each accommodating c50 patients and the requisite staff. They were completed in 1906 and were for laundry workers (no 18) and needleworkers and dressmakers (19, 20, 21).The annual report for 1906 described these villas thus;

> 'Internally in the finishing and decoration of the various rooms, the utmost regard had been paid to economy, while a bright and cheerful effect has been produced by staining and varnishing the woodwork and treating the plaster walls and distemper in various shades. The furnishings are as they ought to be excellent in design, in quality of material and in workmanship, without being in any sense luxurious or extravagant. A feature of these Industrial Homes is the absence as far as this can be attained of arrangements suggestive of an asylum. There is not in any of them a bolt or bar or shuttered window. The doors open with ordinary handles. There is no padded room or single room in which a patient can be secluded from her fellows and liberty and freedom of action are allowed to the utmost extent consistent with safety'. (Bangour Village Annual Report 1906).

VILLA 18

Known as the 'laundry home', this villa was conveniently situated near the laundry as a residence for female patients employed there and in the central kitchen, as well as the laundry staff (Figure 3-26). The villa for 46 females with chronic mental illness, which also would have been used for recuperating patients is one of the largest in Bangour Village (main elevation 95 feet wide). It is oriented with its main elevation facing towards the south-east in order to receive a maximum amount of healthful sunlight. The villa was originally projected to be of two floors only, but pressure to cut costs led to a decision to increase the numbers accommodated and a consequent lessening of the domestic aspect of the building. Nevertheless the villa exhibits a number of domestic features, the canted bays on either side of the main elevation, the verandah spanning the middle three bays (shadow visible in Figure 3-26), the wall-head dormers—a characteristic feature of Scottish domestic architecture, pedimented bays, grouped windows and angled chimney stacks. The building exhibits height variation between various parts and some bays project slightly. The variation in roof line, heights, canted bay windows and projecting structural bays adds to an overall sense of articulated surfaces and lines, which although subtle, softens the building's uniformity as institutional space. The main elevation bears comparison with Edinburgh's stone tenements, which are often three and four storeys high. The interior, however, is laid out as a single, unified domestic villa with living accommodation

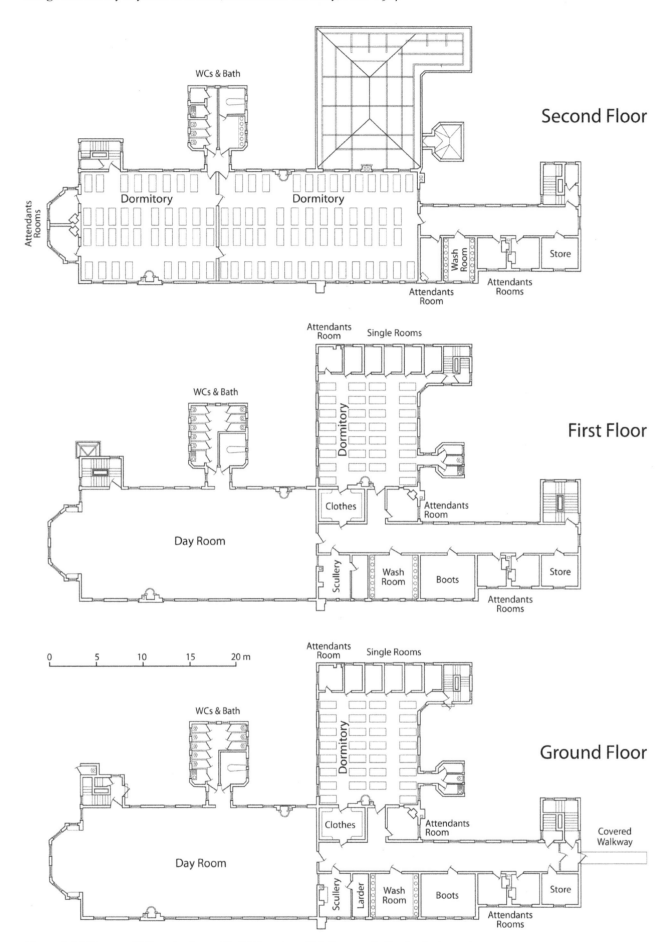

Figure 3-26. Bangour Village Asylum: villa 18 (laundry villa). Source: Author's photograph.

on the ground floor and sleeping and bathroom facilities on the upper floors (Figure 3-27).

The downstairs accommodation consists of a dining room with bay window, an L-shaped day room with bay and double doors opening out onto the verandah and

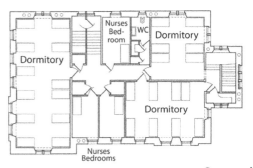

Second Floor

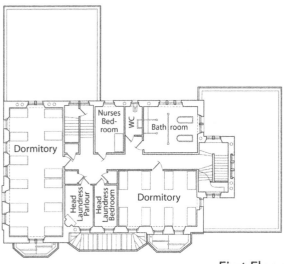

First Floor

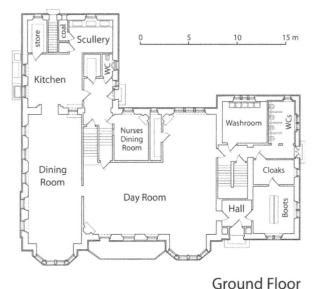

Ground Floor

Figure 3-27. Bangour Village Asylum: villa 18 (laundry villa), plan of ground and first floors. Source: Redrawn by L Mulqueeny of Queen's University Belfast after original plans, NRS RHP49146 National Records of Scotland.

towards the back of the villa, a kitchen and scullery in a single-storey wing. A further single-storey wing to the side contains a boot hall, cloakroom, WCs and washing facilities together with a stair tower which is isolated from the rest of the building to provide an escape route in case of fire. The privileged main elevation is entirely devoted to patient accommodation, but unlike a domestic house the main living areas do not open off a central hallway but open into each other, rendering the control and observation of patients easier. For similar reasons, the staircase to the upper storeys leads directly up from the dayroom rather than from a separate hallway. The large open space required for the dayroom has rendered necessary the use of two cast iron columns to support the ceiling which are not normally a domestic feature. The L-shaped day room which is lit on two elevations allows the room to be some extent cross-ventilated and to receive light from two different directions, the evening sun falling across the rear windows which face north-west. However, it makes for more difficult supervision of patients as not all corners of the room could be seen from one point. The contemporary photograph (Figure 3-28) shows that the room was sparsely, but very comfortably furnished in a restrained domestic style with a wide variety of furniture, upholstered seats, woven armchairs, bentwood chairs, occasional tables and numerous potted plants. A grand piano and a large bookcase complete the decorations. Although a domestic appearance has clearly been striven for, there are some features that betray the room as institutional, the carpets, an expensive and difficult to clean item, are small for the size of the room leaving a large expanse of exposed floorboards and there are no pictures on the walls of any description. No curtains hang from the windows, allowing more light to enter and reducing the hiding places for dirt. Particularly notable is the wall treatment which incorporates panelling and a relatively elaborate egg and dart moulding along the cornice, highly suggestive of a bourgeois domestic interior, which has been incorporated despite the unnecessary expense and the potential to trap dust and dirt. On the first and second floors the sleeping accommodation for patients is divided into five dormitories, two of 12 beds, two of eight beds and one of six beds.[6] The largest dormitories, which stretch from front to back of the house can to some extent be cross-ventilated through the single paired windows. Other dormitories, however, although well supplied with windows, cannot be cross-ventilated. This villa, and all other 'industrial' villas was to have practised an 'open door' system with doors being open during the day and locked at night.

Industrial Homes (Male): Villas 23, 24, 25, 27, 28

Five identical homes for men were built on the higher and more northerly ground of the Bangour estate, each of them with accommodation for 50 patients and the necessary staff. The internal arrangements were 'similar to those

---

[6] The first Scottish Commissioners report of 1859 stated that dormitories should contain no more than 14 beds and no less than 6 (avoiding the models of both barracks and prison) (SLC Report 1859: 236).

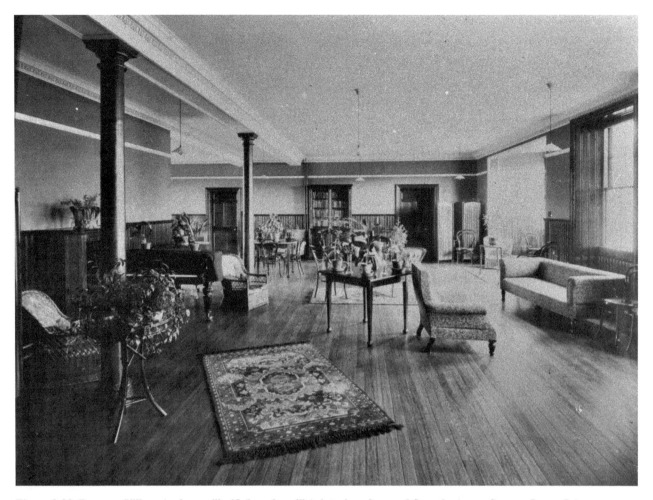

Figure 3-28. Bangour Village Asylum: villa 18 (laundry villa), interior of ground floor dayroom. Source: Image LA LHB44/26/10. Courtesy of Lothian Health Services Archive.

in the women's homes'. These were the first structures to be built on the site and were originally of iron and wood with the walls packed with asbestos and the internal surfaces plastered. However, they were not found to be more economical than stone buildings to construct and maintain, and the experiment was not repeated on the site (Blanc 1908). Two hundred patients and the requisite staff moved in, in June 1904. The newly appointed Medical Superintendent, Irishman John Keay, was among the first to live here. Each of the villas had a verandah erected on the site facing south, about which Keay commented,

'…these verandahs have been most useful. In summer, the female patients practically lived in them during the day, the sewing machines being brought out and work being carried on in them as in a day room. To weakly patients also they are a great boon—those who cannot move about, even the bedridden—are carried out into the verandah and get the benefit of the fresh air and sunshine' (Bangour Village Annual Report 1907).

3.2.6. Medical advisors and superintendents at Bangour and their views on insanity

The two main medical figures associated with Bangour in its early years of operation are Sir John Sibbald, Lunacy

Commissioner from 1870 until 1899 and then advisor to the EDLB until his resignation in April 1904 and John Keay, the first medical superintendent at Bangour, who took over the position in 1903 (EDLB Minutes, 11th January 1904). Sibbald saw the care of the insane as a mark of the progression of civilisation. He felt that a large number of insane patients, 'require little more than kindly care and guidance to induce them to conduct themselves in an orderly and inoffensive manner'. In order to produce this effect, the conditions of an asylum should 'resemble those of a sane community' because the more contented the patients 'the more successfully is their restoration to a really sound state of mind promoted and secured' (Sibbald 1897: 20).

Dr John Keay thought of the patients as being physically weak, 'the insane as a class are weaklings physically as well as mentally' (Bangour Village Annual Report, 1907). He felt that 'unstable, nervous people with morbid heredity and but little self-control' were candidates for drinking to excess and alcohol was a very significant cause of mental breakdown (Bangour Village Annual Report, 1908). But it was not madness itself, but only the tendency which was inherited. People should live 'quiet, unexciting, clean and simple lives. In this way even the "predisposed" person may quite well do his share of the world's work

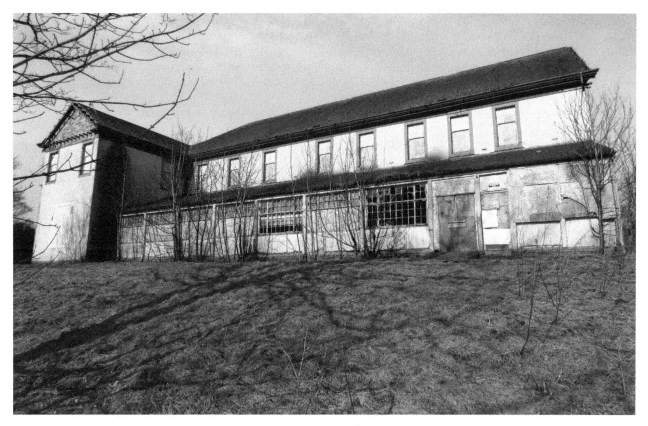

Figure 3-29. Bangour Village Asylum: villa 28 (villas 23, 24, 25 and 27 were identical) Source: Author's photograph.

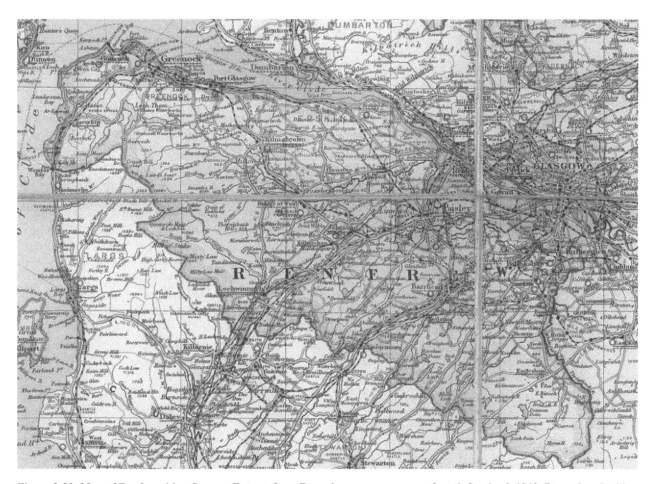

Figure 3-30. Map of Renfrewshire. Source: Extract from Bacon's new survey map of south Scotland, 1910. Reproduced with the permission of the National Library of Scotland.

and pass through life without the semblance of a mental breakdown' (Bangour Village Annual Report, 1908). The causes of madness were seen as largely physical—the two 'moral' or psychological causes often listed in annual reports were 'domestic trouble' and 'worry'. Out of the 212 admissions in 1908, only about 65 were regarded as curable. The urban provenance of many of the patients was seen as an explanation for the large number of 'graver forms of brain disorder and…enfeebled state of bodily health'. The tendency to madness could be acquired by 'foolish, unhygienic living' and those who had acquired it could transmit it to their progeny (Bangour Village Annual Report, 1909). The good health of asylum patients was attributed to the benefit derived from 'the use of the spacious, well-ventilated wards of the hospital and from the more extended use of open air in the treatment of disease in general'. Open-air bed treatment was found to be 'calmative and restorative and of advantage in many directions (Bangour Village Annual Report, 1909).

3.3. Renfrew District Asylum (Dykebar)

3.3.1. Introduction

The county of Renfrewshire extends to the south and west of Glasgow, taking in the south bank of the River Clyde and uplands to the west and south east, the towns of Greenock, Port Glasgow and Paisley where thread-making and shipbuilding industries were located, and rural areas and villages to the south (SLC Report, 1900: 140) (Figure 3-35). A relatively densely populated county, it contained over six per cent of Scotland's population in less than one per cent of its area at the 1911 census (Mort, 1912: 174). Prior to the 1857 Lunacy (Scotland) Act, the poor insane of Renfrew were cared for in the two parochial asylums of Paisley, at Riccartsbar (replaced in 1876) and Craw Road (replaced in 1872) and in Greenock Parochial Asylum (opened 1821 and replaced in 1879). The parochial asylums were administered under the Poor Law and had originally been established as 'lunatic wards' within Poorhouse accommodation (Darragh, 2011:130-131; Farquharson, 2016; SLC Annual Report, 1896:xlix-xlx). Patients accommodated at Craw Road, Paisley were moved to Riccartsbar in 1909, thus combining the two institutions (Figure 3-31) (Farquharson, 2016). Renfrew was also the home of a charitable colony for epileptics which was established in 1903 as part of the Quarrier's Village for Orphans to the west of Bridge of Weir (Figure 3-32).

This pre-existing provision initially made a District Asylum for Renfrew unnecessary in the view of the Lunacy Commissioners, but with rising numbers of insane, by 1900 all the available accommodation was full and the question of additional provision had to be addressed (SLC Annual Report, 1900:xliii). A Renfrew District Lunacy Board was established by order of the Lunacy Commissioners on 26th June 1901 and was to serve all areas of Renfrewshire apart from the parishes of Paisley and Greenock (Figure 3-33). These two parishes continued to provide for their poor insane in the parochial asylums (SLC Annual Report,

100:xlvi; RDLB Minutes, 3rd October, 1901), while all other insane poor in Renfrewshire were to go to the new asylum. Annual Reports for Dykebar show that the majority of patient occupations were industrial/urban rather than rural (Dykebar Annual Reports).

3.3.2. Construction of asylum

Renfrew District Lunacy Board first met on 3rd October 1901. The Board consisted of 14 people, elected by the county council of Renfrew for the most part, and including the former MP for Renfrew, Baron Blythswood and the sitting MP, Sir Charles Renshaw (RDLB Minutes 3rd October, 1901). By 7th August 1902, the Board's offer to purchase Dykebar estate of 539 acres had been accepted and they began to consult the SLC with Dr A Campbell Munro, the County Medical Officer of Health concerning 'alternative types of asylums, their relative advantages and disadvantages and as to their capital cost and expenses of working' (RDLB Minutes, 16th September, 1902). The Board decided against an architectural competition and appointed an applicant who had written to the Board requesting the job, Thomas Graham Abercrombie. Abercrombie was an architect local to Paisley who had designed a hospital block at Paisley Parochial Asylum, and the Royal Alexandra Infirmary at Paisley as well as numerous other public buildings and private residences (RDLB Minutes, 31st October 1902; Dictionary of Scottish Architects). He has been described as the architect to the Paisley thread magnates, and is credited with bringing architectural sophistication to the town, thought to be the 'fruits of his work in America' where he lived as a young man (Bailey et al., 1996:42). In contrast to other Lunacy Boards in this study, the Renfrew District Lunacy Board did not visit England or the continent but took their inspiration solely from asylums within Scotland. A sub-committee visited Murthly Asylum, Perth which had built three villas in its grounds in 1894 in an early attempt at 'colonisation' and Kingseat, Aberdeen, as well as Hartwood, Gartloch, Woodilee and Hawkhead. The Board had completed their visits by the end of December 1902, and decided that the new asylum, for 300 patients, should combine a hospital for senile and acute cases and cases of bodily disease, with the remainder of cases, namely the chronic and convalescent being housed in villas (RDLB Minutes, 23rd December 1902). Administrative sections were to be capable of dealing with a total of 600 patients, in case of expansion. It was originally envisaged to build five villas housing 25 to 32 patients each, three of which would be for patients working in laundry, kitchen or workshops and grounds, and two of which were designated for chronic, noisy or excited patients no longer needing hospital care. A house in the farm buildings would accommodate 30 males and four females and a poultry farm would have accommodation for eight females (RDLB Minutes, 19th January 1903). While the plans of the new asylum were in preparation, advice was sought from Dr L R Oswald, Medical Superintendent of Glasgow Royal Asylum, Gartnavel, who suggested some modifications and was subsequently appointed expert adviser to the Board in the

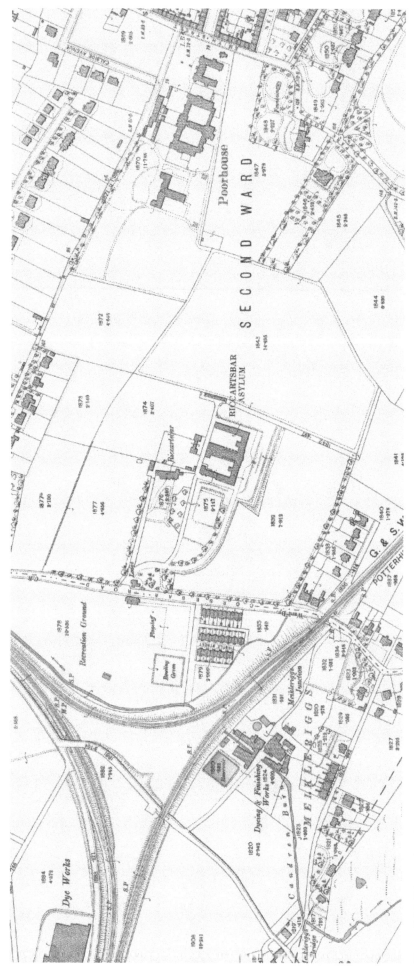

Figure 3-31. Riccartsbar Asylum, Paisley (also showing position of Poorhouse). Source: Ordnance Survey 25 inch to one mile, surveyed 1897. Reproduced with the permission of the National Library of Scotland.

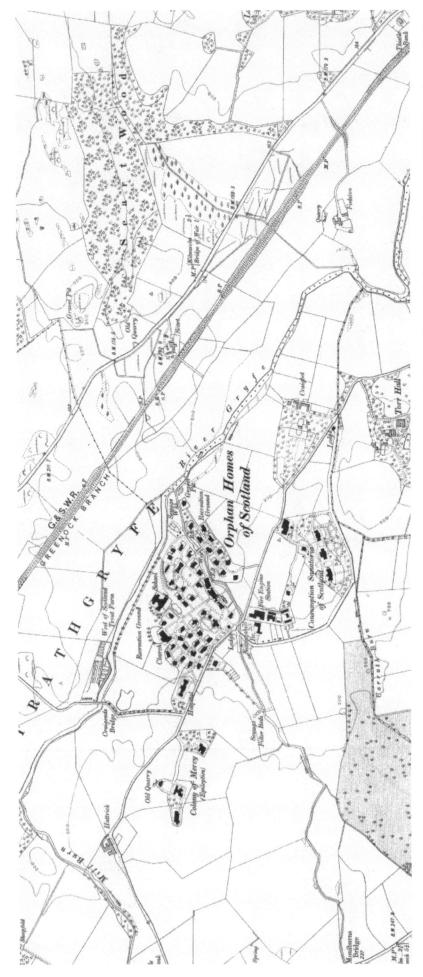

Figure 3-32. Quarrier's Village (Orphan Homes of Scotland) showing small epileptic colony to the west. Source: Ordnance Survey 6 inch to one mile, surveyed 1916. Reproduced with the permission of the National Library of Scotland.

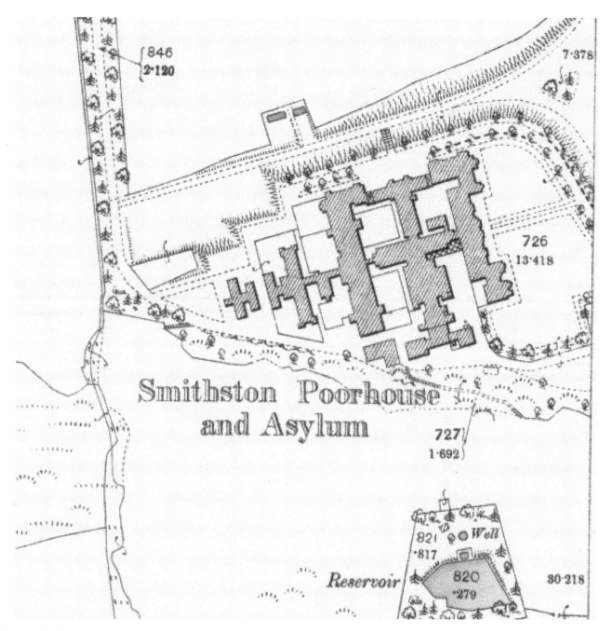

Figure 3-33. Greenock Parochial Asylum and Poorhouse (known as Smithston). Source: Ordnance Survey 25 inch to one mile, surveyed 1897. Reproduced with the permission of the National Library of Scotland.

construction, equipment and working of the new asylum (RDLB Minutes, 5th May 1903). By the time plans were submitted to the Board by Abercrombie, the asylum accommodation was to consist of a hospital of 140 beds which should have large wards, 'as the larger number of beds in each ward makes for economy in administration' (RDLB Minutes, 19th June 1903). The board wanted a large hospital because they thought that,

'The modern idea regarding treatment of the insane appears to be that patients should be treated in hospital in the first instance, with the view of curing the disease in its initial stage, and for this purpose it is necessary to have hospital accommodation for at least one third of patients'.

An infectious diseases block was also to be built, housing eight of each sex and made of wood and iron so it could be burned down in 20 years as 'most of these places ... become saturated with germs'. Dr Oswald requested that a relief map be made of the site, so that the committee would be able to see the situation of the buildings without visiting the site (RDLB Minutes, 19th June 1903). Although the Board had originally thought to build the asylum from brick and tile, it was subsequently decided, for reasons that are not recorded, to build with 'stone from Locharbriggs quarry, or some equally good red sandstone' and to use 'good green slates' rather than tiles. This increased the cost of the asylum by eight to ten per cent for mason work alone (RDLB Minutes, 8th June 1903).

The Lunacy Commissioners suggested some modifications to the plans in August 1903, which appear to have included a recommendation to make the buildings of 'as simple and inexpensive a character as possible' (SLC Report, 1904: liv). By 4th August 1904, the Lunacy Commissioners had approved plans for the new asylum (RDLB Minutes, 17th February 1904). These plans altered slightly as the months proceeded. By early 1905, the RDLB had decided to build: a central hospital for 48 patients, a reception block for ten patients of each sex, two villas for 47 patients each, male and female, needing special supervision, one male villa for 47 quiet patients and one female villa for 40 laundry workers (RDLB Minutes, 27th February 1905) (Figure 3-34). Also to be built were a laundry, power house, workshops, administration block, kitchen and stores for 500 patients, medical superintendent's house, a lodge and houses for married attendants. A request was made to the architect by the RDLB that the original style of the reception block be altered to make it more simple, and contractors were appointed to excavate and build up to damp course level in October 1904, the work commencing in December of the same year (RDLB Minutes, 3rd October 1904). In September 1905, the RDLB appointed contractors to construct the asylum buildings from damp proof course upwards (RDLB Minutes 5th September, 1905). Finishing materials were much discussed during 1906, and it was decided that maple rather than cheaper softwood should be used for flooring all the buildings, but

that yellow pine could be used for finishing and panelling (RDLB Minutes, 19th March 1906; 27th April 1906). A long-running discussion about slates concluded with the decision that grey Burlington slates (less costly than the green Elterwater slates originally chosen) should be used. In coming to their decision the RDLB inspected nearby school buildings 'with a view to comparing the effect of the different slates' (RDLB Minutes, 4th May 1906).

On 5th July 1906, the RDLB appointed Dr Robert Dunmore Hotchkis, formerly a Senior Assistant at the Glasgow Royal Asylum, as Medical Superintendent for the new asylum, with the view of benefitting from his advice during the construction of the asylum, which by this time, was well under way, two villas having been almost completed (RDLB Minutes, 5th July 1906). Hotchkis was required to 'consult with the Architect and Engineer and give his advice in connection with the plans, erection, and furnishings of the buildings [and] to visit the buildings regularly from time to time during their construction' (RDLB Minutes, 5th July 1906). Hotchkis received his medical training at Glasgow and Durham Universities (*St Andrews Citizen*, 20th April, 1946).

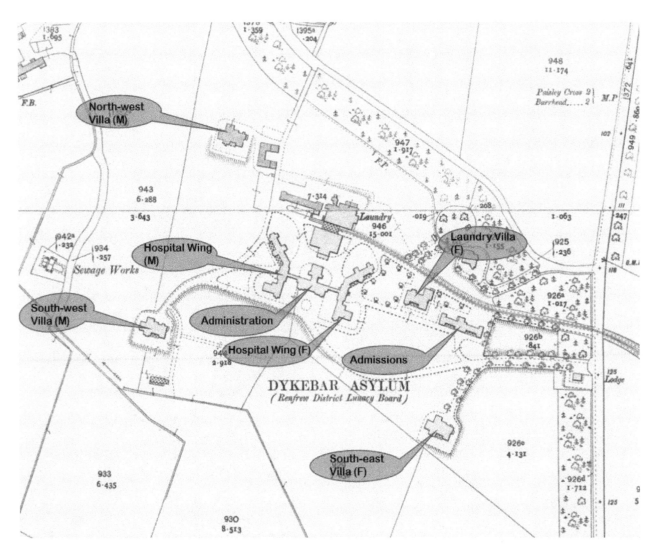

Figure 3-34. Dykebar Asylum showing main accommodation. Source: Ordnance Survey 25 inch to one mile, surveyed 1913. Reproduced with the permission of the National Library of Scotland.

As the buildings were fitted out, some cost-saving measures were instituted including dispensing with a padded room, and substituting cheaper finishing materials in some instances, for instance cement dados were substituted for tiles on the villa staircases (RDLB Minutes, 30th July 1906). However, the RDLB did not agree to substitute less expensive granolithic for terrazzo on the floors of bathrooms, lavatories and WCs. The asylum was to be lit, indoors and out, by electric light and fitted with electric fire alarms and telephones connected by underground cables. Gas was to be used for cooking and laundry purposes (RDLB Minutes, 21st January 1907; 18th February 1907).

On 22nd April 1907, a ceremony was held to mark the construction of the asylum with a memorial stone on the administration building with a glass jar deposited within containing 'certain particulars regarding the Board and the District and also copies of local newspapers, and certain other documents' (RDLB Minutes, 17th April 1907). By 31st May 1907, the RDLB had agreed in consultation with the SLC that they would increase the size of the hospital by 44 beds, making a total of 90, by building two further wings to the rear. At the SLC's recommendation these were to be fitted with 'suitable verandahs…for the out-door treatment of patients' (RDLB Minutes, 31st May 1907). The asylum perimeter was enclosed with iron fences and an entrance lodge and gatescreen were constructed (RDLB Minutes, 31st May 1907). Villas had central heating (by the Reck circulatory system, hot water circulating through radiators) and bathtubs specially made by the suppliers, Shanks & Co (RDLB Minutes, 29th November 1907; 14th February, 1908).

Dr Hotchkis undertook visits to Kingseat and to Bangour Village in order to ascertain 'the best way of proceeding to make arrangements for the furnishing of the Asylum' and he was empowered by the Board to make up a list of the necessary furniture (RDLB Minutes, 14th February 1908; 16th March 1908). The Furnishing Committee went to Bangour Village to inspect the furnishing there, a specification was drawn up and contractors from Paisley were appointed to fulfil it (RDLB Minutes, 17th April 1908; 10thAugust 1908). German silver (a copper/zinc/nickel alloy) dinner boxes for carrying food by waggon from the kitchen to detached buildings were to be made by an ironmongers in Edinburgh who had also supplied these items to Bangour (RDLB Minutes, 30th November 1908). The asylum crockery was to be stamped with the monogram R.D.A. (RDLB Minutes, 7th December 1908).

Dr Hotchkis estimated the staffing needs at the villas to be up to 25 by day and nine by night, with quieter patients requiring less supervision. He felt that staff should be 'of the best sort', as in the villa system 'more responsibility rests with them' and requested that attendants should be 'strictly sober, trustworthy and of a kindly disposition' (GGCA AC18/3/1 Dykebar Letter Book, 3rd June 1909; 13th August 1909). Female nurses were to be employed in the hospital, even in the male wings (RDLB Minutes, 28th December 1908). A hot-house, with forcing pits and

potting sheds and garden were to be built (RDLB Minutes, 28th December 1908). On 24th March, 1909, the asylum was inspected by the SLC and approved and adopted as a District Asylum (RDLB Minutes, 25th March 1909). On 3rd April, the asylum was opened for the inspection of ratepayers, and on 8th April, it was legally opened for the reception of patients, admitting 120 patients between 10th April and 21st May, having a capacity of 296 in total (RDLB Minutes, 24th May 1909; Dykebar Annual Report 1910, 1912). The buildings were fully completed in September of the same year (Dykebar Annual Report 1910).

In 1914 two further villas and a nurses' home were added to the site, but these do not form part of this survey. From 1916-1919 the hospital was taken over by the military authorities as a hospital for acute mental cases and the inmates were sent to other institutions (*Daily Record*, 8th December 1915). The hospital has since continued in use as a psychiatric facility, with large additions made to the site in the second half of the twentieth century (Darragh 2010:139). Of the original buildings on the site, two of the villas are derelict and in poor condition, as is the medical superintendent's house. The hospital/administration building, reception house, recreation hall, service buildings and workshops, the lodge and two of the hospital villas remain in use and although they have been subject to alteration some original features and layouts remain internally.

3.3.3. Site layout and structures

Relative to the other sites in this study, the buildings at Dykebar are of visibly higher quality, being constructed of ashlar sandstone in a relatively ostentatious Edwardian Baroque style. On first inspection, the SLC reported that the asylum was of the 'segregate or village type' and favourably reported on the design and internal fittings and furnishings. They noted the liberal provision of sofas and easy chairs, which afforded 'comfortable seats for the aged and infirm, and will conduce to good conduct and contentment of the other inmates'. They noted that the walls were bare of pictures, but that these would soon be supplied and approved of the fact that a piano had been provided in two of the 'female sections'. They recommended supplying bagatelle tables in the male villas, because this would 'do much to break the monotony of asylum life' (SLC Annual Report, 1910: 135). Of the 224 patients admitted in the first six months, about half of the men were engaged daily in outdoor labour. Most of the asylum acreage was leased out, but the Commissioners were anxious to point out that 'the amount of land considered sufficient for asylum purposes is an acre per male inmate' and approved of the acquisition of a neighbouring farm to provide for the 'beneficial and remunerative employment of the patients'. The asylum farm, once established, was seen as a means of supplying produce and an outlet for patient labour, but also as a means of creating interest and community: 'the fact that the surrounding land is our own, and farmed by our own people, rounds off in a way unfelt before, the life of the Asylum community' (Dykebar Annual Report 1915).

Nineteen attendants and nurses were on duty by day and six by night, giving a ratio of one to 15 by day and one to 48 by night, which the commissioners considered adequate (SLC Annual Report 1910: 135). The buildings were ventilated, both naturally by open windows and by the use of electric fans in hospital wards and villas (SLC Annual Report 1910: 135). Instructions for nurses and attendants noted that Staff are to,

> '...give constant attention to the ventilation of their wards, day-rooms, dormitories, closets, staircases etc and to see that the air is kept free from pollution and as nearly as possible at a temperature of 58 degrees [14 degrees Celsius]. The windows are always to be kept open when the state of the weather makes it practicable to do so' (NRS MC14/4 General Rules and Instructions for Nurses and Attendants, Dykebar, 1912).

The medical superintendent attributed the low rate of TB in the asylum to the 'healthy surroundings and open-air treatment' and also thought that the health of the staff was improved by the absence of corridors (Dykebar Annual Report, 1910).

On admission patients were kept under observation for a few days and then distributed to the different villas, according to their condition (Dykebar Annual Report, 1910). Subsequently, the treatment consisted of outside work for able male patients, while women worked in the kitchen, laundry and at needlework, and rest in bed in the open air for those who were unable (Dykebar Annual Report, 1910). In later years, some female patients were allowed to roll the tennis court, presumably because this was thought to be therapeutic exercise, but outdoor exercise for women was an exception rather than the rule (Dykebar Annual Report, 1915). The Lunacy Commissioners commended the asylum because it did not make use of restraint or seclusion. It was noted that the 'care and surroundings' at Dykebar were of 'such a nature as to promote their physical and mental wellbeing'. (Dykebar Annual Report, 1912). The medical superintendent asserted that the 'great majority' of cases of insanity had a physical cause, including stages of life such as adolescence and menopause and that the causes of insanity were 'intimately connected with the bodily functions' (Dykebar Annual Report 1910, 1911). However, for a large number of patients, no cause could be established, despite the careful questioning of relatives and friends (Dykebar Annual Reports, 1910-1915).

Administration block

The administration block was a three storey building with offices for medical staff, matron and clerk, board room, three mess-rooms, one for officials, one for nurses and one for attendants (Figures 3-35, 3-36). On the first floor were living rooms for official staff, a surgery, lecture-room and other rooms for scientific purposes (pathological research and photography) and on the second floor, accommodation for nurses and attendants (SLC Annual Report 1910: 135).

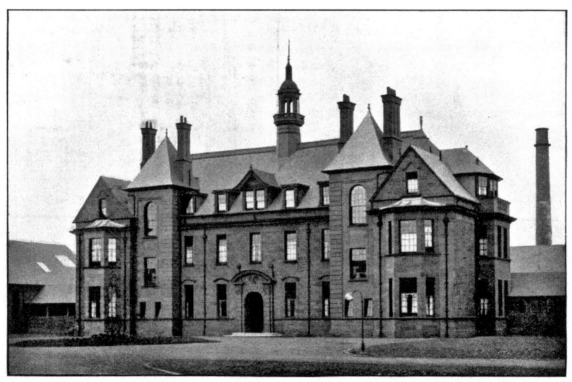

ADMINISTRATIVE BLOCK.

Figure 3-35. Dykebar Asylum: administration block, also containing staff accommodation. Source: AC18/1/1 Dykebar Annual Report, 1910. Copyright NHS Greater Glasgow and Clyde Archives.

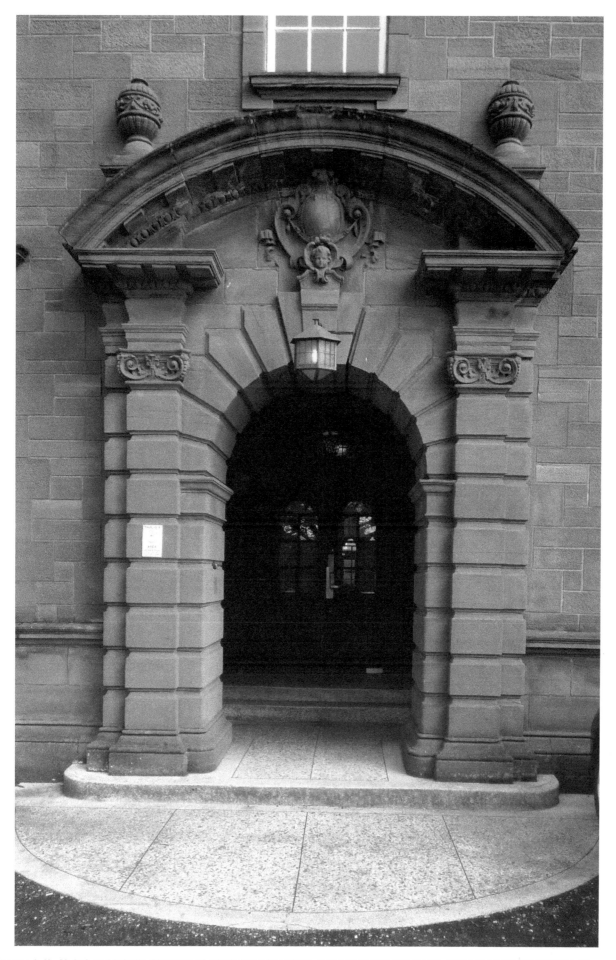

Figure 3-36. Dykebar Asylum: doorway of administration block showing stonework detail. Source: Author's photograph.

Hospital wings

The hospital wings were single storey and connected to the administration block by short, wide fire-proof corridors which were used as visiting rooms (Figures 3-37, 3-38). Each side consisted of two wings, one for sick and infirm cases and the other, to the rear, for acute cases, with a verandah for out-door treatment. The SLC pronounced the hospital wards 'well designed and well lighted … excellently equipped' (SLC Annual Report 1910: 135).

Engine house, laundry, workshops and mortuary.

The workshops were sited near the railway for easier delivery of goods. The mortuary was small in size as the pathological work was carried on elsewhere. It was positioned so that deceased patients could be collected from it for interment in the local cemetery at Hawkhead, by means of a rear entrance and without passing the main buildings of the asylum (GGCA AC18/3/1 Dykebar Letter Book, 15th July 1909). This was probably in order to avoid exciting morbid thoughts in the patients.

Four villas

The villas were three storey buildings, two for men and two for women, accommodating 45 patients in each. Three were on an identical plan (Figure 3-39), the fourth, the laundry villa, being a larger variation (Figures 3-40, 3-41). Described by the SLC as 'plain but pleasing externally and substantially built. It was abundantly evident that every detail as to internal construction had received careful and enlightened consideration on the part of the District Board and of their Architect' (SLC Annual Report 1910: 135). Each villa had a verandah which was used for open-air treatment of those confined to bed (RDLB Minutes, 31st May 1907). Meals were taken in the villas, rather than in a central dining room and this was felt to be one of the advantages of the villa system, in that different categories of patients were not brought together for dining (Dykebar Annual Report, 1910).

- North-west Villa – Male, open villa for convalescent, working patients
- South-west Villa – Male, closed villa for patients requiring continuous observation
- South-east Villa – Female, closed villa for patients requiring continuous observation.
- Laundry Villa – Female, open villa for patients working in the laundry and also providing accommodation for kitchen and laundry maids

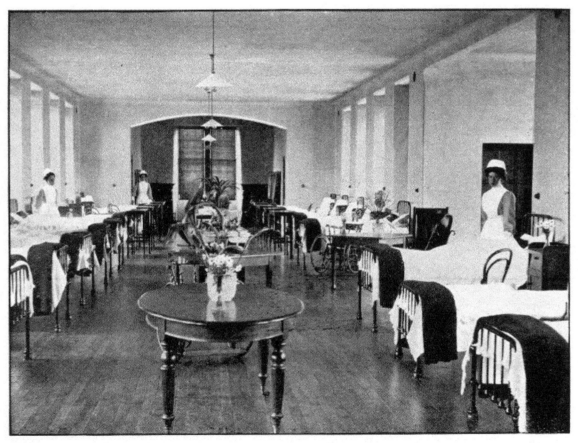

FEMALE ACUTE HOSPITAL.

Figure 3-37. Dykebar Asylum: interior of acute ward, hospital wing (female) Source: AC18/1/1 Dykebar Annual Report, 1910. Copyright NHS Greater Glasgow and Clyde Archives.

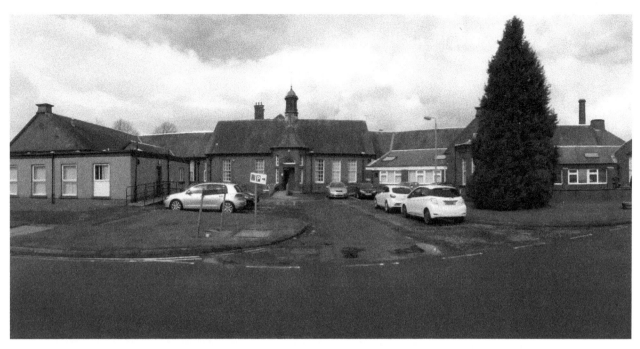

Figure 3-38. Dykebar Asylum: exterior of hospital wing (female - former verandahs now filled in). Source: Author's photograph.

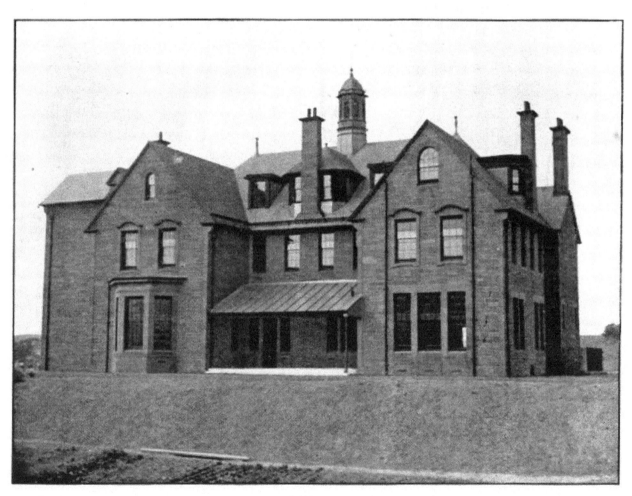

VILLA.

Figure 3-39. Dykebar Asylum: villa. Source: AC18/1/1 Dykebar Annual Report, 1910. Copyright NHS Greater Glasgow and Clyde Archives.

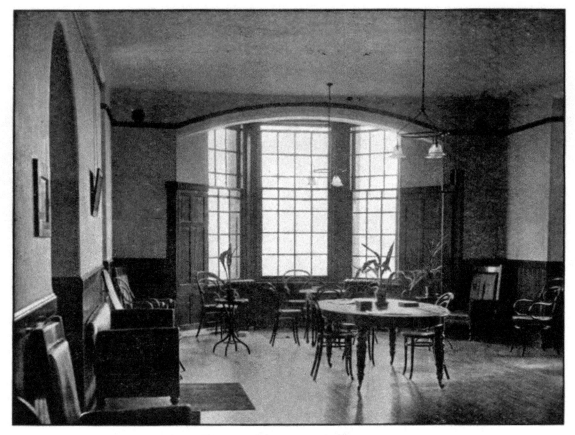

PART OF INTERIOR OF VILLA.

Figure 3-40. Dykebar Asylum: villa interior (unidentified, possibly laundry villa). Source: AC18/1/1 Dykebar Annual Report, 1910. Copyright NHS Greater Glasgow and Clyde Archives.

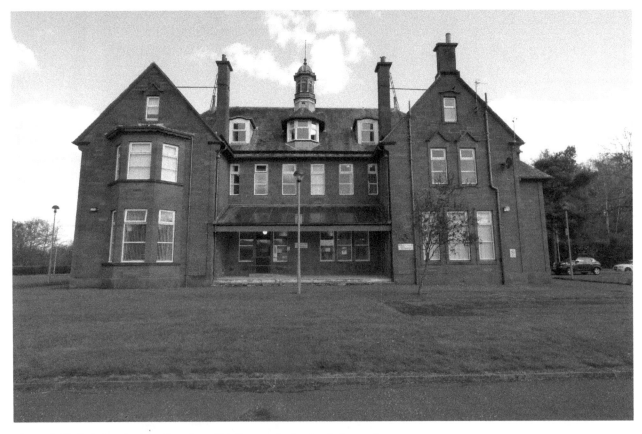

Figure 3-41. Dykebar Asylum (laundry villa) Source: Author's photograph.

4

Study Sites: Ireland, England and Germany

This chapter continues the site biographies and building descriptions of the previous chapter with portraits of the villa colony at Purdysburn, near Belfast; the pavilion asylum at Whalley in Lancashire, where the construction of a colony asylum was considered, but ultimately rejected and of Alt Scherbitz in Germany which provided the inspiration for the majority of village and colony asylums in this study.

4.1. Belfast District Lunatic Asylum (Purdysburn)

4.1.1. Introduction

The first asylum to be built in Belfast was located on the outskirts of the city at Grosvenor Road and was constructed under the terms of the Lunacy (Ireland) Act 1821 (Figure 4-1). Completed in 1829, it was on a radial K-plan, identical to several other asylums around the country, and designed by Francis Johnston, architect to the Board of Works (Figures 2-40, 2-41, 4-2) (Dictionary of Irish Architects). The asylum was described as 'concealed from view from the road by towering walls and a high gateway', access only being obtained by 'giving the proper password to the gate attendant' (*Belfast Newsletter*, 16th October 1896). It was of a design that was later considered 'prison-like', accommodation consisting of numerous small cells, and the windows being small and 'heavily barred' (Belfast Corporation, 1929; BDLA Annual Report 1898, 1903). Initially for 100 patients, additions were made in the 1830s, 1850s, 1870s and 1890s as numbers grew (Dictionary

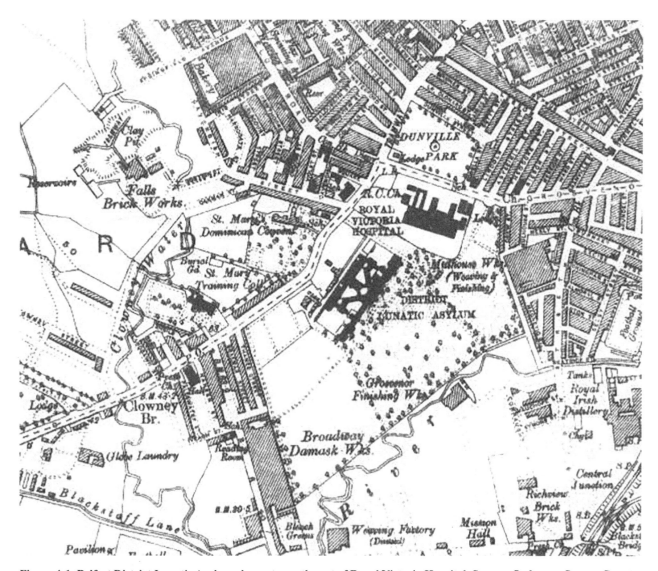

Figure 4-1. Belfast District Lunatic Asylum shown to south-east of Royal Victoria Hospital. Source: Ordnance Survey County Series 25 inch to one mile surveyed c1900.

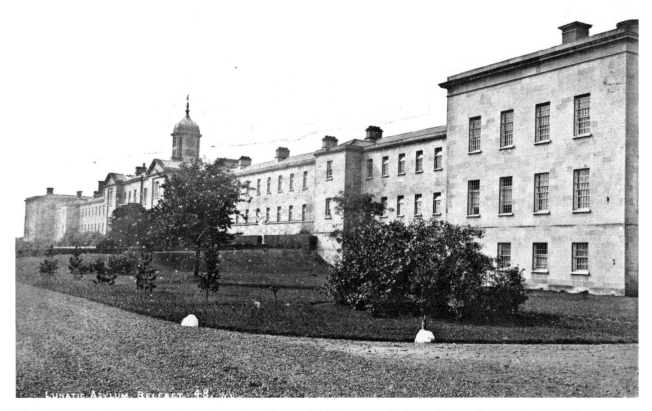

Figure 4-2. Belfast District Lunatic Asylum, c1900. Source: NLI Lawrence photograph collection L_CAB_00048. Image reproduced courtesy of the National Library of Ireland.

of Irish Architects). Although County Down became a separate lunacy district in 1868, and County Antrim followed suit in 1897 (pursuant to the Belfast District Lunatic Asylums Act, 1892) each county building their own asylums, Belfast Asylum continued to be seriously overcrowded (*Belfast Telegraph*, 23rd February 1909; Belfast Corporation, 1929). With the asylum housing 628 patients in 1893, the decision was taken to relocate, both because the old accommodation was overcrowded and unsuitable and because a larger site would give greater potential for future expansion (Dictionary of Irish Architects; Delargey 2002:217-218; *Belfast Newsletter* 11th September 1894; ILC Report 1897:18). A site of 295 acres became available at Purdysburn and was purchased in 1895, although the price, £29,500, was felt in some quarters to be very high. Part of the land, 65 acres, was used to build an Infectious Diseases hospital (opened 1906 with 145 beds), to the great consternation of the asylum authorities, because of the removal of land that should have been for the 'employment and recreation' of the insane and because the hospital was thought to pose a health risk to the asylum patients (*Weekly Irish Times* 13th January 1912; BDLA Annual Report 1900). The Medical Superintendent, William Graham, felt that even the sight of it might arouse 'morbid feelings' in his patients and retard their mental recovery (BDLA Annual Report 1900). However, £6,000 was recouped by the asylum authorities as a result (*Belfast Telegraph* 23rd February 1909).

The existing mansion house on the Purdysburn site was initially used as an auxiliary asylum to deal with the overflow from Grosvenor Road. Adaptations so that the asylum would house 160 patients cost £10,000 (*Belfast Newsletter* 15th January 1895; *Belfast Telegraph* 23rd February 1909). However, the ultimate aim was to build a new asylum in the grounds of Purdysburn which would replace the old asylum at Grosvenor Road (BDLA Minutes July 1895). Dr William Graham was appointed the Medical Superintendent of Belfast Asylum in 1897 (*Belfast Newsletter*, 21st August 1897). Formerly the Medical Superintendent of Armagh Asylum, Graham had obtained his medical degree at Queen's College, Belfast, followed by surgical training in Edinburgh and further specialised training in London and Europe (*JMS*, 1918:(64) 114-4). A competition to design a new asylum was instigated and in 1897 the plans of Jackson & Tilley were selected, Anthony Thomas Jackson having worked for the BDLA on extensions to the asylum at Grosvenor Road and on modifications to the mansion at Purdysburn (Dictionary of Irish Architects; ILC Report 1897: 18). The design consisted of two buildings, a main asylum for 550 patients of the recent, acute, epileptic and chronic classes and a separate hospital for 256 recent, acute, sick and infirm cases, the buildings being partly single storey, partly two storey, with three storey blocks for chronic patients (BDLA Annual Report, 1899). Experimental excavations took place on the site in 1898, but construction of the new asylum was postponed because the Local Government (Ireland) Act was about to come into force, transferring responsibility for asylums to local authorities. Similar legislation had been passed in England, Wales and Scotland by Acts of 1888 and 1889.

Meanwhile, William Graham had been stressing the value of the Purdysburn site as a refuge from noise and excitement and a means of providing 'plenty of fresh air, exercise and salubrious surroundings' and a greater degree of freedom for patients (BDLA Annual Report 1898). It was believed at this period that 'city life, with its high pressure and frequently unhealthy surroundings' was productive of more mental disease than 'rural life with its fresh air and agreeable conditions of existence' (*Belfast Health Journal*, May 1901). Graham was of the opinion that the site would be ideal for an epileptic colony, as had been established in England, the continent and the US (BDLA Annual Report 1898). Graham believed the colony plan to be more suitable for this category than an asylum or hospital because the needs of epileptics included mental improvement, industrial education and physical development as well as medical treatment (BDLA Annual Report 1898). Graham cited epileptic colonies at Chalfont St Peter (opened 1894 as a series of wooden huts but which eventually comprised five dwellings, each housing 25 epileptics and a central administrative building) and epileptic colonies in Massachusetts, Maryland, Ohio, California and New York in which the epileptics were 'happily employed in useful pursuits' (BDLA Annual Report 1898). In suggesting a colony for epileptics, Graham was here echoing the orthodoxy of the day which held that a colony was suitable only for quiet, harmless cases and was inappropriate for the majority of the insane. In 1899, Jackson & Tilley's asylum plans were sent to G T Hine, consulting architect to the English Lunacy Commissioners for his comments. Hine had consulted with William Graham about the design, and suggested the erection of one or two small villas on each side (i.e. male and female 'sides' of the asylum) for convalescents 'without going to the extreme adopted in the villa system', giving as 'extreme' examples, Alt Scherbitz, some American asylums and Bangour village (BDLA Annual Report, 1899). Hine's designs for London County Council at this period, usually included a number of villas in addition to the main asylum. However, in 1901, William Graham changed his position entirely on the form of the new asylum and suggested jettisoning the existing plans by Jackson & Tilley, whether or not they were modified according to Hine's recommendations, and adopting the 'villa colony' that had been seen by Hine as 'extreme' (BDLA Minutes 1901:116-7). He appears to have been inspired by the LAB's report on continental asylums which was published in 1900 and is the only published source in English before 1901 to use the term 'villa colony' when discussing the German model of colony asylum (Report of a Lancashire deputation, 1900). Although William Graham does not specifically mention Alt Scherbitz in the annual reports and minutes, perhaps because of Hine's characterisation of it as 'extreme', it is clear from a local publication '*Belfast Health Journal*' that Alt Scherbitz was

the model that was followed at Purdysburn. The *Belfast Health Journal* carries a drawing based on a plate from the LAB report depicting an Alt Scherbitz villa, and gives a brief description of Alt Scherbitz, stating that this is the system being adopted at Edinburgh and Aberdeen and the system that has been proposed by William Graham (*Belfast Health Journal*, May 1901). On 11th February 1901, the BDLA committee decided to adopt the 'villa colony' system for the new asylum, dropping the earlier plans by Jackson & Tilley.[1] Graham lauded the decision of the committee calling the villa colony, 'the fruit of the highest scientific study in the care of the insane, [which] springs from the two dominant principles of our time— exact and accurate knowledge , and a love of humanity' (BDLA Annual Report, 1911). For Graham, the villa colony represented the height of 'hygienic efficiency' and an elevation of the living conditions of the poor insane and he concluded that it was 'impossible to exaggerate the significance of this work as an historical contribution to asylum care and management' (BDLA Annual Report, 1911, 1913). He praised the layout on economic grounds, claiming that the accommodation would be simpler and internal arrangements less detailed, but it is clear that when Graham highlighted cost-saving measures, he was partly playing to his audience, as in a paper in the *Journal of Mental Science*, Graham makes clear his contempt for the 'parsimonious and pettifogging spirit' that led public authorities to recommend cheaper accommodation for the insane (Graham, 1901: 688). He also praised the villa colony in terms of treatment, saying that it allowed for more complete classification of patients, so that noisy patients would not be an annoyance to quiet ones and it would promote more individual treatment of patients by staff, because of the more home-like conditions. He concludes, 'It is almost impossible to calculate the beneficent influence that would be exercised on a patient by association with an attendant, himself mentally sound and skilful in his care and attention' (BDLA Annual Report, 1900). Once the patients had been moved in he expressed his delight at the transformation they had experienced in their surroundings, 'No longer with vision confined in narrow limits, they can enjoy the ever-shifting scenery of earth and sky; they can breathe the fresh upland air— in a word, they can experience the healing influences of Nature, the great Mother of us all' (BDLA annual Report, 1913). Nature had qualities of reality, simplicity, purity, regularity, order, power and vitality which dissipated the wandering confusions of the abnormal mind (BDLA Annual Report, 1913).

A layout for the new asylum along villa colony lines was produced by the City Surveyor, showing suggested villa sites and accommodation for 1,000 patients in 20 detached two-storey buildings. The layout shown at Figure 4-3 is possibly the design that was produced at

---

[1] A 2015 publication (Carpenter et al., 2015:213), makes several errors in relation to the early history of the construction of Purdysburn, principally as regards the nature of the asylum, the architects (not ultimately Jackson & Tilley, as stated), and the role of G T Hine as advisor and architect, which was more significant than the authors suggest.

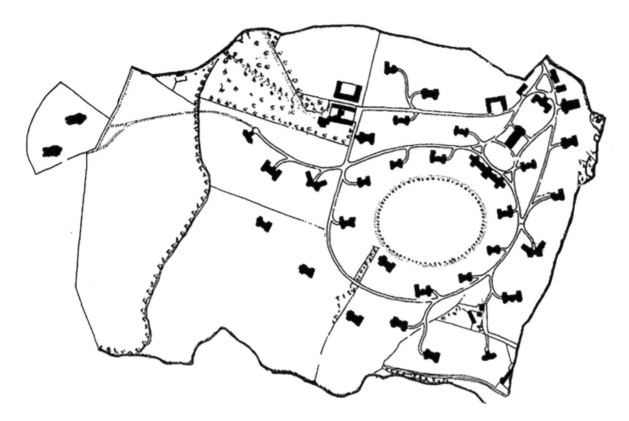

Figure 4-3. Layout design for Purdysburn. Date of design unknown, but produced prior to 1902 and the start of building work, as the orientations and positions of villas are not as actually constructed. Source: Reuber, M (1996) The architecture of psychological management: the Irish asylums (1801-1922) *Psychological Medicine*, Vol 26, pp1179-1189. Reproduced with the permission of Cambridge University Press and Professor Markus Reuber.

this stage. Applications for the position of architect were submitted by various firms and Graeme Watt & Tulloch were selected by ballot and given instructions to provide drawings for two villa buildings to accommodate 50 patients each. Graeme Watt & Tulloch was a partnership of Robert Graeme Watt and Frederick Henry Tulloch whose previous work had consisted mainly of commercial buildings in Belfast (Dictionary of Irish Architects). Frederick Tulloch appears to have been the partner who was responsible for the designs at Purdysburn. The villa was to exhibit 'architectural character without undue extravagance' and designs were to be produced by the architect in consultation with the Medical Superintendent (BDLA Minutes 1901). Following this decision, further land was purchased contiguous to the Purdysburn estate which included a farmhouse, at a cost of £7,250 (*Belfast Telegraph* 23rd February 1909). The farmhouse was made ready for the reception of 30 patients and was known as villa 1 (Figure 4-5).

The architect, Frederick Tulloch, decided to visit asylums on the continent before producing plans. Once the plans were submitted, a dispute arose within the committee about where to position the WCs within the villas. The Chairman wanted the WCs to be placed in a separate sanitary annexe as was then the norm in asylum and hospital wards. However, William Graham objected strongly to this, citing 'increased expenditure, asymmetry and disfiguration of the buildings and inconvenience

for administrative purposes'. He thought that a separate annexe would destroy the homelike character of the buildings and that proper supervision of the patients would be impossible (BDLA Minutes 1901: 332). The argument was temporarily won by Graham, but ultimately the majority of the villas were built with a semi-detached sanitary annexe. The new buildings at Purdysburn were thought to be the first villas of their kind in the United Kingdom and therefore comparison with other sites was not possible (BDLA Minutes 1901:332). Building of the two villas (villas 2 and 3 in 4-4) commenced in 1902.

In late 1903, the committee decided to visit, with the architect, Aberdeen asylum at Kingseat, which was nearing completion and Crichton Institution Dumfries whose 'Third House' was also built along villa colony lines. Villas 2 and 3 were completed and occupied in late 1903 (BDLA Minutes 1903: 209). In 1904 plans were supplied by the architects for two new villas with separate sanitary annexes, and a south facing verandah. These plans were objected to by Graham on the basis that the proposed villa was smaller in size that villas 2 and 3 and the layout did not lend itself to supervision. The placement of furniture and fireplaces was also problematic. The closets were so far from the dayroom that an attendant would need to accompany the patients, the visiting room was in the body of the house and had to be accessed through the main hall and attendant's rooms on the first floor were placed so that no supervision could be exercised over the dormitories.

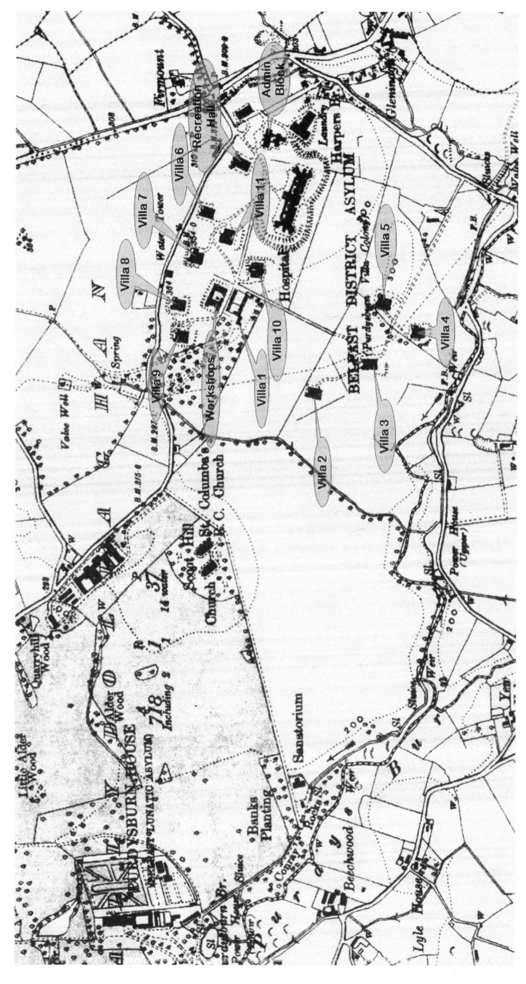

Figure 4-4. Purdysburn House and Purdysburn Villa Colony. Source: Ordnance Survey County Series 6 inches to one mile, surveyed 1920–21. Labels added by author.

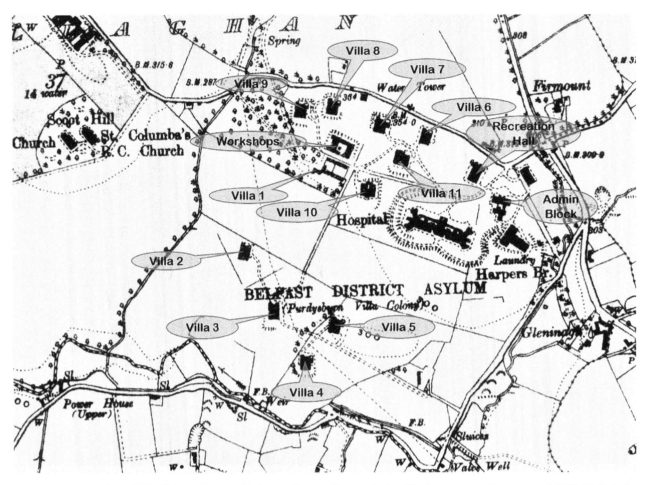

Figure 4-5. Purdysburn Villa Colony. Source: Ordnance Survey County Series 6 inches to one mile, surveyed 1920-21. Labels added by author.

Due to these and other objections it was decided to erect duplicates of villas 2 and 3, despite the fact that variety in the structure of the villas had been thought desirable, but ultimately these two new villas were built with sanitary annexes (BDLA Minutes 1904: 249).

Two more small farms were purchased in the ensuing months, at a cost of £1,880, bringing the asylum estate to a total of 379 acres, and villas 4 and 5 were constructed on one of these (BDLA Minutes 1904: 356-381; *Belfast Telegraph* 23rd February 1909), construction being completed in 1906 (BDLA Minutes 1906: 127). The purchase of additional land for the asylum was resisted by some councillors who argued that city patients were 'untrained to agricultural pursuits' but it was generally agreed that 'open-air exercise and labour were the best curative powers in connection with sanity' and so the purchase ultimately passed (*Belfast Newsletter* 14th January 1902). The total cost for five villas, four of which were newly built, was £20,122 (*Belfast Telegraph* 23rd February 1909). In 1906 it was decided to consult with G T Hine on a complete villa colony scheme (despite his earlier reservations about such a plan), with Hine preparing preliminary plans and handing these over to the local architects Graeme Watt & Tulloch to prepare working designs, Hine to advise on all points of detail and construction and on all engineering matters. G T Hine visited Purdysburn and went over the

site with William Graham the same year (BDLA Minutes 1906: 142). Hine then produced an overall layout for the remaining buildings and scale plans of each floor showing positions of fittings and windows. Frederick Tulloch and Hine were to split the architects' fees between them, with Hine receiving extra fees for visits to Ireland (BDLA Minutes 1906: 190-199). In early 1907, it was decided to erect four further villas and administrative buildings. Preliminary plans of the administrative buildings were drawn up by Hine and approved after revision by William Graham (BDLA Minutes 1908: 302). Hine's plans of the churches and recreation hall were approved and Graeme Watt & Tulloch began to prepare working drawings (BDLA Minutes 1907: 286-293).

In 1908 approval was sought for a loan to build an admin block, recreation hall, protestant and catholic churches, a hospital, laundry and boiler house, mortuary, farm buildings, stores, workshops and four villas, an acute villa, an observation villa and two repeats of the previous villas at an estimated cost of £83,000. The administrative buildings were to cater for an ultimate total of 1,300 patients (BDLA Minutes 1909: 30). The laundry and workshop sites were fixed so as to effectively separate the sexes (BDLA Minutes 1908: 342). Some levelling of the land was needed for the sites of hospital and recreation hall and it was proposed to have this carried out by staff and patients (BDLA Minutes

1908: 350). Graham suggested that the utilitarian nature of levelling the hospital site was of great therapeutic benefit to the patients, giving the workers 'a sense of achievement and a certain interest, and even enthusiasm, seems to drive out false notions and feelings by filling life with a positive and healthy content' (BDLA Annual Report 1908). Graham saw digging in the soil, the 'permanent source of recreative energy', as the best type of work for all mental illnesses because contact with 'mother earth … gives steadiness, poise, balance' (BDLA Annual Report 1908). Hine visited the site again, with the committee, and satisfaction was expressed with the buildings already constructed (BDLA Minutes 1908: 350-352). Construction work began in 1909 and an inquiry was held in Belfast City Hall in which witnesses were questioned about whether the amount of land needed for the asylum was excessive. Witnesses concurred that a large farm for the patients was necessary 'having regard to modern ideas', although they were under some pressure to account for this as workhouse patients and patients in the old asylum had made do with much less land. A councillor wanted to know why the villa colony had been chosen instead of the block system, and was told that 'the villa colony system had yielded results beyond their greatest hopes'. However, there was strong objection to spending so much ratepayers' money particularly when lunacy was understood to be the result of 'rascality and immorality', although the expenditure was eventually sanctioned (*Belfast Telegraph* 23rd February 1909). The churches were completed in 1910, and the same year a further 38 acres of land was purchased (further purchases of land brought the estate to 500 acres in extent by the 1920s), and it was agreed to construct a further two villas, duplicates of the existing villas, for male patients (BDLA Minutes 1910:189; Belfast Corporation, 1929). The building scheme, initially housing c530 patients (a further 200 patients were housed in the mansion house and other buildings on the estate), was completed in 1913, and G T Hine was invited to come and see the asylum in April 1913. Hine stated that the buildings were 'second to none in the Kingdom' while costing at least £50 per bed less than English or Scottish asylums (BDLA Minutes 1913: 24-30). The Asylum Committee then wished to obtain an additional loan of £88,500 to build villas for a further 400-500 patients but no further construction took place at the site until the inter-war period (*Belfast Newsletter* 2nd March 1912; Belfast Corporation, 1929). The original asylum at Grosvenor Road, having served as a War Hospital during WWI, was demolished in 1924, at which time Purdysburn Mental Hospital became the sole facility for the poor insane in Belfast. Purdysburn (now known as Knockbracken Healthcare Park) remains in use as a psychiatric hospital to the present day, but housed only around 150 patients in 2013 compared to the 2,200 patients resident in 1970 when patient numbers were at their height (Hamilton & O'Donnell, 2013).

4.1.2. Site and layout

Purdysburn Villa Colony was situated approximately 4 miles south of Belfast city centre, on a south-facing undulating site. A boast was made that there 'are not any bars on any of the windows nor is there a wall round the Estate' and that 'the entrance gates are always open' (an entrance lodge and gatescreen were added during the 1920s) (Belfast Corporation, 1929). The buildings discussed in this research were all added during the course of two main phases of development, from 1902-1906 and from 1909 to 1913. The villas were all built for 50 patients and were laid out on what was described as a 'crescent-shaped' plan surrounding the hospital building (Belfast Corporation, 1929) (Figure 4-5). Accommodation was organised within the villas with dayrooms on the ground floor and dormitories on the upper floors. Dormitories ranged in size from four to 16 beds and there was a 'single room' with two beds. However, the single room was not considered part of the regular patient accommodation and was not counted in bed numbers. Villas 10 and 11 were of a completely different design, as set out below. Cross lighting was an important feature of the villas, with light coming in on both sides in most principle rooms. It was later stated that 'light is now being regarded as an all-important factor in mental and physical healing' (*Belfast Newsletter*, 21st October, 1929). There were no barred windows or bolted doors and patients were 'free to wander at liberty', with a number being 'on parole' and therefore free to leave the asylum grounds (*Belfast Newsletter*, 21st October 1929).

4.1.3. Selected buildings

Villa 1

Pre-existing farmhouse on the site, adapted for the use of patients in 1902 and housing 30 male patients who were employed caring for the livestock at the farm and within the dairy. The matron also lived in this building (PRONI HOS/32/1/9 Belfast Mental Hospital, 1924).

Villas 2-3

Constructed 1902-3. These villas for 50 female patients were built to an identical plan by architect Frederick Tulloch (Figure 4-6, 4-7).

Villas 4-5

Constructed 1904-6. These two villas were built to a plan similar to that of villas 2 and 3 but with a sanitary annexe, also to designs by Frederick Tulloch and provided accommodation for 50 female patients each. The female patients in these villas (and villas 2 and 3) were chronic and convalescent patients who were employed in the laundry and at needlework and dressmaking (Figures 4-8, 4-9) (PRONI HOS/32/1/9 Belfast Mental Hospital, 1924).

Villas 6-9

Constructed during the second phase of 1909-1913. Three of these villas were identical to villas 4 and 5 (with

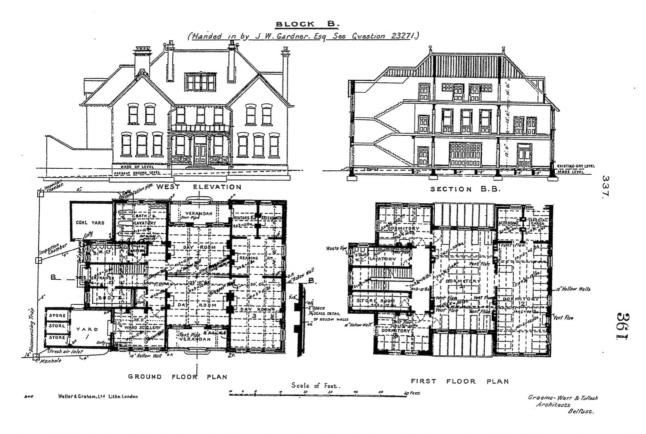

Figure 4-6. Purdysburn Villa Colony: elevations, plans and sections of colony villa. Source: *Royal Commission on the care and control of the feeble-minded volume III* (1908). Image from ProQuest's House of Commons Parliamentary Papers. Permission provided by ProQuest LLC.

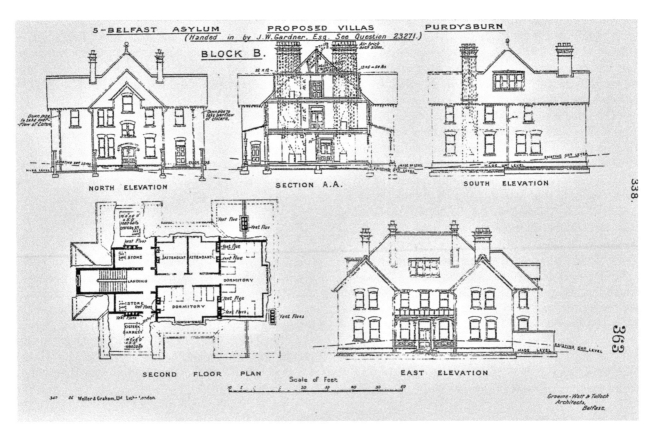

Figure 4-7. Purdysburn Villa Colony: elevations, plans and sections of colony villa. Source: *Royal Commission on the care and control of the feeble-minded volume III* (1908). Image from ProQuest's House of Commons Parliamentary Papers. Permission provided by ProQuest LLC.

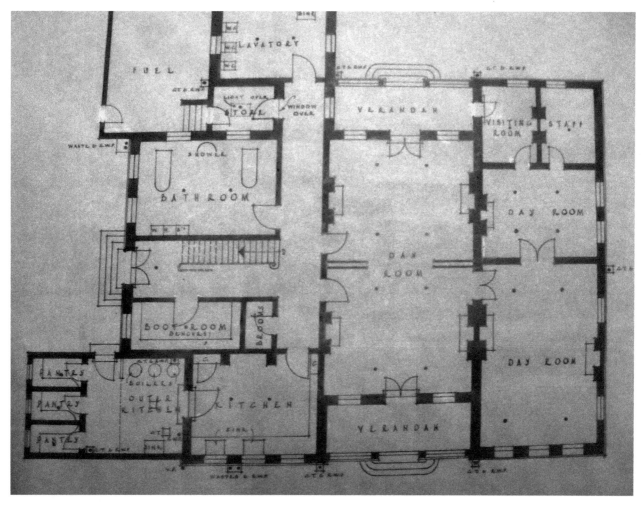

Figure 4-8. Purdysburn Villa Colony: ground floor plan of villa with sanitary annexe (undated). Source: Author's photograph of plans held by Estates Department, Knockbracken Healthcare Park.

sanitary annexe), and villa 6 was identical to villas 2 and 3 (without sanitary annexe). These were villas for 50 male patients each, occupied by patients who were classified as chronic, convalescent, 'feeble-minded and dements' (PRONI HOS/32/1/9 Belfast Mental Hospital, 1924).

Villa 10

Constructed during second phase 1909-1913 for male 'acute' patients and designed by G T Hine (Figure 4-9). The accommodation consists of south facing dayrooms on the ground floor and service rooms to the rear with two large dormitories on the upper floor, and six single rooms (Figures 4-11, 4-12).

Villa 11

Constructed during the second phase 1909-1913 for male patients under observation and designed by G T Hine (Figure 4-10). The accommodation consists of south-facing dayrooms and verandah with service rooms to the rear on the ground floor and a large upper dormitory of 44 beds and six single rooms (Figure 4-13).

Hospital

Constructed during the second phase 1909-1913. The hospital accommodated 50 patients of each sex, males to the west and females to the east, in dormitories of 18, 14 and 14, with four single rooms. The wards were organised around a central 'Winter Garden' lit by a conservatory roof and sanitary facilities were placed in separate annexes. A south-facing dayroom completed the accommodation. Verandahs extended across the south-facing elevation of the building and also wrapped around two sides of one of the ward extensions, providing south-east facing and south-west facing outdoor shelter. Patients in bed were pushed out onto the verandahs when weather was 'favourable' (Belfast Corporation, 1929). Nurses could reach the wards without passing through them by means of a covered way, which extended across the rear of the hospital (Figure 4-14, 4-15).

4.1.4. Medical superintendent at Purdysburn and his views on insanity

Relative to other sites in this study, at Purdysburn there was an unusually complete relationship between the Medical

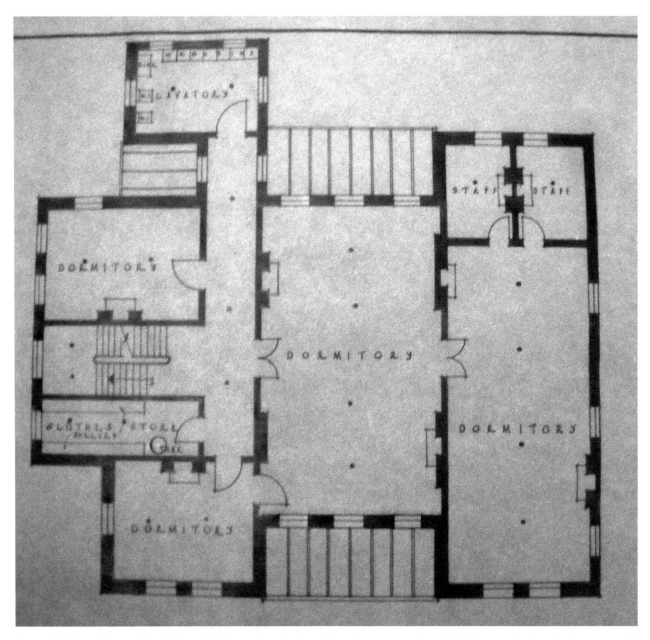

Figure 4-9. Purdysburn Villa Colony: first floor plan of villa with sanitary annexe (undated). Source: Author's photograph of plans held by Estates Department, Knockbracken Healthcare Park.

Superintendent and the building of the colony asylum. It was William Graham's idea to drop the pre-existing plans for the asylum, and to build a villa colony instead. Graham saw the project through to its completion, overseeing and contributing to the design, building and management in the early years before his premature death in 1917. At sites in Britain, the Medical Superintendent was appointed when the project was well under way, and medical advice was usually given in the early stages by a Medical Superintendent from another asylum (Renfrew; Whalley) or by a Lunacy Commissioner (Bangour; Kingseat).

Although William Graham was appointed after the Purdysburn estate had been purchased, he was delighted with the acquisition, noting that fresh air, exercise and salubrious surroundings was one of the most effective ways to benefit 'the diseased brain' (BDLA Annual Report,

1898). The interest provided by such an environment could be an important factor, he asserted, in increasing the contentment of patients. Getting the patients away from excitement and noise and allowing them freedom was beneficial (BDLA Annual Report, 1898). Graham referred to insanity as 'a symptom of a disease of the brain—an organ which is just as liable to suffer from derangement as is any other organ of the body' and in this view of psychiatric illness as somatic, he was in step with the medical thinking of the day (BDLA Annual Report, 1898). However, he also said that psychic causes, such as worry, needed to be taken into consideration, despite the root of mental disease in the 'breakdown or perversion of cells of the brain' (BDLA Annual Report, 1901). In later years, Graham was impressed by Freud's psycho-analytic approach and began to give greater weight to psychic factors, but this did not influence the period of Purdysburn's

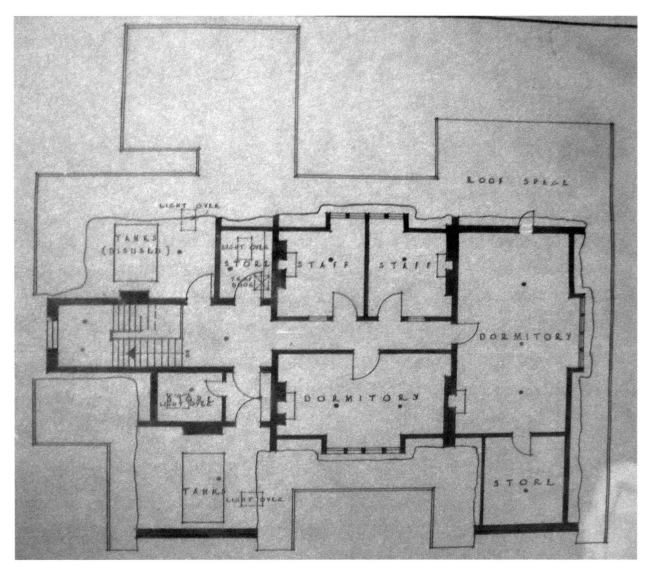

Figure 4-10. Purdysburn Villa Colony: attic floor plan of villa with sanitary annexe (undated). Source: Author's photograph of plans held by Estates Department, Knockbracken Healthcare Park.

construction, during which time Graham was adamant that mental illness was a disease of the nervous system (BDLA Annual Report, 1912). Humanity was subject to physiological crises such as birth, puberty, maternity and menopause and at these times or times of mental strain, 'an unfavourable environment or pernicious training' could bring on insanity (BDLA Annual Report, 1901). Graham also put forward the widely-held belief that mental disease was a uniquely terrible affliction, which required a special response from society. It was uniquely human to express sympathy and compassion towards the suffering—indeed not to do so would represent a retrogression to a lower stage of humanity (BDLA Annual Report, 1901, 1906).

Graham advocated a four part method of treatment, comprising: avoidance of excitement, freedom of movement, occupation and adherence to 'hygienic laws'. A model asylum should pay attention to environmental factors, such as ventilation, cleanliness, harmonious decoration, heating, lighting, plumbing and water supply and the regime should offer good diet and healthful

agricultural pursuits (BDLA Annual Report, 1898, 1899). Graham thought that a colony would give the facilities for 'mental improvement, industrial education and physical development, as well as for proper medical treatment' (BDLA Annual Report, 1898). The outcome of good treatment in an asylum was patients who improved more rapidly and were cured more quickly but also who were more tractable, amiable and mild, took more interest in their surroundings, were more contented, more cheerful and showed greater zest for life (BDLA Annual Report, 1898, 1899).

Although Graham attributed mental disease to heredity in large part, often counselling against 'marriage with neurotic persons', he also stated that the tendency could remain dormant unless there were 'exciting and preventable causes' which he attributed to the 'violation or neglect of physiological law' which stemmed from principles of morality and hygiene. Intemperance was another cause (although this could be the symptom of degeneracy of the brain and nervous system), as was physical weakness which

149

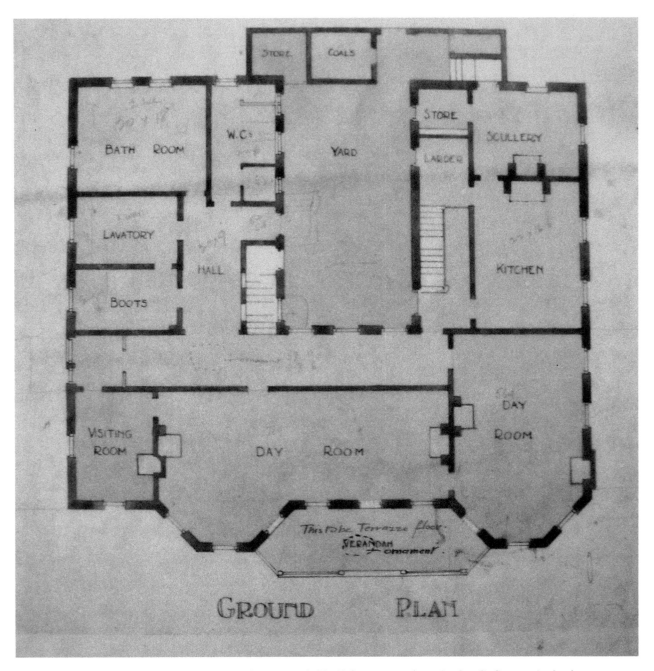

Figure 4-11. Purdysburn Villa Colony: ground floor plan of villa 10 for acute patients (undated). Source: Author's photograph of plans held by Estates Department, Knockbracken Healthcare Park.

allowed emotional disturbances to become established and meant that the insane were especially prone to infectious disease (BDLA Annual Report, 1899, 1903; Graham, 1901:,695). Physical diseases in one generation could appear as insane predispositions in another and therefore, treatment of diseases such as TB could also be seen as a means of preventing insanity (BDLA Annual Report 1910).

Graham asserted that insanity was linked to poverty, and that increases in the insane were 'mainly in the ranks of the poorest and most uneducated of the people; hence we may assume that the bulk of mental derangement is due to neglect or violation of fundamental hygienic laws' (BDLA Annual Report 1900). Poverty and the environments

associated with it, were therefore, a prime cause of mental illness. Either external factors or internal factors such as unhealthy nutrition could give rise to 'toxins' which could act on the nerve cells of the brain and nervous system and give rise to insanity (BDLA Annual Report 1900;1902). Prevention of mental illness consisted in 'sound training: physical, mental and moral'. Important causes were diet, drink and the 'very air we breathe', 'the unhygienic conditions of life' and 'defective morals and lack of self-control'. Exercise in the open air was not only beneficial in itself, being the 'ideal employment for the mentally disturbed' allowing them to receive the 'solidarity, the reality, the order and cohesion which are wherever Nature is', but allowed the 'deleterious products of respiration' to be removed from the asylum buildings by natural

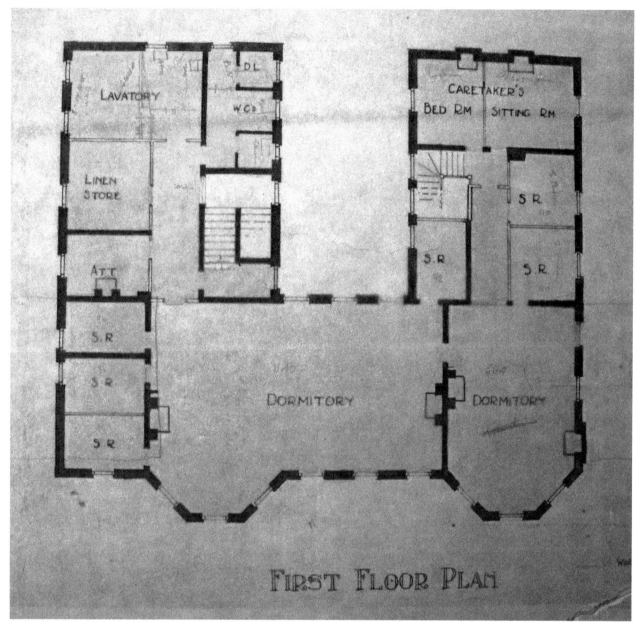

Figure 4-12. Purdysburn Villa Colony: first floor plan of villa 10 for acute patients (undated). Source: Author's photograph of plans held by Estates Department, Knockbracken Healthcare Park.

ventilation (BDLA Annual Report 1901, 1911). Airy day-rooms and dormitories were essential, where elaborate decoration was not (Graham, 1901:697). Graham believed that so-called 'chronic' patients could sometimes be cured 'after many years' derangement through the quiet of a rural life and a pleasant and cheerful environment' (Graham, 1901:689). Graham attributed a 'process of degeneration' among the poorer classes in Scotland to defective food (such as stewed tea, stout, artificial drinks, white bread, canned and concentrated meats) and environment, describing the 'lower quarters of our great cities' as inhabited by 'thin, stunted anaemic figures' (BDLA Annual Report 1902, 1903). Graham correlated physical degeneration with a progressive 'mental enfeeblement' within society, and called for hygienic conditions in 'the home, the school and factory' to be improved in order to stem the tide of insanity (BDLA Annual Report 1902).

Graham advocated physical exercise and a return to nature to redress these problems, suggesting that nerve cells weakened by the transgression of physiological law could be passed on to progeny (BDLA Annual Report 1902). He was particularly concerned by the great increase in general paralysis of the insane, which it was thought was often caused by an earlier contraction of syphilis.[2] The connection of syphilis with mental disease at this period gave a moral dimension to 'physiological laws', suggesting that physical, moral and mental degeneration were inter-linked. An inherited weakness

_____

[2] Although it was accepted by the early 1900s that GPI was often connected to syphilitic infection, the theory that it could also be caused by 'stresses of civilisation' continued to be promulgated alongside and it was not until 1912 and the discovery of spirochaetes in the brain tissue of general paralytics that GPI became fully recast as neurosyphilis (Hurn, 1998:135-140)

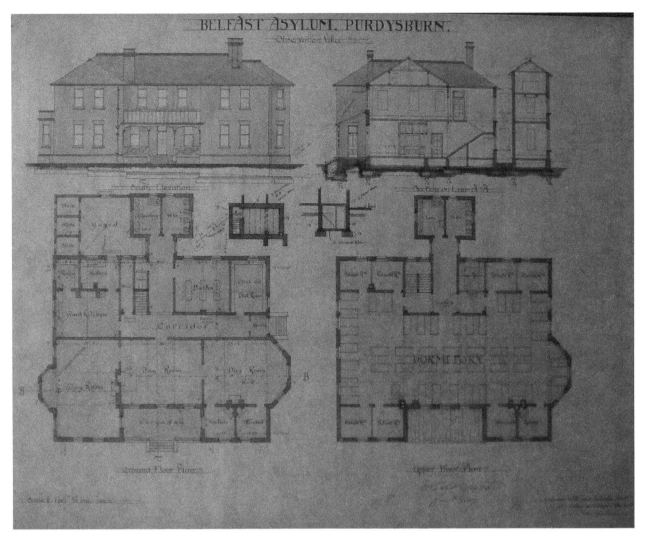

Figure 4-13. Purdysburn Villa Colony: plans and elevations of villa 11 for patients under observation (undated). Source: Author's photograph of plans held by Estates Department, Knockbracken Healthcare Park.

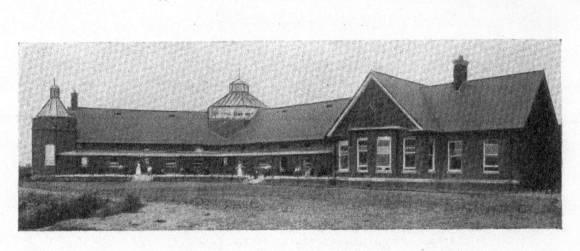

A section of the Hospital Block.

Figure 4-14. Purdysburn Villa Colony: hospital wing showing verandah and roof of winter garden. Source: PRONI HOS/32/1/9. Reproduced with permission of the Deputy Keeper of the Records, Public Record Office of Northern Ireland.

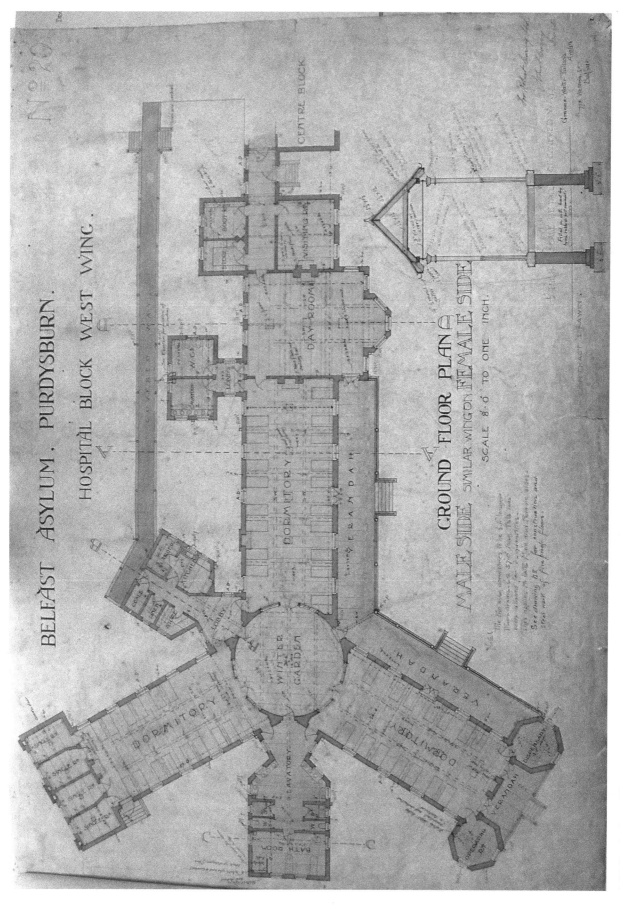

Figure 4-15. Purdysburn Villa Colony: plan of hospital wing. Source: Author's photograph of plans held by Estates Department, Knockbracken Healthcare Park.

might draw to itself 'whatever is harmful in the daily environment of life' by which Graham was probably referring to drinking, poor diet and 'vicious moral environment' (BDLA Annual Report 1903, 1905). A 'reversion to a lower stage of development' could also be due to an early upbringing in a 'tainted environment' (BDLA Annual Report 1905). Graham seemed to claim a two-way relationship between mental weakness and unhealthy practices and environments in that each may lead to the other. Alcoholism, for instance, could be a cause of changes that could be inherited (although Graham was elsewhere agnostic about the possibility of the transmission of acquired characteristics) but most cases were due to a degeneracy producing a 'weakness of brain and nerve which leads to a want of self control' (BDLA Annual Report 1903). Vice of any kind involved a 'profuse waste of vitality' which 'must end sooner or later in mental and physical bankruptcy' (BDLA Annual Report 1905). Although there had been a steady increase in the numbers of insane in Ireland, Graham pointed out that the increase had been in first admissions and that theories that the insane were accumulating in asylums rather than being cured could not account for the increase. Graham attributed the problem to the emigration and lower reproduction rates of the 'middle classes' which included for him the well-to-do artisan and farmer leaving those classes who did not have 'healthful existence' within their reach and were reduced to 'starvation, disease, stunted development and moral degradation' (BDLA Annual Report 1903).

Poverty was a cause of intemperance because of overwork and mental and physical stress. Graham pointed to 'long hours, unrelieved by a touch of lightness, the extreme specialism that marks industrial life, the utter absence of what the French call the 'joy of living' and the increasing anxiety in view of sickness or old age' as causes of despair leading to insanity (BDLA Annual Report 1905). As preventive measures against insanity Graham counselled that reproduction of the unfit should not be sanctioned, the sale of alcohol should be restricted and over-crowded, unhygienic, unaired tenements should be replaced by homes which would enable 'men and women to live decently'. Places of recreation, baths and gymnasiums should be increased and children should be given physiological education (BDLA Annual Report 1905). Graham held insanity, idiocy, imbecility, epilepsy, hysteria and neurasthenia to be closely allied and springing from the same neuropathic disposition (BDLA Annual Report 1906). Early admission to the asylum was thought to facilitate a cure and therefore prevent suffering and be more economical (BDLA Annual Report 1907).

Therapeutic work was of the greatest importance to patients because it 'regulates the psychic functions, trains the attention, gives rise to new and healthy complexes of thought, and tends to destroy that mental egotism which too often complicates the psychic disturbance' (Graham, 1911:622). A colleague of Graham's offered the opinion that the attention which was given to the general

environment of the insane, 'the buildings which housed them and the interests which were provided for them, offered them healthy suggestions' with the aim of replacing the 'painful and morbid suggestions' that affected those of unsound mind. Graham concurred that the villa colony brought patients 'into the healthy currents of normal social life' (BDLA Annual Report 1912).

4.2. Sixth Lancashire County Asylum (Whalley)

4.2.1. Introduction

Most asylum authorities in England, built one or two asylums during the course of the nineteenth century, typically a building intended for a few hundred patients that was then extended for up to 1,000 patients as the century progressed. Lancashire, Yorkshire and London asylum authorities were exceptions to this rule, each building a relatively large number of asylums (London County Council built ten by 1910, and Yorkshire, West Riding built five, with a further two in North and East Ridings), the latest of which were at least double the size of most other county asylums. The first asylum to be built in Lancashire was constructed under the permissive Act of 1808 and was opened in Lancaster in 1816 (Figure 4-16). The building was on a corridor plan and was intended for 150 patients. However, it was extended multiple times and by 1910, the original asylum together with a later building on the same site were catering for 2,573 patients (ELC Report 1910: 258-265). Lancashire's second and third asylums were Rainhill and Prestwich which were both opened in 1851 and were of the corridor plan (a later (1884) annexe at Prestwich is of a circular corridor design) (Figure 4-17). Rainhill and Prestwich were built for 400 and 500 patients respectively but both held several times this by 1910 (1,975 and 2,709 patients each) (ELC Report 1910: 258-265). The fourth asylum built, Whittingham in 1873, demonstrates the change to pavilion styles in asylum planning and was arranged as a series of pavilions in a horseshoe shape with administrative buildings at the centre. However, in this early style, some pavilions were orientated away from maximum sunlight. Whittingham was built for 1,000 patients and housed double that by 1910. The fifth asylum, opened at Winwick in 1902, was a very large building, designed for 2,050 patients, and utilising the then-prevailing compact arrow plan (ELC Report 1910) (Figure 4-18).

Winwick Asylum is orientated in a north-south direction so that all pavilions face SSW or SSE, and are stepped back in echelon, giving dayrooms the benefit of sunlight and views, although the arrangement of pavilions means that views are somewhat obscured for pavilions to the rear, and totally obscured for chronic patients in blocks 8 and 9. Patient accommodation for chronic patients was organised with dayrooms on the ground floor and dormitories above. These dormitories were exceedingly large (between 47 and 63 beds) and the pavilions appear to have been three storeys high, so that over 100 patients were accommodated in each one.

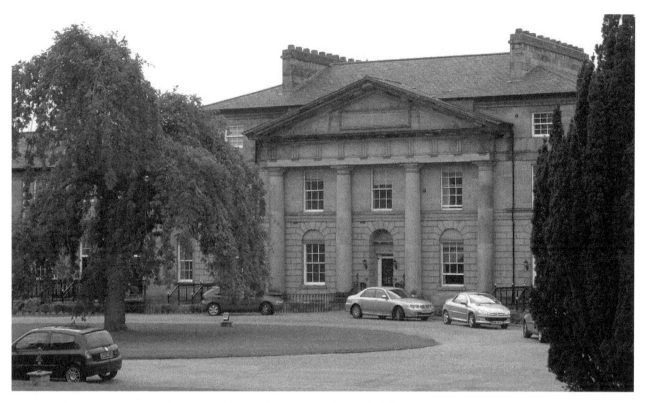

Figure 4-16. Lancaster County Asylum, original building dating from 1816. Source: www.countyasylums.co.uk, reproduced with permission.

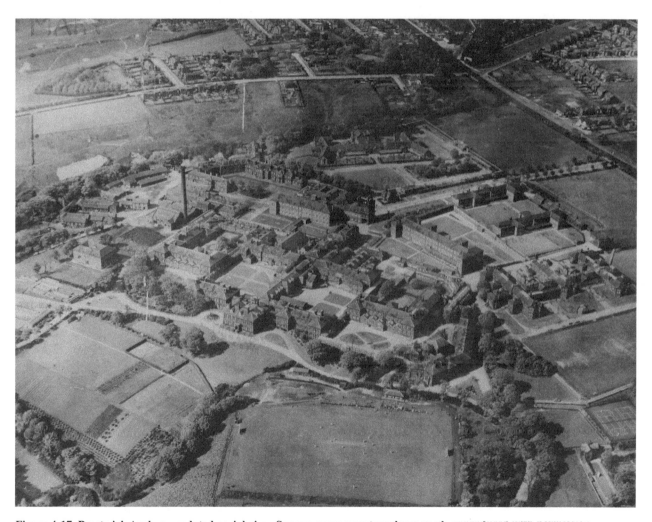

Figure 4-17. Prestwich Asylum, undated aerial view. Source: www.countyasylums.co.uk, reproduced with permission.

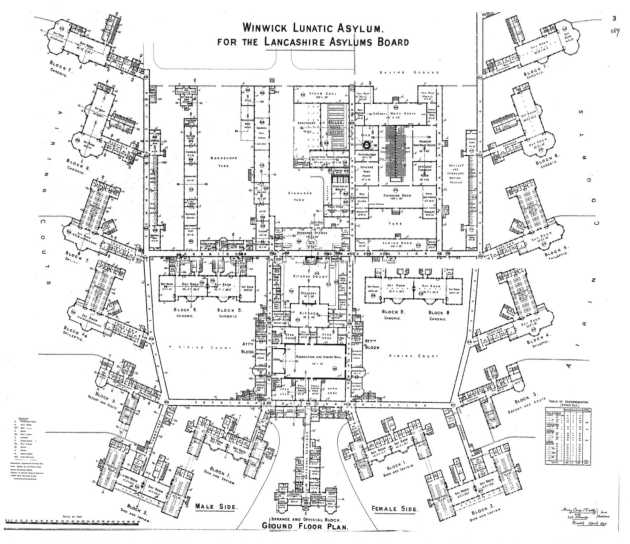

Figure 4-18. Winwick Asylum (Fifth Lancashire Asylum): ground floor plan. Source: *Commissioners in Lunacy, fiftieth annual report to Lord Chancellor*, 1896 (Supplement) (plan fitted together by author from separately printed sections). Image from ProQuest's House of Commons Parliamentary Papers. Permission provided by ProQuest LLC.

4.2.2. Construction of asylum

A sixth asylum for Lancashire was first discussed before the opening of the fifth asylum at Winwick. Numbers of insane in county asylums in Lancashire increased by more than 500 per cent in four decades (from 1,587 in 1859 to 8,655 in 1900) (Report of a Lancashire deputation, 1901: 70). In August 1898, a committee was appointed by the LAB to investigate further accommodation for 'imbeciles and epileptics' and to visit asylums in Britain and Europe. Some members of the board did not want this trip to go ahead and a vote in its favour was only narrowly carried (LAB Minutes 25th August and 24th November 1898). In 1900 a deputation, comprising Alderman Jenkins, vice-chairman of the LAB, Dr David Mackay Cassidy, a Scot who was Superintendent of Lancaster asylum and Dr Joseph Wiglesworth, Superintendent of Rainhill, was appointed. By September 1900, the committee had visited several sites in Europe and had produced a printed report (*Manchester Courier* 4th September, 1900; Report of a Lancashire Deputation, 1900). They visited ten sites in Germany, including Alt Scherbitz, four in France and one in Belgium.

The LAB deputation were impressed by German and French pavilions, and their architectural 'lightness of effect', but the disposition of pavilions, close together with their long axes parallel and opposite to each other, was criticised for circumscribing views and making the spaces between pavilions too confined. The lack of embellishments was also thought to present 'a somewhat bare appearance'. German colony asylums gave patients much more freedom and the absence of restraint was noted. At Alt Scherbitz the deputation noted that the villas were grouped together 'but so surrounded by trees and shrubs that they are partially hidden and the contiguity, slight as it is, is not perceived'. The villas were in the Italian style and were decorated with ivy and climbing plants. No two were exactly alike and 'there are no connecting galleries or passages of any kind between them'. They had plenty of 'acute and excited cases' but 'there are no walls at Alt Scherbitz', the closed houses only being surrounded by wooden palings. The exercising grounds were full of shrubs and flowering plants and all had good views of the gardens and grounds. The colony was distinguished by 'the segregation of the inmates into small communities, where they live in a more domesticated and home-like style than would be possible in a large building, and the disuse, during the day time, of locks and keys'. The houses were of differing styles and were scattered around rather than being on a regular plan round the sides of a square or on a curved line (Report of a Lancashire deputation, 1900).

The deputation concluded that the housing of patients in large asylum pavilions was too abnormal, the departure from the conditions of ordinary domestic life was too abrupt and they were too vast to be conducive to real comfort and happiness. They thought that patients would prefer to live within a small circle, rather than in enforced association with others. This would allow for greater division between interests and illnesses and smaller numbers meant that the attendant would be more interested in his charges. 'Individuality is lost in a crowd and the increasing loss of the sense of individuality in a lunatic goes *pari passu* with a loss of initiative and mental energy, in short, of mind'. The colony was a better environment for patients because it increased personal initiative and made conditions more normal. They could become familiar with attendants assigned to each villa, making for more intimate living conditions, 'the smaller the groups the better'. The deputation asserted that the cost of building a villa asylum was less and that there was no difference in maintenance costs, ultimately recommending the 'villa-colony' system as the 'principle of construction for the new projected asylum' (Report of a Lancashire deputation, 1900).

In 1901 the committee decided that the need for acute provision was such that the new site should be allocated to curable rather than incurable cases (LAB Minutes, 29th August 1901; 28th November 1901). By February 1902, some sites had been visited and the Committee commented on their advantages and disadvantages. What was being sought was level land at a high elevation at a good price. It should not be too far from a railway, should not be cold or bleak, hilly or irregular, lacking in water, have a soil that was composed of clay or was badly draining, and should not be too near the sea or too high (because it would be exposed to cold). One site was rejected because the chimneys of Oldham were in full view (LAB Minutes 27th February, 1902).

Once located in May 1902, the site at Whalley was deemed suitable due to its gentle slope to the south and its good drainage. Water could be supplied from the water mains and the clay soil, which had been seen as a disadvantage during the search for a site, was now touted as an advantage because it would mean less excavation for the foundations (LAB Minutes, 22nd May 1902). The site was 233 acres (at a cost of £25,630) with an additional 68½ acres from a different farm (at a cost of £6,000) for a railway siding, and was 175 to 200 feet above sea level. It was judged to have 'very fine, expansive views' and regular contours with woods providing shelter to the north. The clay was seen as a possible building material for brick construction of the buildings and a decision was made to purchase on 7th November 1902 (LAB Minutes,

7th November 1902; *Manchester Courier*, 8th November, 1902). Strong objections were raised to the purchase by some councillors and by local residents, leading ultimately to the holding of a Board of Enquiry in 1905. Alderman Miles said it was 'the very last place in the world where he would build a residence for himself' because it was low and had a clay soil and, by implication, bad air. Others countered that the site was in fact high, suggesting that little consensus existed about what was healthy in terms of sites (*Manchester Courier*, 8th November 1902). A Mr Carter objected that the site was 'too low and would be found to be conducive to phthisis and other tubercular diseases among the patients, who were generally in an enfeebled state of bodily as well as mental health'. It was near a river which was practically an open sewer (the river Calder) and the site was not dry (due to the clay subsoil). The nearby road was also said to be too busy for patients to exercise on safely (*Lancashire Daily Post*, 8th June 1905). The local aristocracy and clergy objected on the grounds of the potential reduction to the price of their property and the association of the name of Whalley with an asylum (Cornwell, 2010: 10).

In late 1903, Henry Littler, the County Architect and designer of previous institutions, in particular Whittingham, the fourth Lancashire Asylum, was appointed the designer of the new asylum. The Chairman of the LAB was of the view that chronic patients 'could be dealt with in less expensive buildings and cared for at a much less cost' than those suffering from acute mania who needed asylums 'of a curative nature' and therefore wanted Whalley to be an asylum for chronic patients (LAB Minutes, 26th November 1903). But there were objections that an asylum filled with incurables offered no hope for its inmates and this idea appears to have been dropped (*Lancashire Evening Post*, 31st August 1903).

In 1904, it was resolved to set up a sub-committee for building the new asylum at Whalley and to send the architect to visit asylums in Germany, Scotland and England (namely Galkhausen, Wuhlgarten, Uchtspringe, Alt Scherbitz, Gabersee, Am Stettin, Aberdeen, Bangour, Montrose, Dumfries, Bexley and Stone (the first eight being colony asylums and the latter four providing villas supplementary to the main accommodation). The architect was sent to Germany because his first design for the colony, placing two thirds of the patients in a main building and the remainder in villas, was deemed too conservative, as the Board wanted more of the accommodation to be provided in villas. On returning from his visit Henry Littler declared that his hesitation about the villa system had been removed and he was confident that 'the surroundings of the Villa or detached building have a beneficial and quietening effect upon the condition and health of the patients' (LAB Minutes, 23rd September, 1904; 17th November, 1904). The Whalley Committee decided to build an asylum on the 'colony system' on Mr Littler's return and the lunacy commissioners approved this plan. The architect assured the committee that a colony system would only be very slightly more expensive to build and Dr Cassidy also assured them that the cost of running it would be similar to a traditional asylum. They proposed to build an asylum for 2,000 patients (this was larger than the German asylums which were from 800-1300 patients), the main concern being that the food could not be easily distributed from a central kitchen to such a large number, but it was thought this drawback could be overcome.

The colony design produced by Littler (no drawings survive) consisted of a wide avenue running east to west and dividing the asylum into two sections, to the south would be a Medical Section and a colony of villas for each sex and to the north would be administration buildings, kitchens and engineering departments, large pavilions for chronic cases and two small villa colonies for working patients. The medical section was to consist of an admission hospital for 100, a general hospital for 120 and a TB hospital for 100. Two observation villas housing 45 each and two acute villas housing 40 each were to be placed near the admission hospital. The RC church was to be placed to the south of the Admission hospital and between the acute villas 'thus effectually separating the sexes'. To the south-east and the south-west of the medical section were to be eight villas with 45 patients in each villa. On either side of the central administration buildings were to be six pavilions and two large villas for chronic, infirm and epileptic patients, providing 'suitable and economical accommodation for 700 patients'. The pavilions were for 100 patients and the villas for 50 patients, suggesting that the chronic patients were to have cheaper accommodation where larger numbers of patients were placed together. The church and the recreation hall were to be situated in this area between pavilions and admin buildings. On the north side of the avenue were to be located eight villas for 45 patients each, intended to be occupied by the 'quieter and working patients' and close to the laundry, workshops and kitchens where patients' labour would be required. Littler suggested that the design was 'an entirely new departure in the planning of the English Asylums' (LAB Minutes, 23rd September, 1904). By May 1905, it was again proposed that Whalley should be built as an asylum 'of cheap construction to accommodate cases other than of the acute and dangerous class' (LAB Minutes, 25th May, 1905). But this proposal appears to have again been dropped in favour of accommodating chronic and harmless cases in the workhouses at the expense of the Asylums Board.

The construction of a villa colony was dropped at this stage of deliberations and it was decided to build on the Whalley site, a more conventional reception hospital for 100 patients, an administration block large enough to deal with 2,000 patients and attached wards for about 500 acute and curable cases. The question of adding villas for 600 patients to the site at a later stage was left open (LAB Minutes, 30th August 1905). In comparing the villa and block systems, the LAB were doubtful that more cures would be effected or that 'the general condition of the patients would be substantially improved' by the villa system, and so did not want to recommend the increased

expenditure which had been put at £15 to £30 more per bed (approximately 10 per cent). They did think that 'for certain classes of curable cases, the more home-like surroundings of a villa may result in a greater probability of a cure to the patient than treatment in a large ward'. But they decided to postpone adding villas to the site until greater experience had been obtained of the villa system elsewhere (LAB Minutes, 23rd August 1905). In October 1906 the plan for the new asylum was accepted by the LAB.

The new asylum was to accommodate 1,180 and consisted of a reception hospital, administration block with recreation hall, kitchens and stores to the rear and five wards on each side of the central buildings, catering for sick (100), infirm (140), two acute (100 each), and a further ward for the 'general class of patients' (100) for men and women (Figure 4-19). It was stated that the most southerly position was chosen for the reception hospital and that the wards were only two storeys high, arranged so that the day rooms would face the south 'and ample space between each block will be given for light and air'. Although not explicitly stated in the LAB Minutes, Littler's design bears a strong resemblance to the (much-criticised) asylums for the imbecile poor built by the Metropolitan Asylums Board at Caterham and Leavesden, which both opened in 1870 housing 1,510 patients each (Taylor, 1991:142). The arrangement of the wards was intended to shorten the length of corridors, simplify the drainage and reduce the cost of water pipes, heating pipes and electrical mains (LAB Minutes, 18th October 1906). When the plan was submitted to the Lunacy Commissioners, they remarked that the scheme had 'advantages in concentration and economy of working' and that 'the cost should work out at less than certain other asylums of different design that have of late years been erected—a matter to which they attach the greatest importance and desire to promote in every way compatible with efficiency' (*Lancashire Evening Post*, 27th February 1907). The first construction on the site, of the branch railway, began in May 1907 (LAB Minutes, 16th May 1907). Meanwhile the LAB continued to deliberate on ways of providing more cheaply for 'chronic harmless lunatics, for whom there is no hope of cure', and met with the Home Secretary and representatives of the Local Government Board and the Lunacy Commissioners to discuss possible solutions. They contrasted the incurables with those who could be cured by 'special medical treatment, environment and diet' (LAB Minutes, 16th May 1907).

The LAB set about the process of initiating brickmaking on the site in December 1907, estimating that 20–25 million bricks would have to be produced, at 200,000 per day, taking two years (LAB Minutes, 9th December 1907). In 1908, the LAB decided to build the main buildings 50 yards south of the position formerly proposed, in order to use the best building land on the estate and to increase accommodation for patients to 1,260. This would leave less room for villas in the future and it was proposed to reduce the villa accommodation that might be built

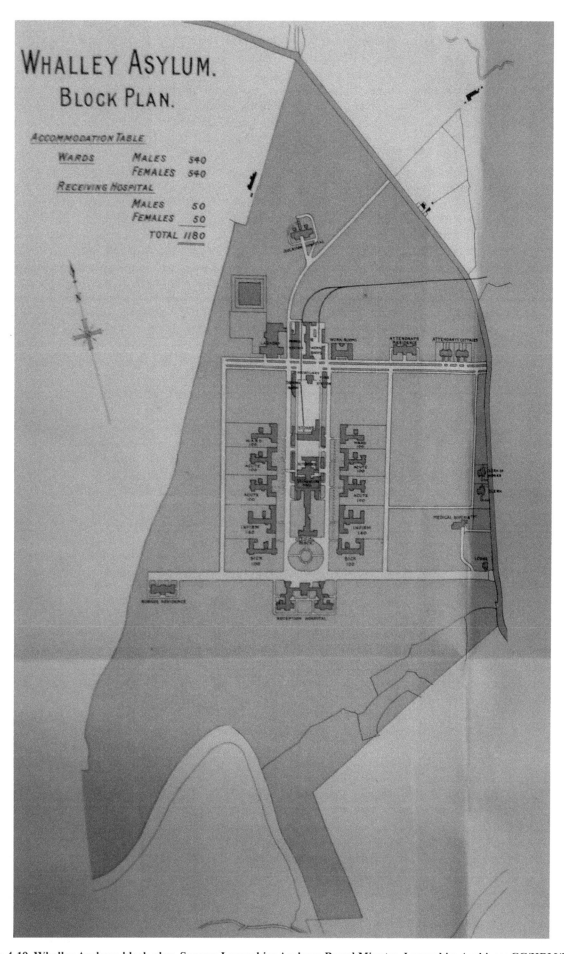

Figure 4-19. Whalley Asylum: block plan. Source: Lancashire Asylums Board Minutes. Lancashire Archives: CC/HBM/2, 29 Oct 1906.

to 400 patients (rather than 600)(LAB Minutes, 22nd February 1907). The first buildings to be constructed on the site were attendants' cottages, a house for the clerk of works, a house for the clerk and steward and two lodges and these buildings were completed in early 1910 (LAB Minutes, 24th February 1910). Final approval was given to the detailed plans of the main buildings in May of the same year, by the Lunacy Commissioners and the Home Secretary and Messrs R Neill & Sons were appointed the contractors, for the sum of £355,846. Engineering contractors were also approved at a cost of £30,408 (LAB Minutes, 11th May 1910; 18th August 1910). The Board also decided to buy two further parcels of land to give another access point and to facilitate enlargement of the local sewage works (LAB Minutes, 17th November 1910). In 1911 the Board decided to take advantage of an offer from the contractor to complete the asylum on the block system for 2,000 patients, and therefore to finally completely abandon the proposal to add villas to the site. The remaining accommodation consisted of four ward blocks, for chronic patients, which were to be three storeys high and house 157 patients each and two two-storey blocks for working patients housing 56 patients each (Cornwell, 2010:20; LCA DDX 1254/1/1/8 Whalley Asylum plans, 1912).

However, the contractors stopped work on 21st October 1911 and declared bankruptcy. New contractors were appointed to complete the work at a cost of £359,507 and they commenced work in May 1912. Despite a strike among joiners and bricksetters in July 1913 the building of the asylum proceeded to schedule (*Burnley Express* 5th July 1913).

In February 1915, it was announced that the government had taken over Whalley asylum for use as a general military hospital (*Manchester Evening News*, 26th February 1915). Although not completed, the hospital opened formally for the reception of wounded soldiers on 14th April 1915, when it was described as 'this newest and most modern asylum' (*Burnley Express*, 17thApril 1915). After some initial confusion about the name of the new hospital it remained 'Queen Mary's Military Hospital' until 30th June 1920, when the War Office handed it back to the LAB. It was then decided to use the asylum as a certified institution under the terms of the 1913 Mental Deficiency Act which required the LAB to provide accommodation for so-called 'mental defectives' and the hospital was renamed 'Calderstones Institution' (Figure 4-20) (Cornwell, 2010: 88-89). Although this was intended to be a temporary measure, the new designation became permanent, and by 2017 the hospital was the only specialist hospital for learning disabled patients in England, although it has since been earmarked for closure. Most of the former hospital buildings have now been demolished and replaced by housing. However, the reception hospital, the administration building, and the female sick and infirm blocks survive in a somewhat altered condition.

4.2.3. Site and layout

The asylum was built on the pavilion plan, using a variation that has been coined 'dual pavilion', that is consisting of two rows of pavilions arranged one behind the other, either side of the central administration buildings. This plan was first used at Caterham and Leavesden (by the Metropolitan Asylums Board, both opening in 1870), to construct large asylums for chronic cases and was repeated at Banstead in Middlesex, which was intended for a similar category of patients, but by 1905 was compelled also to receive acute patients (opened 1877) (Taylor, 1991:39). However, Whalley differed in several ways from these three asylums. Firstly, the wards at Whalley were somewhat further apart (on average c20 metres further apart than those at Leavesden) so increasing access to light, air and views (distances were calculated by author using measurement tools for historic maps at digimap.com). Wards at Leavesden were generally built to house 160 on three floors so were somewhat larger than the acute and sick wards at Whalley (*The Builder*, 25th July 1868).

Female wards at Whalley were to the west and male wards to the east, all connected to the kitchens and to each other by means of a corridor which was lit by electricity and open at the sides to admit light and air (Cornwell, 2010: 64). Each ward had a grassed airing court surrounded by iron hooped safety railings, six feet six inches in height. Hedges and trees were planted to disguise these, and the airing courts were patrolled by staff to prevent violence and escape attempts (there were on average six escapes per month) (Cornwell, 2010:17). The asylum was approached through a gated entrance with accompanying lodge, along a driveway, and it is likely that the majority of the estate perimeter was fenced (Cornwell, 2010:19).

4.2.4. Selected buildings

The main structures on the site were as follows:

Administration Block

The administration block (Figure 4-21) is located at the centre of the site on the axis dividing female from male accommodation, as was usual in the traditional asylum layout. An enclosed corridor led from the rear to the recreation hall and further to the rear were the kitchens, stores, communal baths, sewing rooms and mortuary.

Admissions Hospital

This building (Figure 4.22) housed 50 patients of each sex, in a combination of five-bed and 15-bed dorms and single rooms, with south-facing dayrooms. Initial processing of patients took place in a receiving room with attached bathroom, where they were prepared for photographing. Visitors were received in the central block in dedicated rooms for each sex. The hospital also contained living

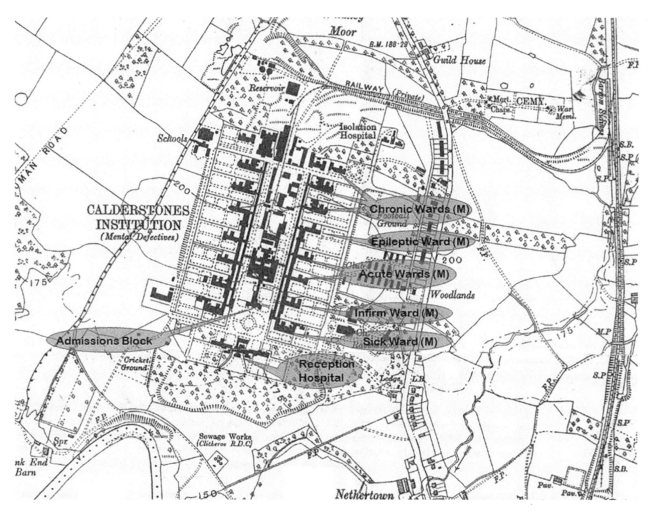

Figure 4-20. Calderstones Institution (formerly Whalley Asylum): labels added to show administration block, reception hospital and main wards (as constructed) on male side. Female side was identical. Source: 1:10 560 County Series 3rd Revision [TIFF geospatial data], Scale 1:10560, Tiles: lanc-sd73nw-4, Updated: 30 November 2010, Historic, Using: EDINA Historic Digimap Service, <https://digimap.edina.ac.uk>, Downloaded: 2021-05-17 16:54:09.469. © Crown Copyright and Landmark Information Group Limited 2021. All rights reserved. 1932.

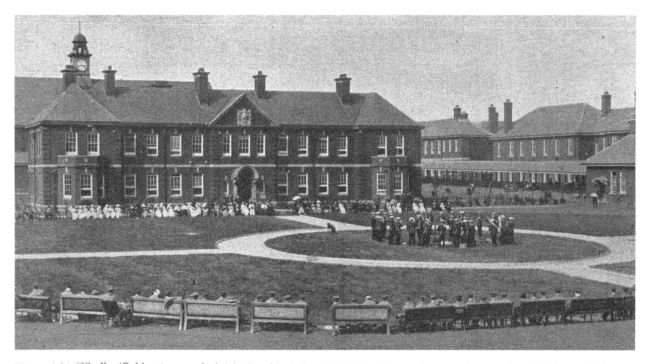

Figure 4-21. Whalley/Calderstones: administration block. Source: www.countyasylums.co.uk, reproduced with permission.

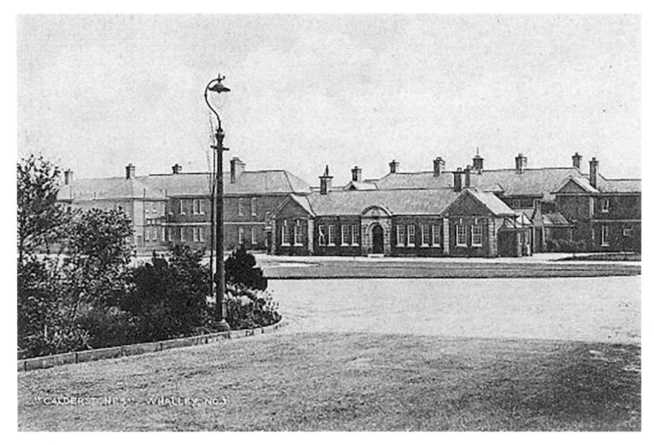

Figure 4-22. Whalley/Calderstones: admissions hospital. Source: www.countyasylums.co.uk, reproduced with permission.

accommodation for the Assistant Medical Officer, the Matron and the Head Attendant and mess rooms and sitting rooms for nurses and attendants.

Sick and Acute Wards

The first five wards on each side of the central spine, originally intended for curable patients, of the category, sick, infirm or acute were of a similar character. These were two-storey buildings with south-facing dayrooms and double-height bays, the three sick and acute wards catering for 100 patients, and the 'infirm' and 'epileptic' blocks on each side housing 140. The pavilion for 'sick' patients appears to have been constructed with a full-length verandah to the south, but other blocks did not originally feature verandahs (LCA DDX 1254/1/1/8 Whalley Asylum plans, 1912; OS Map 1932). The blocks were joined by an aerial walkway at second floor level constructed from a steel framework with a concrete floor and timber sides, roofed with asphalt, and window openings covered with wire mesh (Cornwell, 2010:20). The sick ward consisted of 18 single rooms with dayrooms and larger dormitories (number of beds not marked on plans) on each floor. The two acute wards were similarly arranged with single rooms for up to 30 patients and four larger dormitories for 17/18 patients. The infirm ward had fewer single rooms (20) and larger dormitories (four with 30 beds each) (Figure 4-23). The remaining ward, whose purpose was unassigned in the original design, was designated an epileptic block during the construction and contained dayrooms and dormitories

on each floor with two large dormitories of 61 beds each and 18 single rooms (LCA DDX 1254/1/1/8 Whalley Asylum plans, 1912).

Chronic Wards

These four wards (two for each sex) were somewhat larger than the sick and acute wards and provided 10 single rooms, and four dormitories of 29, 29, 36 and 54 beds. Accommodation was arranged with dayrooms and dormitories on ground and first floors, with dormitories only on the third floor (Figure 4-24). Two further wards for working male and female patients were positioned at the rear of the asylum near the laundry and workshops. These housed 50 patients each and were arranged on a more domestic plan with a single large dayroom below and a large dormitory for 50 patients above. These wards for working patients were detached from the corridor system.

4.3. Alt Scherbitz Provincial Asylum (Die Provinzial Irrenanstalt zu Alt Scherbitz)

4.3.1. Introduction

The colony asylum of Alt Scherbitz was constructed over several decades on a large acreage of agricultural land between the German cities of Leipzig and Halle in what was then the province of Saxony (Figures 4-25, 4-26). The asylum appears to have very quickly come to international

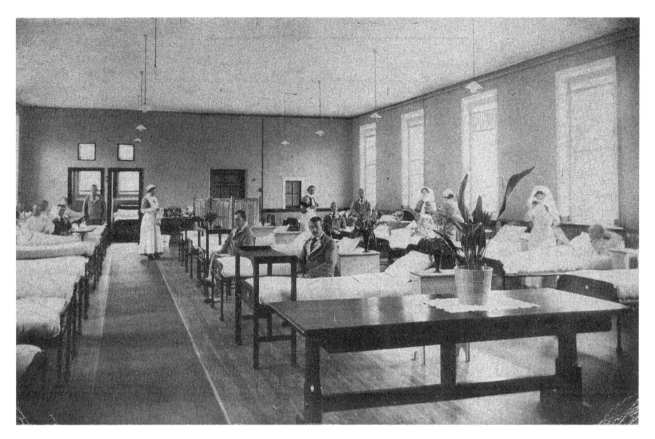

Figure 4-23. Whalley/Calderstones: interior of infirm ward dormitory c1915 Source: www.countyasylums.co.uk, reproduced with permission.

notice and was the inspiration for colony asylums all over the world including Scotland, in the period before the First World War. It is credited as the model for asylums in Brazil (1898), Argentina (1901), Norway (1904), Italy (1908), New Zealand (1912) and Tokyo (1919) as well as many examples in Germany and the Austrian empire where the colony design was almost universally adopted (Eraso, 2010; Hashimoto, 2013; Skålevåg, 2002; Topp, 2007). Alt Scherbitz was a standard stop on tours of the continent for asylum officials and doctors hoping to see the latest developments in asylum care for the insane in the late nineteenth and early twentieth centuries.

The asylum was founded in 1876 by Professor Dr Johannes Moritz Koeppe, who was succeeded on his death in January 1879 by Dr Albrecht Paetz, his assistant (Sonntag, 1993: 26-29). Although *Ackerbaucolonien* or agricultural colonies for the insane had been established in many places in Germany in the 1860s, these were always annexes to the main institution, usually physically separated from the 'closed' asylum and catering only for relatively small numbers of physically able patients. The *Ackerbaucolonien* were a phenomenon that had grown out of a nineteenth century European pedagogical and utopian tradition of combining agricultural education, training or work with 'family-style' accommodation. The immediate precursor for the *Ackerbaucolonien* was the French colony for the insane at Fitz-James, established in 1847 on a farm of c590 acres. This catered for selected patients from the closed asylum at Clermont-en-Oise (about a quarter

of the total number, the majority of them fee-paying and, therefore, non-labouring). Labouring patients were accommodated in medium-sized buildings containing dormitories of 20 to 30 beds each (Burdett, 1891; Labitte, 1861; Letchworth, 1889).

At Alt Scherbitz, Koeppe wanted to develop the idea of an agricultural colony much further by extending the amount of land to at least, ideally, 1,000 acres for 400 patients and dispense with the 'closed' asylum by accommodating all patients on a single site. The large expanse of land would then allow a wider variety of agricultural occupations than was possible in a smaller institution (Besser, 1881). Koeppe saw considerable benefits for the physical and mental health of patients in outdoor work:

'The Broken Down learn to have confidence again; the Sleepless again feel fatigue; the Scholar finds a soothing distraction; those in the field of ideas obtain stimulation in a whole new world of creativity; experiencing successfully the joy of working together. Otherwise anxiously guarded at every step, the patient here at work feels free from rules and regulations ... his blood circulation improves and he begins to take in food in a more normal ratio' (Besser, 1881). Patients having been chosen for work to which they were particularly adapted, small-scale accommodation was to be provided for them close to the location of their work e.g. the stables, orchards, bee hives, flower gardens etc. Paetz, in continuing Koeppe's work, stated that the chief advantages of the *Irrenkolonie*

163

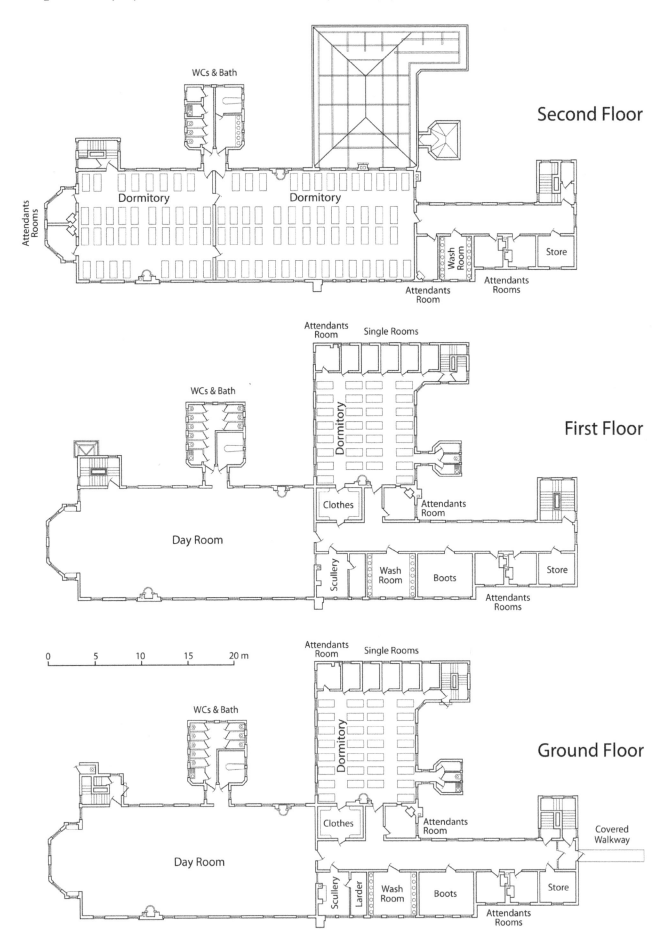

Figure 4-24. Whalley/Calderstones: plans of chronic block. Source: Redrawn by L Mulqueeny of Queen's University Belfast after original plans of Whalley Asylum dated 1912, LCA DDX 1254/1/1/8, Lancashire Archives.

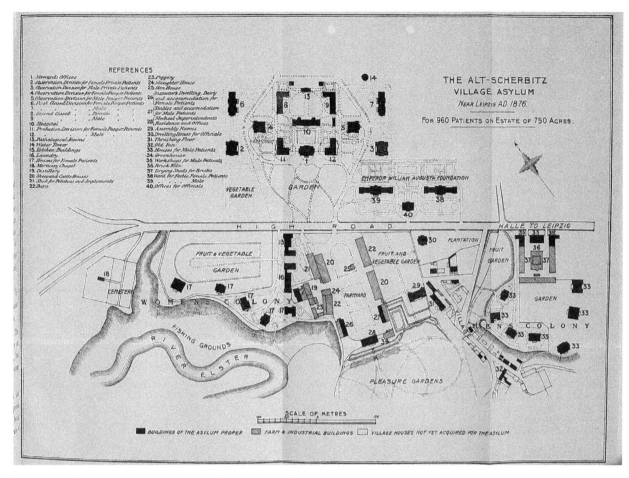

Figure 4-25. Alt Scherbitz: plan of layout. Source: Sibbald, J (1897) *On the plans of modern asylums for the insane poor.* **Edinburgh: James Turner & Co.**

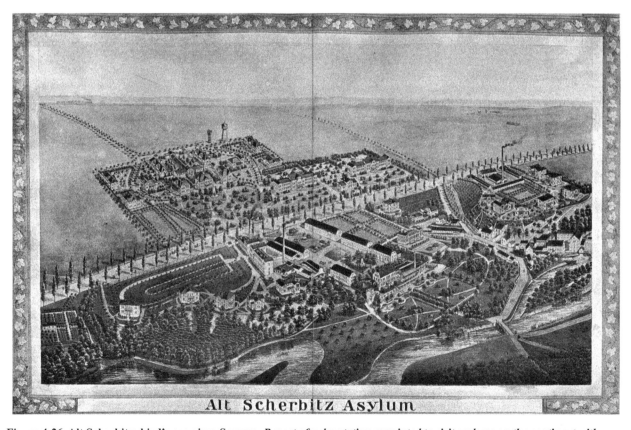

Figure 4-26. Alt Scherbitz: bird's eye view. Source: *Report of a deputation appointed to visit asylums on the continent with recommendations regarding the building of a new (sixth) Lancashire asylum* **(1900). Preston: Lancashire Asylums Board.**

were 1) the combination of agricultural colony with central institute on a large estate, in contrast to the closed institutions of the *Ackerbaucolonien;* 2) the renunciation of corridors, walls and all other restrictions; and 3) the first implementation in Germany of the Scottish 'open door system' as a general principle (Paetz, 1893). At Alt Scherbitz around 90 per cent of the patients worked, the percentages lowering to 70-80 per cent for older patients, which was far in excess of the usual numbers of working patients at asylums. Most villas at Alt Scherbitz contained only 30 to 40 patients and 2/3 of the patients were held in 'open-door' accommodation, signifying a much greater freedom for patients than was the norm (Paetz 1893). Dr Paetz promoted Alt Scherbitz assiduously, not only in his annual reports but also at the International Medical Congress at Copenhagen (1884), naturalist meetings in Magdeburg and Wiesbaden (1887) and the Congress of the German Association for Poor Relief and Charity (1889). Paetz gave a lecture 'Über die Bedeutung der Arbeitskolonien für die Behandlung der Geisteskranken' [On the importance of labour colonies for the treatment of the mentally ill] to the Berlin Psychiatric Association in 1885 and in 1886, he spoke at the Annual Meeting of the Association of German Psychiatrists on the 'open-door system' in Scotland (Sonntag, 1993).

4.3.2. Construction of asylum

The site of the asylum, comprising a large manor-house, and an associated village, flour mill and distillery on an estate of 700 English acres (less land than originally projected), was purchased for one million marks or approximately £50,000. It was originally planned to accommodate 450 patients here, although patient numbers grew to 960 by the mid 1890s, following gradual additions to the site. Buildings, furniture and electric light cost £86,090, making the total cost per bed including land £142, relatively cheap compared to British asylums (*JMS* 1894 40: 487-499). Prussian asylums for the insane were, at this time, managed by the provincial government who appointed superintendents and medical directors and were responsible for oversight and inspection. The asylum was opened in 1876 with 40 patients who were initially accommodated in the old manor house (this building later became the director's house and is still present on the site), while the main asylum buildings were constructed.

The site has been described as a 'river valley' and indeed the asylum is spread out along the north banks of the River Elster. However, the site is slightly elevated above, and slopes gently down to, the course of the river itself which has cut a channel below the level of the surrounding land. The land is largely level (indeed, an airport has been built just north of the asylum in recent years) and lacks the elevation and views that would have been considered optimal for an asylum in Britain.

The foundation stone for the 'Central Institute' or medical section, designed by Dr Koeppe in conjunction with the Royal Surveyor, Kilburger, was laid on 15th August 1876, and the initial building works were completed by 1878 when the building committee dissolved. However, construction work continued throughout the final decades of the nineteenth century. Between 1883 and 1884, the Emperor William Augusta Foundation buildings (38, 39, 40) were built to commemorate the Emperor's golden wedding with funds raised by public subscription. The following year a recreation hall was constructed. By the late 1880s the asylum consisted of buildings 1, 4, 5, 8, 9, 11, 12, 13, 38, 39, 40 and villas A, B, C on the women's side and A, B, C on the men's side. Further villas (men's D, E, F, G and women's D, E) and buildings 2,3, 6 and 7 had been added by 1897 and a separate church was built in 1913 (Sonntag, 1993).

An assistant doctor (Herting) at Alt Scherbitz later wrote of the period 1889 to 1899, that 'Es war eine Zeit der Hochflut der Besucher' [There was a high-tide of visitors at this time]. Herting sought to explain the attraction of Alt Scherbitz in his diary notes, 'Keine Planken, keine Palisaden, keine Gitter, keine Handschuhe … ganz offene Villen, überall Parkettboden, Blumen, Spiegel, weiße Tischtücher, Licht, Luft' [No planks, no fences, no bars, no [restraint] gloves … very open villas; everywhere - hardwood floors, flowers, mirrors, white tablecloths, light, air](Sonntag, 1993: 31).

The earliest published account of Alt Scherbitz to appear in English was in the *Boston Medical and Surgical Journal,* by notable American neurologist George Miller Beard, who visited Alt Scherbitz as part of a tour of European asylums, calling it 'the institution that is now exciting so much attention in Germany' (Beard, 1880). He praised the asylum (among others) for the use of 'non-restraint' and labour as a therapeutic agent.

The asylum was further publicised among the international psychiatric community in 1889 on the publication of *The Insane in Foreign Countries* by William P Letchworth who was President of the New York State Board of Charities. The author visited a number of asylums in the British Isles and Europe and his account of Alt Scherbitz, which is the last institution to be described, indicates that it is seen as providing exceptional facilities. He writes, 'Of the many asylums for the insane in Europe, there is none more interesting than that of Alt Scherbitz … Here has been wrought out a system in which are incorporated some of the best and most modern methods of caring for the insane in England, Scotland, France and other countries.' (Letchworth 1889: 279) By the time of Letchworth's visit in the 1880s, the asylum had been expanded to accommodate 600. The patients to be provided for were the 'apparently curable' but also the 'incurable and dangerous insane' of the province of Saxony. Patients who could pay were expected to do so, and wealthier patients were permitted to have their own attendants. Patients of three classes were admitted, the first class paid 1,200 marks a year, second class 600 marks a year and third class 240 marks a year, the third class also receiving clothing in addition to maintenance (although later accounts indicate that those who could not pay had their fees covered by outside bodies). The provincial government made up any shortfall between payments and the actual cost. (Letchworth 1889:283).

Letchworth's book was briefly reviewed in the *Journal of Mental Science* on its publication in 1889 and attention was drawn to the description of Alt Scherbitz, the detached layout of the buildings and the high numbers of patients employed in outdoor or indoor work (JMS 1889 35:232-233). In 1891, Dr Hack Tuke, descendant of a noted psychiatric dynasty and editor of the *Journal of Mental Science*, recorded his visit to the 'now celebrated' Alt Scherbitz, describing it as an example of the 'pavilion' or 'cottage' plan. Tuke also records that the, 'impression received on approaching the institution is an agreeable one and conveys no idea of the object for which it is designed... When one thinks of some of the gigantic and monotonous structures which have grown up in England as county asylums, one is thankful, indeed, that the spirit, under the influence of which such cumbrous piles of buildings have been too frequently erected, was far away, and could not desecrate this pastoral scene' (*JMS* 1891 37:465-473). By the time of Tuke's visit the asylum had grown to 700 patients and accommodation was projected for 1,000. One third of the patients were in the central institution and two thirds in the villas. The average cost per bed was £50. Of the 700 patients, 630 were 'either paid for by the parish or were in very poor circumstances'. The remaining 70 were divided into two classes paying £80 or £40 per year. The main difference in accommodation is seen as the class of furniture, which varied between first and second class. The male villa A for these patients is described as being built 'in the style of a Swiss chalet'. A description is given of some of the individual villas and it is noted that the 'open-door system is carried out' in most of the villas. The emphasis is on the pleasant grounds, the segregated layout and the employment of the patients. Tuke compares Alt Scherbitz to two similar institutions in the US, Kankakee and Willard and also a private Scottish institution, Craig House.

In 1892, Burdett published his influential *Hospitals and Asylums of the World* in four volumes with plans. The very lengthy review in the *Journal of Mental Science* criticises the book's omissions, stating that, 'We should have expected to see [a plan] of Alt Scherbitz, and to have had the increasingly-adopted principle of segregation, of which this asylum is the type, more prominently brought forward' (*JMS* 1892 38:271-275).

The Presidential address of the annual meeting of the Medico-Psychological Association, delivered on 12th June 1894 by Conolly Norman, Medical Superintendent of Richmond District Asylum in Dublin and editor of the *Journal of Mental Science*, drew attention once again to Alt Scherbitz. Norman called it 'so successful a new departure that one cannot doubt but that it will be the model asylum of the future...Instead of vast buildings,

modelled on a prison, a barrack or a monastery; instead even of semi-detached buildings connected by passages, the entire institution consists of groups of houses entirely detached and every one surrounded by its own garden' (*JMS* 1894 40:487-499). Norman describes the colony buildings as 'constructed to resemble, as far as possible, the ordinary houses of the neighbouring country'. The cost of the asylum was felt to be moderate. Norman concludes, 'This bold departure from the conventional ideas of asylum architecture and asylum management seems...to form the coping-stone to the great structure of non-restraint, the foundations of which were laid by Pinel and Tuke more than a hundred years ago. It is to be hoped that...this last reform may soon be accepted, and that we shall not see many more of those vast and costly buildings erected which one of our number long since truly designated as "gigantic mistakes"' (this was Yellowlees, a Scottish medical superintendent). Dr Hack Tuke commented on the address and recommended all connected with asylums to study Alt Scherbitz and advised 'the younger men especially to include in their autumn holiday a visit to Alt Scherbitz, where they would find Dr Paetz most happy to give them every information'.

Dr Albrecht Paetz, the medical Director of Alt Scherbitz published in 1893 a full-length monograph in German on the hospital and its therapeutic regime, (Paetz 1893). However, it was not until 1895 that this book was reviewed in the *Journal of Mental Science*, the reviewer commenting that he had been waiting for the book to be published in English, due to its importance, but a translation had not been forthcoming. According to the reviewer, Paetz saw a layout of 'detached pavilions' as 'an essential vital development of the principles of non-restraint' (*JMS* 1895 41:697-703). Asylums were becoming less prison-like and 'approximating more closely to the conditions of ordinary life'. Systematic employment was seen as the 'necessary complement of non-restraint'. Work must be adapted to the individual patients' capabilities and must be 'of a nature having some interest' i.e. patients were not to be employed in pointless activities such as digging holes and filling them again, as was common in institutions for the poor. The varied fertility of Alt Scherbitz was seen as giving varied occupation and this was important because the monotony of institution life 'serves to cripple the intelligence and depress the spirits'. Classification was also easier, which made individual care more possible. In closed asylums the 'unfortunate mean' were left to 'struggle unassisted against the tendency to dementia'. Paetz felt that the beneficial effect of work was lost if the patient had to return behind bars afterwards, or if the attendant was only there to issue commands. The reviewer concludes, 'The feature which will strike the average English observer in Alt Scherbitz is that there is no asylum there, or that the asylum exists only as a theoretical entity. No building of those which are grouped together under this name contains more than about forty patients. Even the central institution consists of ten pavilions'. Connecting corridors were dispensed with because they gave an 'air of confinement' and the reviewer affirms that 'the asylum of the future will consist of groups of entirely detached houses which will present the freedom and the homeliness so often spoken of and so unattainable in the colossal institutions of the past'.

After a visit to Alt Scherbitz in the late 1890s, the Scottish Lunacy Commissioner John Sibbald claimed that all the buildings were like private houses externally and internally. There was no wall around the central institution or the colony and the only enclosed spaces were gardens. (Sibbald, 1897: 24). The lack of a general heating apparatus, houses being heated by stoves or low pressure steam in single rooms, was thought to make the houses more domestic in feel. Food was distributed to each house from a central dining room by wagon. A recreation hall was used for religious services and entertainments and was set apart, making it seem that the patients were out of the asylum when they went to it. A billiard room was attached for the men. There were no corridors in the asylum (which would have given a prison character) and every house had its own front door. Most of the doors were unlocked during the day, in accordance with the open door system—33 per cent of the patients were in locked houses and 67 per cent in open houses. Escapes and suicides were lower than at other asylums and no 'untoward sexual incident' had ever occurred among the patients. Sibbald concluded that Alt Scherbitz 'seems to me to be the type of asylum that conforms most completely to the most modern and the best idea of what an asylum ought to be' (Sibbald, 1897: 31).

Under the influence of Dr Sibbald, a deputation from the Edinburgh Lunacy Board also made a visit to Alt Scherbitz (among other asylums in Britain and the continent) and their report was published the same year as Dr Sibbald's (1897) although their visit was subsequent to his. The deputation claimed that Alt Scherbitz was 'altogether different from anything the deputation ever saw before', particularly since there were no walls or railings and no porter's lodge or gateway (Report of an Edinburgh deputation, 1897: 15). The deputation was told that the attendants lived in complete community with the patients having no separate sitting and bed rooms and living 'in some measure as in a family circle' (Report of an Edinburgh deputation, 1897: 16). They describe the central institution, 'with its pretty ivy-covered houses', as giving the impression 'of a thriving suburb of London or some English town' (Report of an Edinburgh deputation, 1897: 17). There were no padded rooms and attendants did not walk about with keys jangling at their belts. The houses were praised for having 'none of that dead uniformity of design which produces monotony' (Report of an Edinburgh deputation, 1897: 19). It was also noted that the houses all had a southern exposure, facing SE, S or SW (although the demands of symmetry in the central institution suggest that orientation to the south was not the first consideration, and indeed they do not all face south). All were of two storeys (the later villas, which are of three storeys may not have been completed at this point) and the entrances were above the ground, the basement providing cellars and heating arrangements. The houses

and grounds were all arranged so as to make observation easier, e.g. there was no vestibule where patients entered. Each house had a verandah which opened into the main dayroom for the use of patients, and there was a separate entrance for attendants and stores. Sick patients were wheeled out onto the verandah on fine days to get the benefit of sun and air. 'The stair to the main apartments is contiguous to the main room, not guarded or shut off in any way' (Report of an Edinburgh deputation, 1897: 20). Floors were of wood or parquetry laid on asphalt and windows were of 'thin plate glass' with fairly large panes, supervision being found sufficient to prevent breakages. Furniture and furnishings were as plain as possible 'though good and comfortable' without ornamental cornices. 'One reason given for simplicity of design and the absence of ornamentation is that decoration is apt to excite the patients' (Report of an Edinburgh deputation, 1897: 20). The china, glass and earthenware were not unbreakable and were the same as in private houses. The washing room consisted of a board with a row of china basins that were filled from a tap at the end of the row and waste water thrown in a gutter at the back. Each house had a large garden where the patients were free to walk, only in the closed houses was the outer door locked but 'well-behaved' patients could move in and out even there. The closed houses had a special window lock developed by Dr Paetz consisting of external blinds that could be raised or lowered from within the house by a cord or chain in a casing with a box at the bottom. The box was locked with a key where the end of the cord was fastened. In the small kitchen in the villas it was possible to do 'sick-cooking', a cup of tea or coffee or boil an egg. They note that all the coffins needed in the asylum were made in the carpenter's shop. There was no sewerage system at Alt Scherbitz, all closets were earth but the introduction of such plumbing would be easy due to the absence of corridors. The deputation concluded that Alt Scherbitz was 'the logical development of the 'open door' system first introduced in Scotland', and had been made possible 'by the introduction of electricity. The telephone is in use all over Alt Scherbitz, and communication is instantly possible between any two parts of the asylum' (Report of an Edinburgh deputation, 1897: 27-28).

A deputation from the Lancashire Asylums Board visited Alt Scherbitz, among other asylums in Germany, Belgium and France and published their report in 1900, describing Alt Scherbitz as the 'forerunner and the best known of the segregated or village colony type of asylums'. They indicated that Dr Paetz made extensions and improvements between 1888 and 1891 which were 'designed principally for the perfecting of the system of family life in small communities' (Report of a Lancashire deputation, 1900: 27). The dormitories were arranged with one central large room opening into two or more smaller, so as to facilitate supervision. The brick the buildings is made of is noted to be of somewhat coarser quality than in other German asylums. The villas were said to be in the Italian style, and were less ornamented than other asylums but had more natural decoration by ivy and climbing plants. The administration building was described as elegant and tasteful. Each of the observation buildings was entered from a verandah into a large dayroom which also functioned as a dining room with smaller dayrooms to each side. The connection between the three principal dayrooms was by glass-panelled doors, which were usually left open. Doors to dormitories were also glazed. The superficial and cubic space for patients in these buildings seemed ample. Windows of single and stronger isolation rooms were glazed with thick plate which could not easily be broken. (Report of a Lancashire deputation, 1900: 27-35).

The attendants slept in the dormitories with patients, an arrangement which the deputation thought was 'no longer practicable' in England. They felt that in England sleeping rooms for attendants would be required for those on duty at night and detached blocks with recreation rooms for those off duty. Private villas were furnished with sofas, chairs, writing tables and other tables in various forms, and flower stands. Walls in the private villas were papered and in the others they were oil painted up to six feet and distempered above with a stencilled frieze and adorned with pictures and mirrors. Dayroom floors were of hard wood, polished with sometimes a pattern or parquet border. Beds were of iron with a straw palliasse and horse

hair mattress and pillow and a bedside table between every two beds. Beds for epileptics had high wooden sides and very sloping firm pillows. Baths were of enamelled iron and the water was heated in copper cisterns. In summer as many as possible bathed in the River Elster. Dr Paetz felt that natural ventilation by doors and windows was the best.

The deputation contrasted the segregated plan in the US where villas were arranged on a regular plan round the sides of a large square or on a curved line, with Germany where houses were various and more scattered. Dr Paetz told the deputation that the smaller houses were better liked than the larger ones. The deputation thought that dormitories for those requiring observation at night should be made larger and connected with other rooms by larger openings, not mere doors. They noted the danger of publicity and outcry in England after any accident or suicide and implied that safety measures might have to be more stringent if the plan were adapted for England but concluded that they 'have no doubt that before any future new asylum is commenced in this country the arrangement of that at Alt Scherbitz should be most carefully considered'. They concluded their report by recommending a villa colony system for the new asylum for Lancashire (Report of a Lancashire deputation, 1900: 27-35, 63-69).

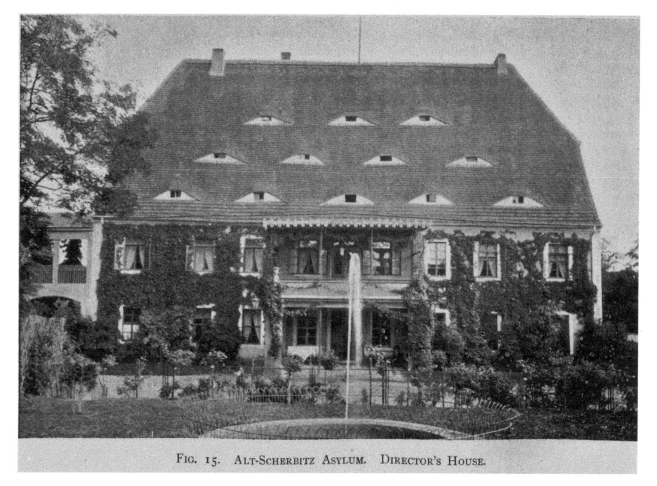

FIG. 15. ALT-SCHERBITZ ASYLUM. DIRECTOR'S HOUSE.

Figure 4-27. Alt Scherbitz: manor house, originally used as patient accommodation and later as the director's house. Source: *Report of a deputation appointed to visit asylums on the continent with recommendations regarding the building of a new (sixth)* **Lancashire asylum (1900). Preston: Lancashire Asylums Board.**

4.3.3. Selected buildings

Letchworth was keen to note that the central buildings 'are entirely separate from one another, having no corridor connection'. Dr Paetz asserted that isolation of patients was avoided and there were no cribs in use or any padded rooms. If patients tried to tear off their clothing they were put in strong garments buttoned at the back, but still had free use of all their limbs. He regarded non-restraint as a guiding principle, 'Every sort of restraint by force is strictly interdicted as being against the fundamental principles of the asylum. The patients enjoy the largest imaginable freedom, the asylum representing the non-restraint system in its widest sense. Restraint is easy to dispense with if one earnestly wishes to dispense with it' (Letchworth 1889: 286). Nurses/attendants averaged about one to ten patients and they lived with the patients, sleeping in the dormitories. The central institution was heated by hot air and the 'isolating apartments' by hot water pipes. In the villas, porcelain stoves were used and supplemented by open fires, which aided heating and ventilation. Water was elevated by a force-pump and distributed by gravitation. Earth closets were provided and the waste used on the farm. Employment suited to the mental and bodily condition of the patient and relaxation in the form of indoor and outdoor games was advocated as a means of cure. Women were employed in the kitchen, the wash-house and the dairy and many worked in the sewing-room making clothes and repairing items for the institution. Some worked in the garden or the fields. Most men did agricultural work or trades, but some who were acute cases, the physically incapacitated or extraordinarily excited did not work (there does not appear to have been an exclusion from work on a class basis—at least this is not mentioned). Patients worked in the brick and tile yards and others worked as joiners, masons, wagon-makers, blacksmiths, carpenters, smiths, shoemakers, tailors, saddlers, bookbinders, stone-masons, painters, basket-makers and clerks. There were occasional leisure excursions for patients and swimming took place in the River Elster (a bath-house was built on the river bank). Letchworth summarises, 'At this institution one is favourably impressed with the absence of barriers, the freedom from restraint, the kind treatment accorded the patients, the thorough supervision of the large numbers occupied in the various employments, the general atmosphere of cheerfulness and quiet, and the cleanliness and country-life aspect of the place…Without any attempt at ambitious architectural display or costly interior furnishing, there is, apparently, in this institution everything essential to the comfort of the insane. The whole system of care and treatment seems adapted to insure highly satisfactory results; and yet a stranger passing along the highway and catching glimpses of the asylum buildings through the trees and shrubbery, would hardly suspect from their unpretentious character and their arrangement upon the estate that the place was a public hospital and asylum for insane people.' (Letchworth 1889:291-2)

Administration Building (1)

The administration building (number 1) (Figure 4-28) contained a reception room, a conference rooms, the superintendent's office, an accountant's office, a treasurer's office and porter's rooms. On the second floor were the living and other apartments of the second physician and of the accountant. A spire and clock were added in the 1890s (Letchworth, 1889: 284).

Hospital (10)

For patients suffering from more serious bodily diseases and housing 18 patients of each sex (Figure 4-29, 4-30). Behind the administration building, 'completely hidden by trees' was the mortuary. An exceptional feature of the hospital was a room at the end of each ward with two doors, one opening into the ward, one into the entrance hall. This was used for patients at the end of their life, so that they 'may not be seen dying by the other patients' and could be removed without passing through the ward. The upper storey of the hospital contained rooms for two attendants on each side and store rooms. The hospital was connected by a covered walkway to the mortuary.

Reception Stations (later Observation Division) (4) and (5)

In 1889 (building uses altered slightly over time), buildings 4 and 5 were used as 'reception stations', women to the west, men to the east (Figure 4-31). Acute curable cases stayed here while incurable patients were transferred to other departments. They were built to accommodate 15 patients each and are described as 'plain but comfortable buildings' which 'within and without resemble private dwellings'. The doors were unlocked and 'there is no suggestion of irksome restraint'. The head female attendant lived in the women's observation station and an assistant physician in the men's building (Letchworth, 1889: 284).

Observation Stations (later Probation Division) (11) and (12)

Buildings 11 and 12 were observation stations for patients who were not acute but needed special observation 'because they were not sufficiently capable of self-control nor reliable enough for reception in the colonial stations' (Figure 4-32). They were built for 35 patients, with furnishing that was 'ample and comfortable'. Open fires were allowed in these buildings. The windows were largely unlocked, the only exception being one with a lockable sash in a room that was 'less under the attendant's eye'. Frosted panes were fitted in windows that looked onto accommodation occupied by the opposite sex. At the back of the buildings were 'shrubbery-planted plots' and in front 'wide porches and the open grounds'. 'Fine views, immediate and distant, are had from both windows and porches'. Curtained couches were provided in the women's

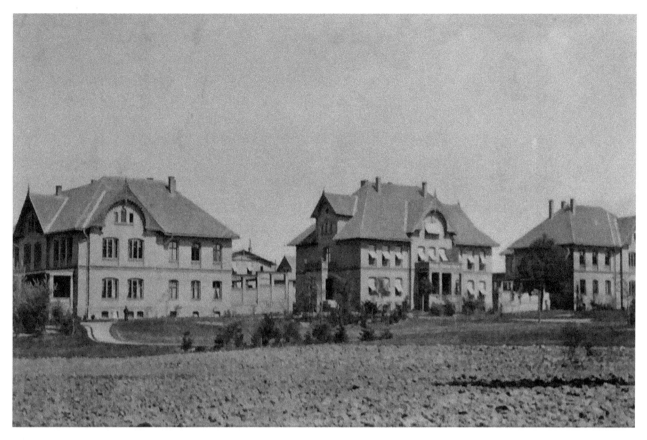

Figure 4-28. Alt Scherbitz: administration building (centre) flanked by observation stations. Source: Author's photograph of image in Alt Scherbitz Traditionskabinett.

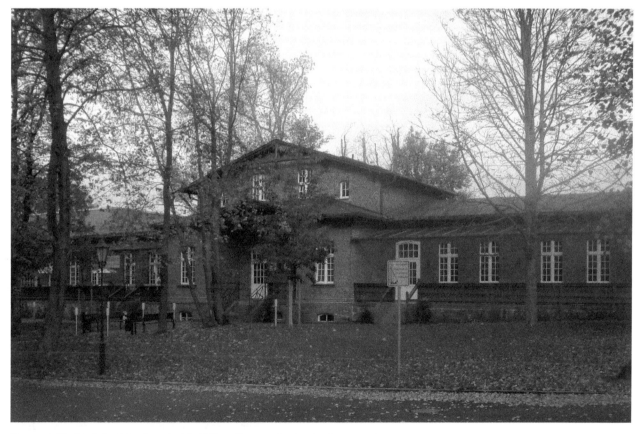

Figure 4-29. Alt Scherbitz: hospital building. Source: Author's photograph.

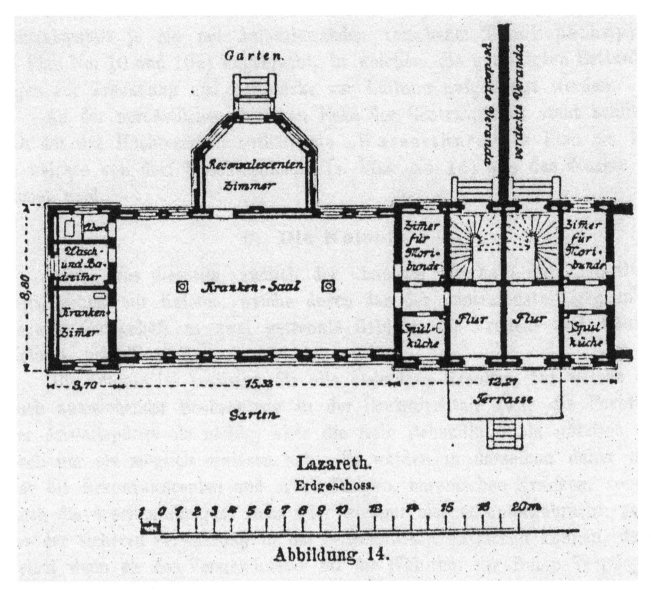

Figure 4-30. Alt Scherbitz: plan of hospital building. Source: Paetz, A. (1893). *Die Kolonisirung der Geisteskranken in Verbindung mit dem Offen-Thür-System: ihre historische Entwickelung und die Art ihrer Ausführung auf Rittergut Alt-Scherbitz.* **Berlin: Verlag von Julius Springer.**

side for patients who desired occasional rest. Flowers were placed in the rooms and windows, 'there is also an abundance of health-giving light'. There were plain chairs and sofas in the sitting-rooms and each station had separate sitting and dining rooms. Six single rooms were set apart for higher class patients. Sleeping apartments were 'mostly on the associate plan' (i.e dorms rather than single rooms) and had iron bedsteads, each with a temporary foot-board, straw, india fibre or horse-hair mattress over which was placed a second mattress, blanket, blanket cover, bolster and pillow. The oiled wooden floors were uncarpeted. The walls shutting off the grounds from the observation court were removed because they were found unnecessary (Letchworth 1889: 284-286).

First Closed Division (6) and (7)

Built c1890 to house 51 patients each (Figures 4-33, 4-34, 4-35). The closed divisions were constantly under

lock and key during the day time and contained seclusion rooms. Patients who might escape, be violent or who were 'untrustworthy' stayed here. The first division were more easily managed and less restless than the second (Paetz 1893; 96).

Detention Houses (later Second Closed Division) (8) and (9)

Buildings 8 and 9 (no longer present on the site) were used as 'detention houses' for patients who were restless, dangerous or showed a desire to escape (Figure 4-36). To the rear of the detention houses were yards with low brick walls surmounted by pillars which supported an architrave. There were no bars or gratings except on the windows of isolation rooms. The detention buildings 'like the other buildings, have numerous windows, from which there are pleasant outlooks'. The interiors were 'cheerful' and comfortably furnished. Women in the

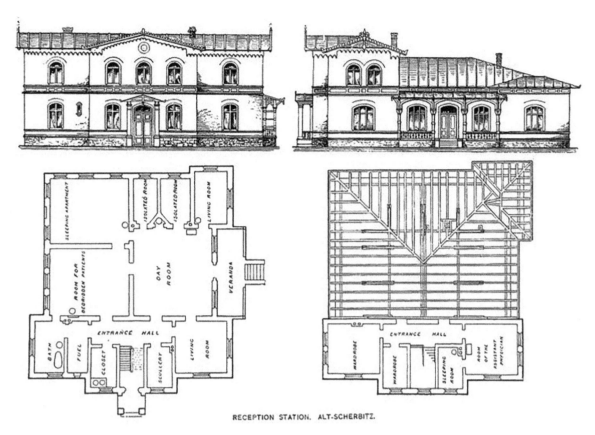

RECEPTION STATION. ALT-SCHERBITZ.

Figure 4-31. Alt Scherbitz: plans and elevations of reception stations. Source: Letchworth, W. P. (1889) *The Insane in Foreign Countries.* **New York and London: G P Putnam's Sons.**

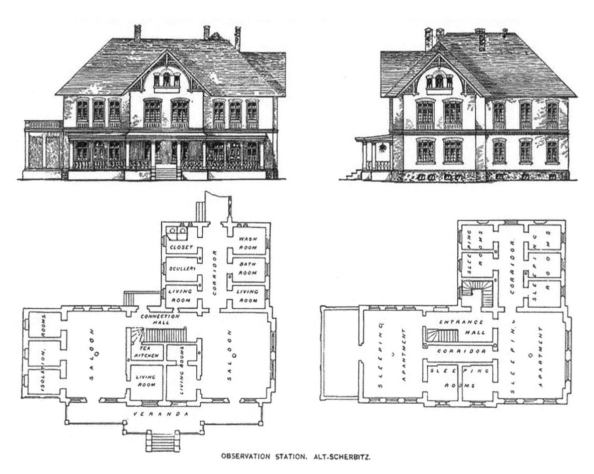

OBSERVATION STATION. ALT-SCHERBITZ.

Figure 4-32. Alt Scherbitz: plans and elevations of observation stations. Source: Letchworth, W. P. (1889) *The Insane in Foreign Countries.* **New York and London: G P Putnam's Sons.**

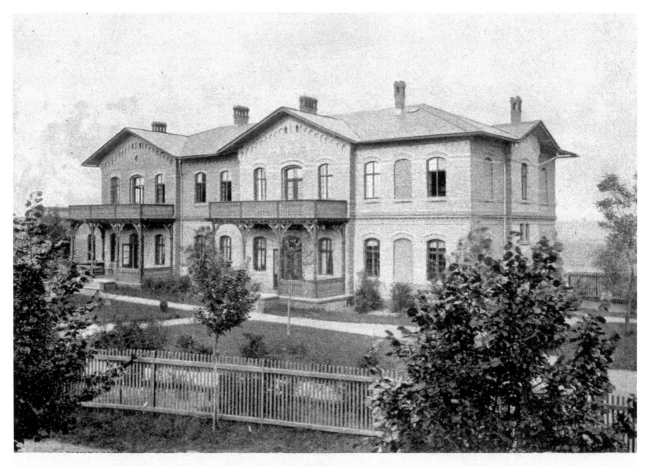

Fig. 21. First Closed House, Central Asylum. Alt-Scherbitz.

Figure 4-33. Alt Scherbitz: first closed division, building 7. Source: *Report of a deputation appointed to visit asylums on the continent with recommendations regarding the building of a new (sixth) Lancashire asylum* (1900). Preston: Lancashire Asylums Board.

female detention house were encouraged to sew or knit. However, Letchworth was not allowed to take notes in their presence 'it being explained that pains were taken to occupy their minds, and every thing likely to prove a cause of disturbance was avoided'. There were 14 isolation rooms, which 'generally stand empty in the day-time' and were used as bedrooms for restless patients at night. Those used for isolating maniacal patients had internal blinds to the windows. Each reception station had two isolation rooms and each detention department five (Letchworth claims this was all that was thought necessary although the plans show additional isolation rooms e.g. in reception stations) (Letchworth, 1889: 285-286).

Private Division (2) and (3)

Built c1890 to house 26 patients each (Figures 4-37, 4-38). For private patients who required special supervision or treatment. These houses were smaller and accommodated fewer patients giving more cubic space per patient. They were furnished as a 'good middle-class private house' with drawing rooms in the female house and billiard tables in the male house.

Pavilions for Infirm cases (Emperor William Augusta Foundation) (38) and (39)

Provision for 60 (later 80) harmless and infirm cases was made in each of buildings 38 and 39 which had dormitories on the upper floor (Figure 4-39, 4-40). An assistant physician occupied building number 40.

Colony (Villas A-G male and A-E female)

Two houses on each side were for private patients and contained from 11 to 20 patients. The other four contained 26 to 42 patients each (there were seven houses on the male side and only five on the female side). The houses were grouped near the farm, laundry, dairy, workshops etc where the patients worked.

It was noted by Letchworth that the villas for men and women were 'widely separated'. There were three classes of cottages or villas. The first and second-class villas were of two storeys and were well furnished, the standard of furnishing depending on the payment made. Letchworth states that the buildings were about 100 yards apart (this is an exaggeration—they are 30 to 40 metres apart at most)

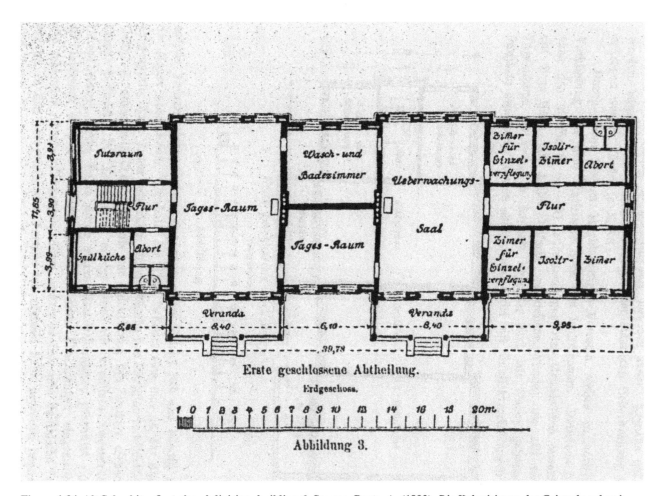

Figure 4-34. Alt Scherbitz: first closed division, building 6. Source: Paetz, A. (1893). *Die Kolonisirung der Geisteskranken in Verbindung mit dem Offen-Thür-System: ihre historische Entwickelung und die Art ihrer Ausführung auf Rittergut Alt-Scherbitz.* Berlin: Verlag von Julius Springer.

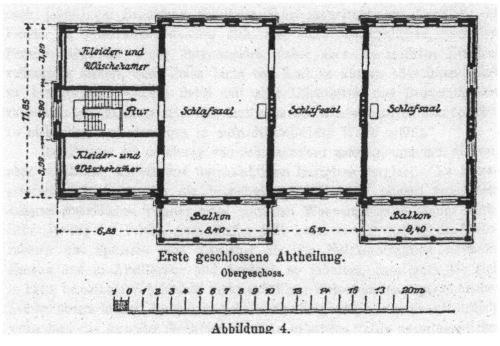

Figure 4-35. Alt Scherbitz: first closed division, building 7. Source: Paetz, A. (1893). *Die Kolonisirung der Geisteskranken in Verbindung mit dem Offen-Thür-System: ihre historische Entwickelung und die Art ihrer Ausführung auf Rittergut Alt-Scherbitz.* Berlin: Verlag von Julius Springer.

175

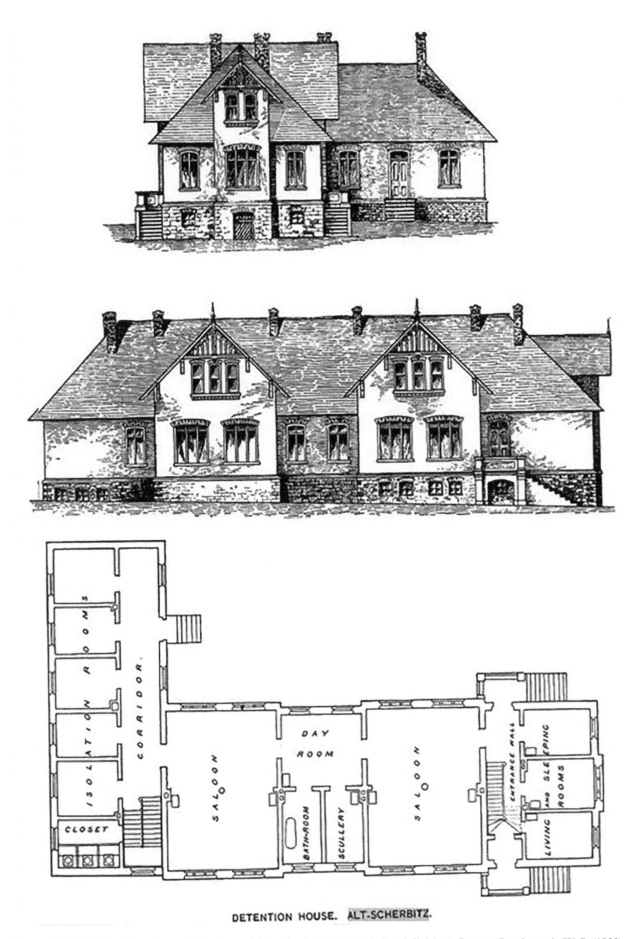

Figure 4-36. Alt Scherbitz: plan and elevations of detention house (second closed division). Source: Letchworth, W. P. (1889) *The Insane in Foreign Countries.* **New York and London: G P Putnam's Sons.**

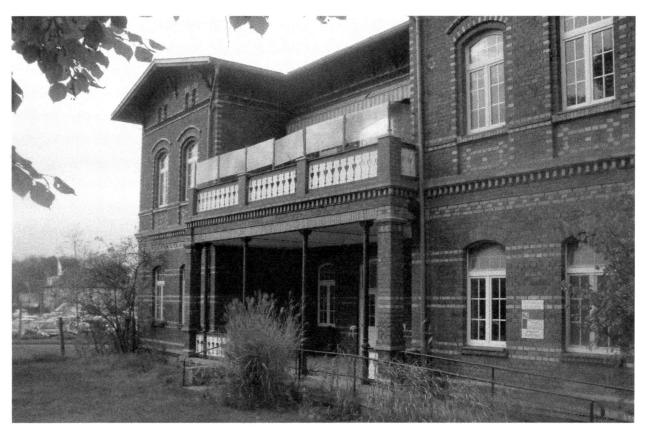

Figure 4-37. Alt Scherbitz: private villa. Source: Author's photograph.

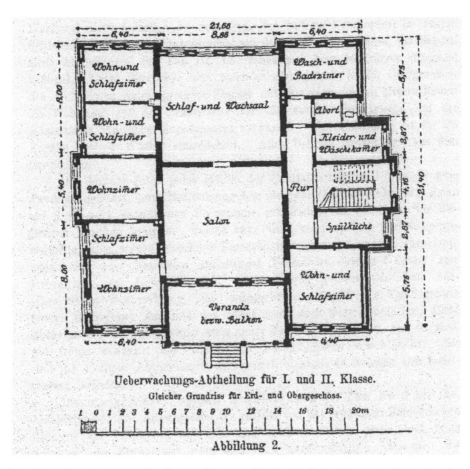

Figure 4-38. Alt Scherbitz: plan of private villa. Source: Paetz, A. (1893). *Die Kolonisirung der Geisteskranken in Verbindung mit dem Offen Thür System: ihre historische Entwickelung und die Art ihrer Ausführung auf Rittergut Alt-Scherbitz*. Berlin: Verlag von Julius Springer.

(Letchworth, 1889: 287). He claimed that glimpses of the river Elster can be obtained from most of them. The villas were separated by neat, low hedges and some had little gardens attached. 'The freedom of the place is shown by open doors, which everywhere meet the eye. It was a pleasant summer day when I was there, and the patients were passing in and out without interference, all, however, being under watchful supervision'. One of the large sitting/day rooms contained a circular sofa in the centre and an ordinary sofa against the wall. There were bright rugs on the floor and flowers and ornaments around the room 'which lent an air of refinement'. Other furnishings included mirrors, pianos, wardrobe, writing-desk, sewing-tables, divans and chests of drawers. Lamps were hung from frescoed ceilings and the walls were coloured. All the cottages were constructed to admit an abundance of sunlight and rested on dry, substantial foundations. The lower floors of the villas housed the sitting or work rooms and the dining room and the sleeping apartments were on upper floors. Letchworth found that it was 'the aim of the management to have every thing relating to the care and treatment of the patients conform as nearly as practicable to home life' (Letchworth 1889: 288).

The women's villas were occupied as follows:

Villa A – 20 patients, 2 attendants, also residence for voluntary physician – 1st and 2nd class (Figures 4-41, 4-42)

Villa B – 11 patients, 1 attendant – 1st and 2nd class (Figues 4-43, 4-44))

Villa C – 26 patients, 2 attendants – 3rd class (Figures 4-45, 4-46, 4-47)

Villa D – 31 patients, 2 attendants – 3rd class (Figures 4-48, 4-49)

Villa E – 41 patients, 4 attendants – 3rd class, also a small hospital ward (Figures 4-50, 4-51, 4-52)

The male villas were occupied as follows:

Villa A – 13 patients, 2 attendants – 1st and 2nd class (Figure 4-53)

Villa B – 11 patients, 2 attendants – 1st and 2nd class (Figure 4-54)

Villa C – 31 patients, 2 attendants – 3rd class (Figure 4-55, 4-56)

Villa D – 32 patients, 2 attendants – 3rd class (Figure 4-57)

Villa E – 5 patients, 1 attendant (1st class) and 3 assistant physicians (Figure 4-58, 4-59)

Villa F – 41 patients, 4 attendants – 3rd class (Figure 4-60)

Villa G – 42 patients, 4 attendants – 3rd class, also a small hospital ward (Figure 4-61, 4-62, 4-63)

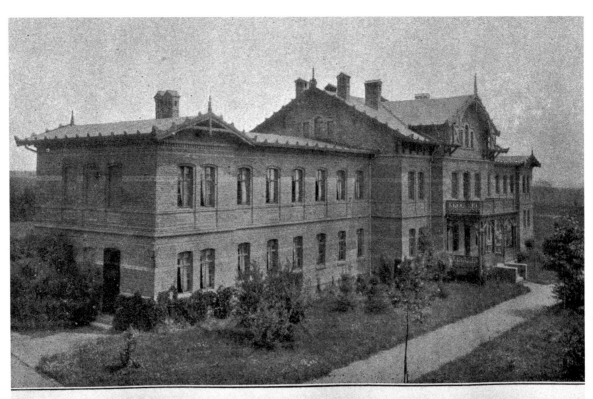

FIG. 32. EMPEROR WILLIAM–AUGUSTA BUILDING. ALT-SCHERBITZ.

Figure 4-39. Alt Scherbitz: Emporer William-Augusta Building. Source: *Report of a deputation appointed to visit asylums on the continent with recommendations regarding the building of a new (sixth) Lancashire asylum (1900).* **Preston: Lancashire Asylums Board.**

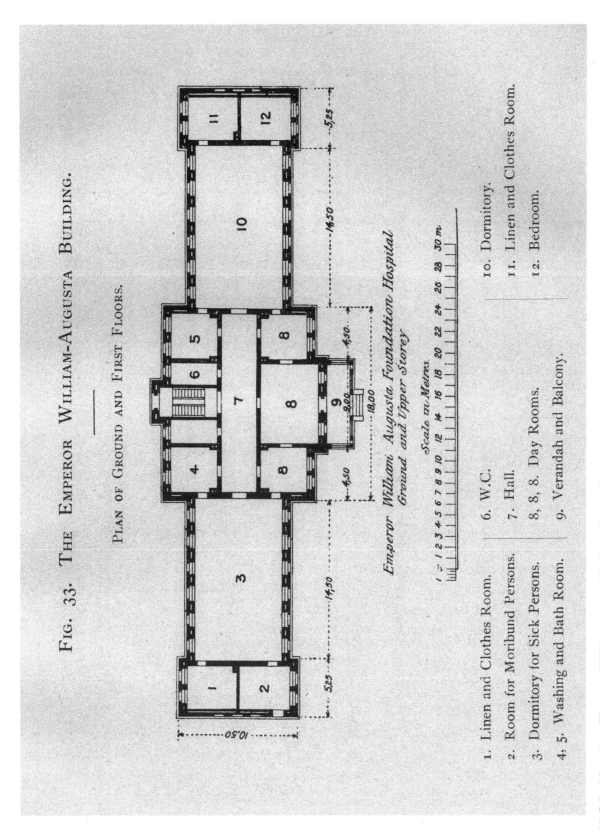

Fig. 33. The Emperor William-Augusta Building.

Plan of Ground and First Floors.

*Emperor William Augusta Foundation Hospital
Ground and Upper Storey*

Scale in Metres.

1. Linen and Clothes Room.
2. Room for Moribund Persons.
3. Dormitory for Sick Persons.
4, 5. Washing and Bath Room.
6. W.C.
7. Hall.
8, 8, 8. Day Rooms.
9. Verandah and Balcony.
10. Dormitory.
11. Linen and Clothes Room.
12. Bedroom.

Figure 4-40. Alt Scherbitz: plan of Emporer William-Augusta Building. Source: *Report of a deputation appointed to visit asylums on the continent with recommendations regarding the building of a new (sixth) Lancashire asylum (1900).* **Preston: Lancashire Asylums Board.**

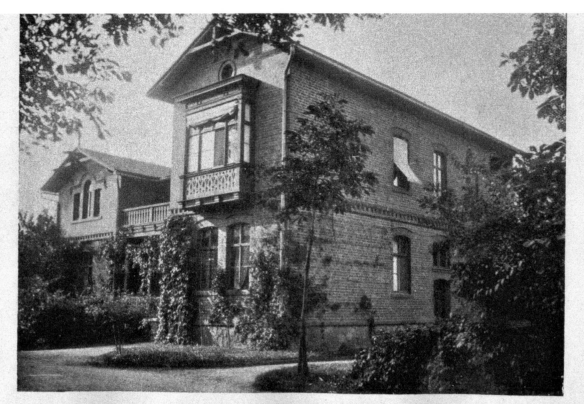

FIG. 30. VILLA IN COLONY. ALT-SCHERBITZ.

Figure 4-41. Alt Scherbitz: female villa A. Source: *Report of a deputation appointed to visit asylums on the continent with recommendations regarding the building of a new (sixth) Lancashire asylum (1900).* **Preston: Lancashire Asylums Board.**

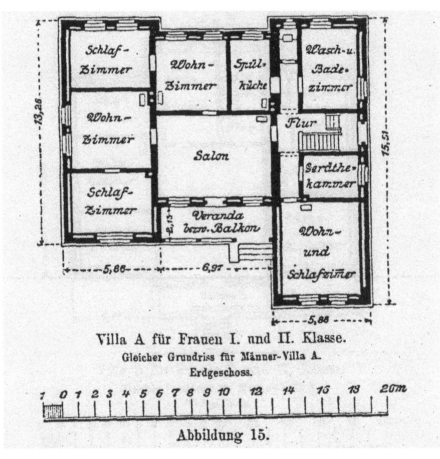

Figure 4-42. Alt Scherbitz: plan of female villa A. Source: Paetz, A. (1893). *Die Kolonisirung der Geisteskranken in Verbindung mit dem Offen-Thür-System: ihre historische Entwickelung und die Art ihrer Ausführung auf Rittergut Alt-Scherbitz.* **Berlin: Verlag von Julius Springer.**

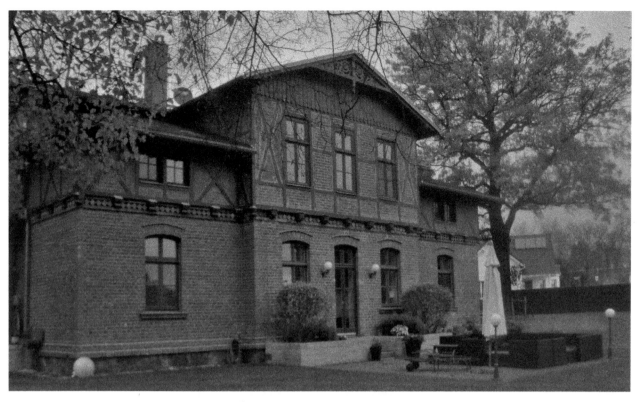

Figure 4-43. Alt Scherbitz: female villa B. Source: Author's photograph.

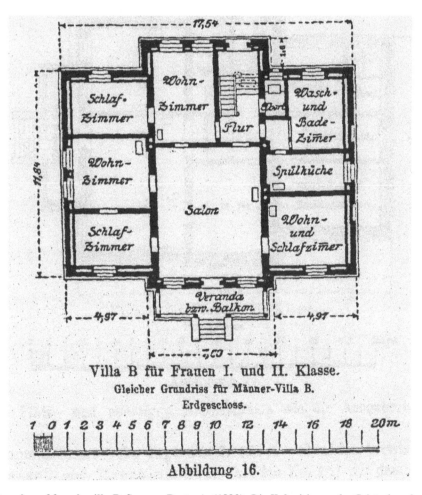

Figure 4-44. Alt Scherbitz: plan of female villa B. Source: Paetz, A. (1893). *Die Kolonisirung der Geisteskranken in Verbindung mit dem Offen-Thür-System: ihre historische Entwickelung und die Art ihrer Ausführung auf Rittergut Alt-Scherbitz.* Berlin: Verlag von Julius Springer.

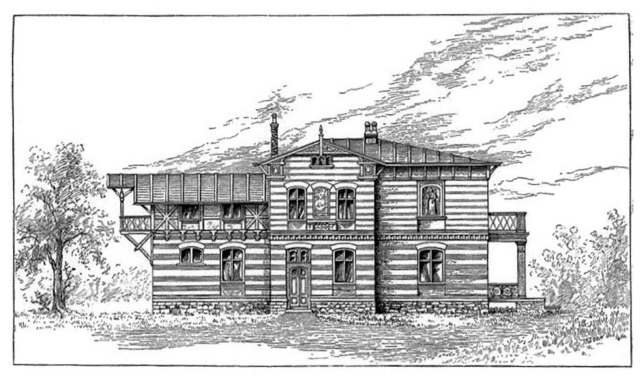

A VILLA FOR PATIENTS. ALT-SCHERBITZ.

Figure 4-45. Alt Scherbitz: elevation of female villa C. Source: Letchworth, W. P. (1889) *The Insane in Foreign Countries.* **New York and London: G P Putnam's Sons.**

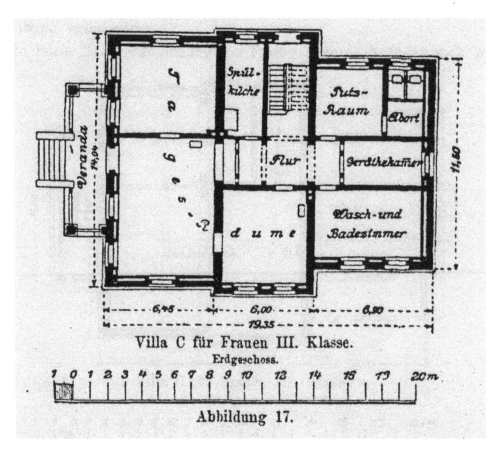

Figure 4-46. Alt Scherbitz: ground floor plan of female villa C. Source: Paetz, A. (1893). *Die Kolonisirung der Geisteskranken in Verbindung mit dem Offen-Thür-System: ihre historische Entwickelung und die Art ihrer Ausführung auf Rittergut Alt-Scherbitz.* **Berlin: Verlag von Julius Springer.**

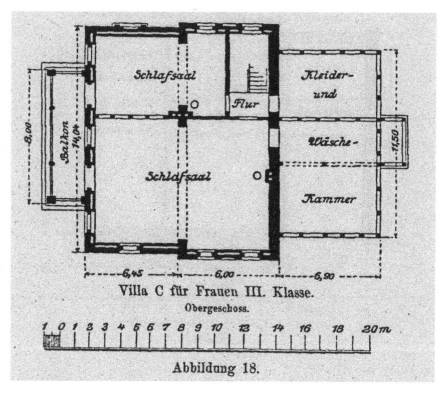

Figure 4-47. Alt Scherbitz: first floor plan of female villa C. Source: Paetz, A. (1893). *Die Kolonisirung der Geisteskranken in Verbindung mit dem Offen-Thür-System: ihre historische Entwickelung und die Art ihrer Ausführung auf Rittergut Alt-Scherbitz.* Berlin: Verlag von Julius Springer.

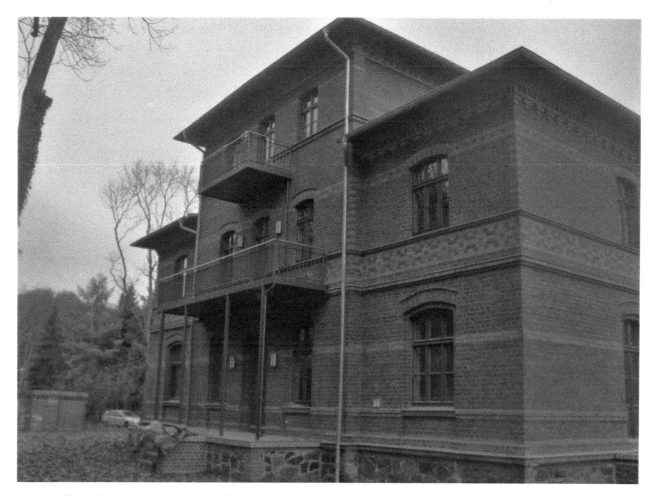

Figure 4-48. Alt Scherbitz: female villa D. Source: Author's photograph.

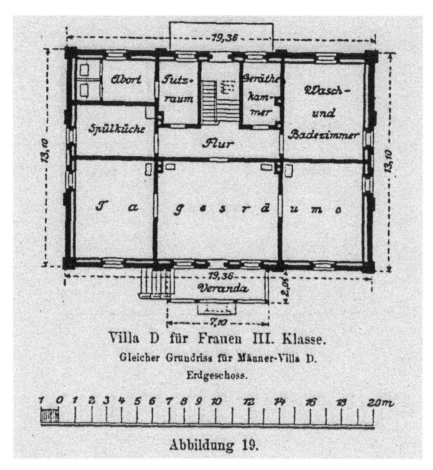

Figure 4-49. Alt Scherbitz: ground floor plan of female villa D. Source: Paetz, A. (1893). *Die Kolonisirung der Geisteskranken in Verbindung mit dem Offen-Thür-System: ihre historische Entwickelung und die Art ihrer Ausführung auf Rittergut Alt-Scherbitz*. Berlin: Verlag von Julius Springer.

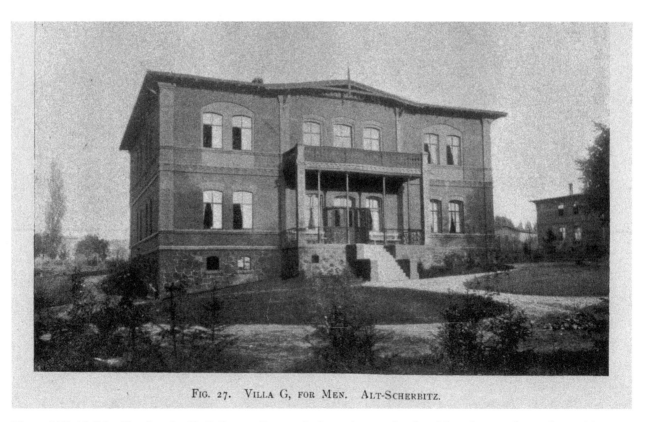

Figure 4-50. Alt Scherbitz: female villa E. Source: *Report of a deputation appointed to visit asylums on the continent with recommendations regarding the building of a new (sixth) Lancashire asylum* (1900). Preston: Lancashire Asylums Board.

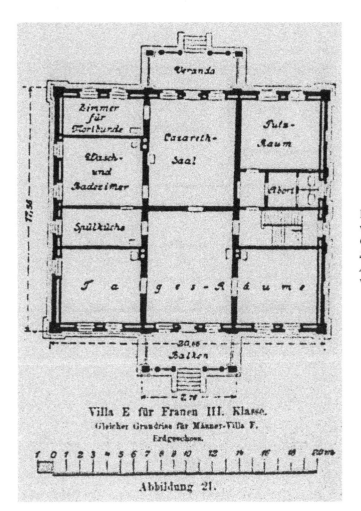

Figure 4-51. Alt Scherbitz: ground floor plan of female villa E. Source: Paetz, A. (1893). *Die Kolonisirung der Geisteskranken in Verbindung mit dem Offen-Thür-System: ihre historische Entwickelung und die Art ihrer Ausführung auf Rittergut Alt-Scherbitz*. Berlin: Verlag von Julius Springer.

Figure 4-52. Alt Scherbitz: first floor plan of female villa E. Source: Paetz, A. (1893). *Die Kolonisirung der Geisteskranken in Verbindung mit dem Offen-Thür-System: ihre historische Entwickelung und die Art ihrer Ausführung auf Rittergut Alt-Scherbitz*. Berlin: Verlag von Julius Springer.

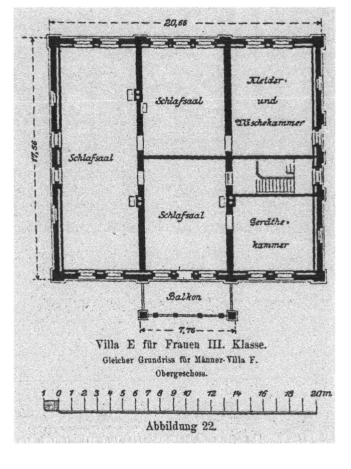

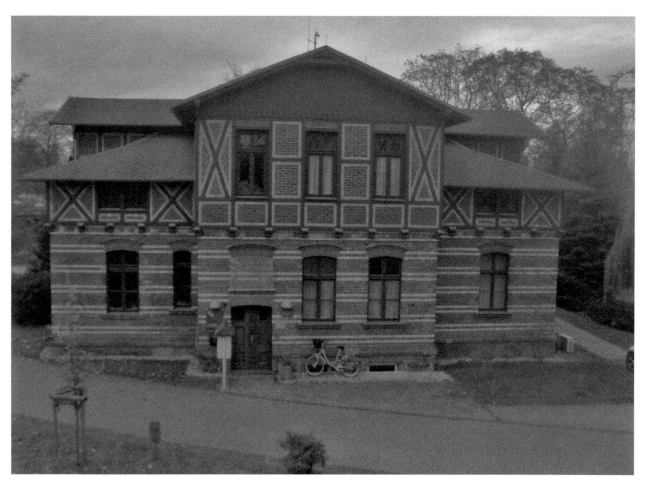

Figure 4-53. Alt Scherbitz: male villa A. Source: Author's photograph.

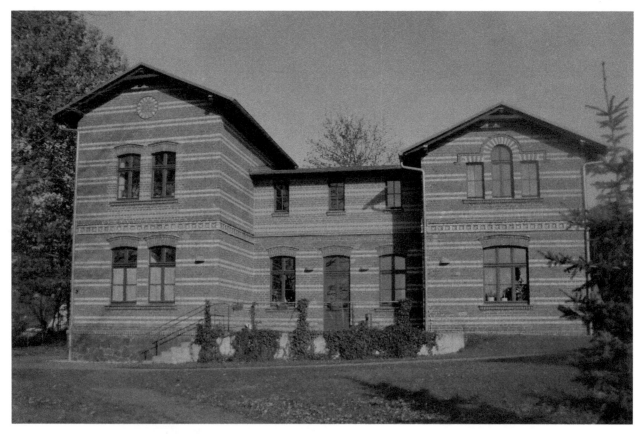

Figure 4-54. Alt Scherbitz: male villa B. Source: Author's photograph.

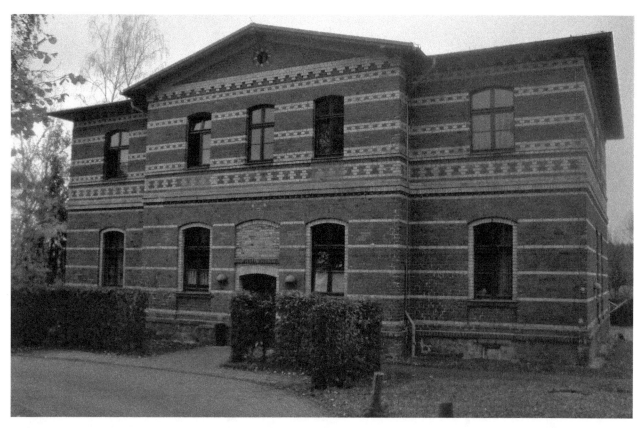

Figure 4-55. Alt Scherbitz: male villa C. Source: Author's photograph.

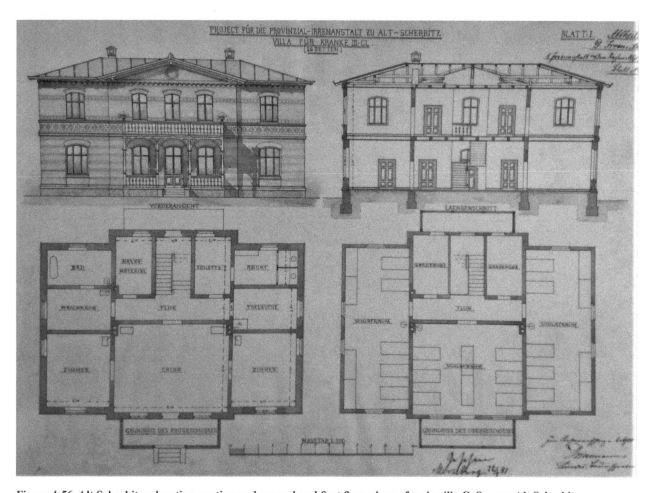

Figure 4-56. Alt Scherbitz: elevation, section and ground and first floor plans of male villa C. Source: Alt Scherbitz Traditionskabinett).

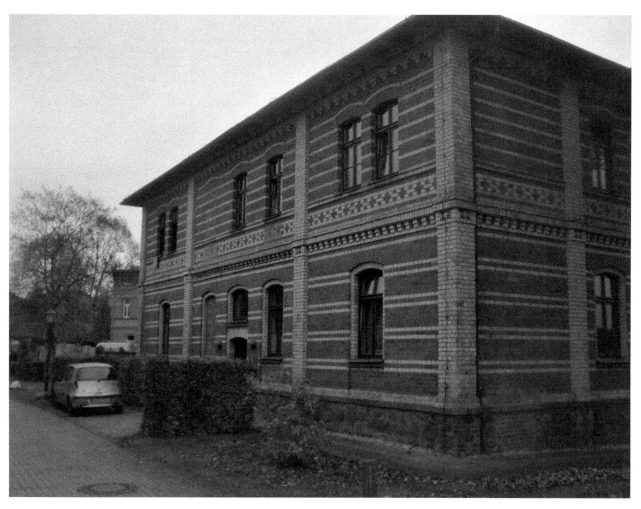

Figure 4-57. Alt Scherbitz: male villa D. Source: Author's photograph.

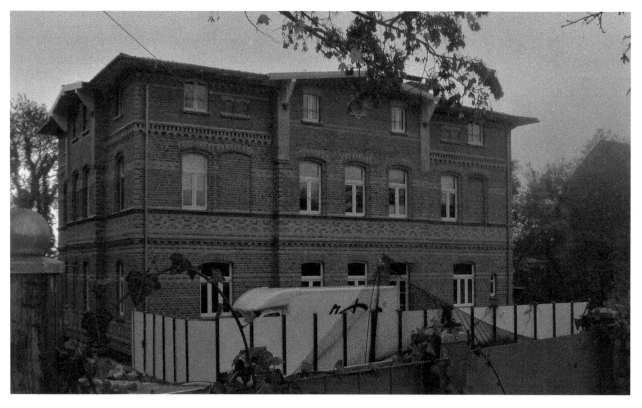

Figure 4-58. Alt Scherbitz: male villa E. Source: Author's photograph.

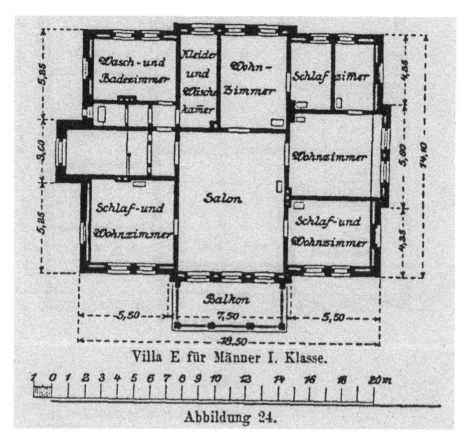

Figure 4-59. Alt Scherbitz: ground floor plan of male villa E. Source: Paetz, A. (1893). *Die Kolonisirung der Geisteskranken in Verbindung mit dem Offen-Thür-System: ihre historische Entwickelung und die Art ihrer Ausführung auf Rittergut Alt-Scherbitz.* Berlin: Verlag von Julius Springer.

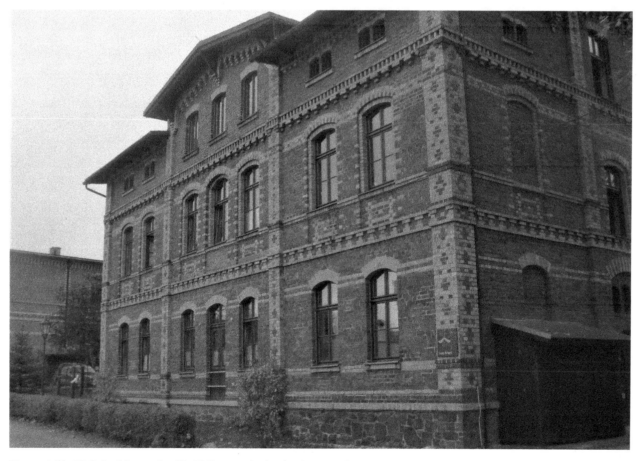

Figure 4-60. Alt Scherbitz: male villa F. Source: Author's photograph.

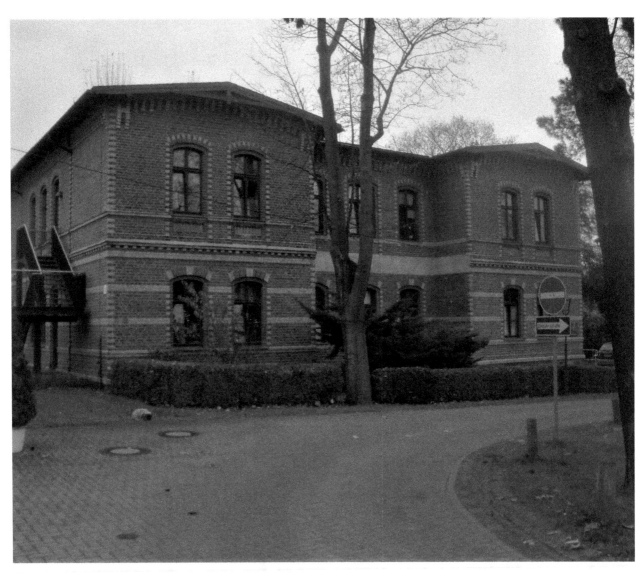

Figure 4-61. Alt Scherbitz: male villa G. Source: Author's photograph.

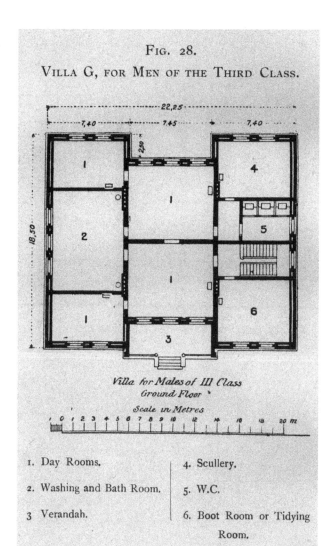

FIG. 28.
VILLA G, FOR MEN OF THE THIRD CLASS.
22,25
7,40
7,45
7,40
2,50
18,50
Villa for Males of III Class
Ground Floor
Scale in Metres
1 0 1 2 3 4 5 6 7 8 9 10 12 14 16 18 20 m
1. Day Rooms.
2. Washing and Bath Room.
3 Verandah.
4. Scullery.
5. W.C.
6. Boot Room or Tidying Room.

Figure 4-62. Alt Scherbitz: ground floor plan of male villa G. Source: ***Report of a deputation appointed to visit asylums on the continent with recommendations regarding the building of a new (sixth) Lancashire asylum*** **(1900). Preston: Lancashire Asylums Board.**

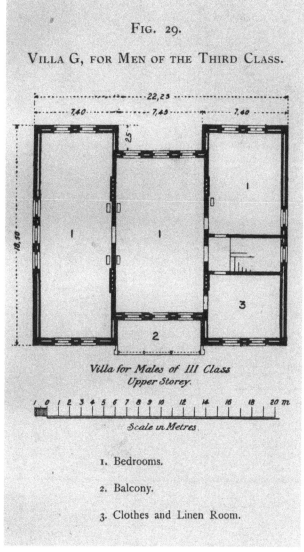

FIG. 29.
VILLA G, FOR MEN OF THE THIRD CLASS.
22,25
7,40
7,45
7,40
2,5
18,50
Villa for Males of III Class
Upper Storey.
1 0 1 2 3 4 5 6 7 8 9 10 12 14 16 18 20 m
Scale in Metres.
1. Bedrooms.
2. Balcony.
3. Clothes and Linen Room.

Figure 4-63. Alt Scherbitz: first floor plan of male villa G. Source: ***Report of a deputation appointed to visit asylums on the continent with recommendations regarding the building of a new (sixth) Lancashire asylum*** **(1900). Preston: Lancashire Asylums Board.**

Locations and Layouts

This chapter will consider the choice of site and the distribution of buildings on each site and the factors affecting these. Colony asylum buildings could be laid out with an unusual degree of freedom relative to topography and to each other and it will be argued that hygienic considerations such as ventilation, were highly important in choosing sites. However, also significant were aesthetic/ domestic concerns, which motivated the asylum builders to create asylum layouts which resembled suburban or rural settlement types. This chapter will use topographical maps to situate each asylum site, showing the detailed topography that affected where individual buildings were sited.

5.1. Factors affecting choice of site

5.1.1. Environment at the turn into the twentieth century

Claire Hickman and Sarah Rutherford have noted that from at least the early nineteenth century, the contemplation of nature was associated with the elevation of mood, tranquillity, order and virtue, and asylums were usually sited with access to the outdoors and to therapeutic views as a prime consideration (Rutherford, 2003; Hickman, 2009, 2013). However, the late nineteenth century saw an intensification of the rural/urban dyad with urban areas, which were rapidly increasing in size as industrialisation took hold, increasingly being seen as productive of disease. Urban areas were associated with the ideology of degenerationism and actively contrasted with the health-giving countryside (Ledger & Luckhurst, 2000: 1-49). It will be argued here that this had a powerful effect on the siting and layouts of the colony asylum which were positioned further and further into rural areas and sought to make greater use of the outdoors in the asylum regime. Not only were asylums pushed further into the countryside, later asylums were also situated at higher, and therefore healthier, elevations.

The environments of the poor were a concern, not only because they affected the health of the poor, but because they were sources of disease that compromised the health of all. In 1898 the infectious diseases of most concern in Belfast, for example, were diphtheria, typhoid, and 'phthisis' or pulmonary tuberculosis, Belfast being particularly badly affected by the latter two. The belief that typhoid was spread by 'sewer gases' - air escaping from drains - was beginning to subside, but alternative theories, such as the idea that germs were transferred into the atmosphere from infected soil 'saturated with the percolations from defective drains, or pervious ashpits', continued to place fresh, clean air at the heart of public health (Lockwood, 1898: 52-3). The spread of diphtheria

was attributed to the crowding together of the 'poorer classes' and the 'lighting, ventilation and overcrowding' regulations with regard to schools were thought to be as yet insufficient. Tuberculosis was thought to be a disease particularly associated with the dwelling houses of the poor, where spitting and poor cleaning practices distributed the bacillus, which was best combated by direct sunlight and 'free oxygen' (Lockwood, 1898: 54). Discourses of public health located communicable diseases in lower class housing, attributing their spread, at least partly, to the ignorance and unhygienic practices of the poor. Disease was to be addressed by education of the poor into cleaner habits and by paternalistic legislation to regulate the spaces in which they lived, worked and were educated.

Discourses of public health constituted the urban poor and their environment as centres of disease in this period. In some senses, this relationship is painted as symbiotic. The poor were mentally, morally and physically unwell because of their poor environment and their poor environment was, at least partially, the result of their mental, moral and physical weakness (Osborne & Rose, 1999: 743). Fears about racial decline and degeneration, excessive reproduction among the working classes and decadence among the upper classes began to achieve coherence in the new racial science of eugenics. This sought to promote the 'best specimens' of every class, those exhibiting 'health, energy, ability, manliness and [a] courteous disposition' and to limit, by social censure, the breeding of less favoured individuals for the good of the 'race as a whole' (Galton, 1904). However, the proponents of reform in the big cities, coming often from an evangelical perspective, represented a different approach, sometimes complementary to the discourse of eugenics but whose emphasis was on environmental progress. It was hoped that improvements in housing and in the general urban environment would address the problems of poverty, disease, social unrest and crime by improving the health of the poor (Rose, 1985: 82).

The 1880s has been seen as marking a greater urgency in the desire to deal with poverty due to a renewed economic crisis. This, coupled with a growth in the tabloid press and increased literacy provided fertile ground for the literature of 'social exploration', which saw adventurers in a colonial mould voyaging into 'unknown territories' to provide the reader with sensationalist and visceral accounts of poverty and moral decline in the slums (Ledger & Luckhurst, 2000: 25-6). The language of the late nineteenth century social explorer uses some striking imagery to conceptualise the poor and their environment. The slums are stinking, full of 'poisonous and malodourous gases', without air, water or light, where 'the sun never penetrates', they are dirty and 'swarming with vermin'. The buildings are overcrowded and fragile, lacking solidity, tottering, toppling and broken down. Such an environment renders the inhabitants passive, lacking in energy, miserable, unable to resist the temptations of drink and vice, whether crime, promiscuity, prostitution or incest. The poor are compared to animals that 'herd together', like 'brute beasts' sometimes literally sharing their accommodation with pigs or other creatures (Mearns, 1883: 4, 15). The rural/urban dyad became, at this period, a cultural trope in which health was correlated with the fresh air and open spaces of the countryside and disease with the industrialisation and slum living of the city.

These two approaches, the eugenicists advocating reproductive control and segregation of the 'unfit' and the social hygienists who linked the physical deterioration of the poor to unwholesome environment, ultimately came together in strategies of social classification which organised the withdrawal of groups such as the insane and 'mentally defective' to idealised hygienic spaces, in the hope of the subsequent re-socialisation of the rehabilitated (Rose, 1985: 82-88). The colony asylum represented an opportunity, not open to traditional asylum forms, to situate individual buildings relative to topography in a way which made full use of variations in land elevations, and also allowed buildings to be positioned at different angles rather than as a symmetrical element in a rectilinear or 'arrow' form. Colony asylums could be situated on uneven land, and at higher (and therefore healthier) elevations than was possible with traditional forms, which, as they became larger, required more extensive areas of relatively level (and therefore usually low-lying) land. Higher altitudes were associated with low temperatures that would kill germs, low atmospheric pressure that would deepen breathing and low levels of aerial pollution and moisture (Worboys, 2000:218). But in addition to this, the air of the outdoors was always seen as preferable to that of indoors, because the air inside buildings caused disease through the breathing of rebreathed air that had low oxygen and high carbon levels (Worboys, 2000: 223)

5.1.2. Ventilation

The siting of asylums in rural areas was directly related to their healthiness with regards to ventilation. Clean, country air was seen as healthier, and higher elevations, where wind travels faster, increased ventilation and helped produce hygienic environments. Absence of good ventilation was directly linked in contemporary minds to poor urban environments and fears of racial degeneration and was associated with the odour of closely confined spaces. Foul air issuing from the lungs was blamed for numerous ailments, including TB and diphtheria, caused by harmful microbes suspended in the breath or exhaled carbon dioxide (Townsend, 1989).

Luckin has referred to a 'moral-atmospheric doctrine', in which the urban wealthy were urged to retreat to areas, such as the country and abroad where the air was healthier in the winter months, an option not available to the

poor, who were trapped in overcrowded, confined slum conditions (Luckin, 2006:250). A number of government reports in the Edwardian era emphasised the importance of ventilation with regard to health. A 1903 report on physical training in Scotland re-iterated the widely held belief that 'the air of Scotland is phenomenally healthy',[1] but lamented the fact that the poorer classes lived in unhygienic and ill-ventilated homes (*Report of the Royal Commission on Physical Training (Vol 2)*, 1903: 235). Health was equated with middle-class villas, and illness with overcrowded working-class tenements, with little access to air;

'Within the town of Leith there is a thickly-populated area, with tenements, and there is a thinly-populated area, mainly occupied by villas. In the thickly-populated areas the residents are chiefly industrial-dock labourers, carriers, iron-founders, and so on. In the thinly-populated area the residents are mainly middle-class merchants, or lawyers or bankers, or shipowners, or others of similar grade. The great mass of infection comes from the thickly-populated areas; it is a comparative rarity to get diphtheria or enteric fever or even scarlet fever in the thinly-populated or villa area.'(*Report of the Royal Commission on Physical Training (Volume 2)*, 1903: 263)

A further report the following year into 'physical deterioration' concluded that urbanization and environment, rather than heredity, was responsible for damaging health, including mental health. Three problems were considered crucial to the unhealthiness of urban areas and these were 1) overcrowding 2) pollution of the atmosphere and 3) the conditions of employment. Good ventilation was at least a partial answer to each of these problems. Overcrowding was seen as 'an important factor in physical and mental degeneration'. It was linked with moral degradation and led to 'filthy habits' which in turn exacerbated the detrimental nature of the environment. Open space and fresh air was a means to address moral, mental and physical illness generated by poor living conditions. However, much city air was too polluted to be of use and had no 'vivifying qualities'. A witness to the committee stated that 'the condition of the air by its direct effect on lungs and skin is the cause of much disease and physical deterioration'. Foul air killed vegetation and made inhabitants unwilling to ventilate their dwellings, leading to 'general gloominess' in some urban areas. Many urban dwellers were working in confined unwholesome factory environments with insufficient ventilation leading to stunted growth and development (*Report of the Inter-departmental Committee on physical deterioration*, 1904: 16-30).

Cubic space of air per patient was a consideration for asylum authorities, and all those responsible for the

---

[1] Scotland was a popular destination for health tourists from the second half of the nineteenth century due at least in part to the belief in the purity of its air (Durie, 2006).

healthiness of public buildings, but no requirements as to cubic space were made in the 1848 'Instructions for the guidance of Architects' produced by Irish Lunacy Commissioners. Scottish Commissioners in 1859 specified that sites for asylums should be elevated, and if possible undulating, 'cheerful in its position, and having a fall to the south'. The buildings were to have 'free access of sun and air' and with principal rooms having a southern or south-eastern aspect, and the Commissioners issued rulings for ceiling heights (generally 11 feet) and superficial area for each patient in dayrooms (20 feet), dormitories (50 feet) and single rooms (63 feet), which effectively guaranteed a minimum cubic area of air per patient. It was also specified that windows must open to allow a free circulation of air and that ventilation should be provided by means of flues, horizontal channels and fireboxes. Plans submitted for approval had to show the means of heating and ventilating each type of room and the general system of ventilation. English instructions to architects are similar, but increased the dimensions allocated to ceilings (12 feet high), to dayrooms (20-40 feet) and specified that detached hospitals for infectious cases must have at least 1,500 cubic feet of space per head (*Sixteenth report from the Board of Public Works,*

Ireland, 1848: 236; *SLC Report (Scotland),* 1859: 115-119; *Commissioners in Lunacy (England),* 1870)

5.1.3. Open-air treatment

Open-air treatment was practised at all the institutions under discussion, but the use of such treatment for the insane has been neglected by previous scholarship which has focussed on its use for the treatment of TB (Bryder, 1988: 23; Bashford, 2004: 63-64; Richardson and MacInnes, 2010: 77). In 1888, an institution was opened at Nordrach-in-Baden in the Black Forest which was based on treating TB patients in the open air. In subsequent institutions this treatment usually took place on verandahs, balconies or in specially constructed shelters (Bryder, 1988: 23-4; Bashford, 2004: 70-1) (Figure 5-1). The first British sanatorium along these lines was opened in Edinburgh in 1889 and Aberdeenshire saw the opening of a similar institution for the tubercular featuring balconies and verandahs in 1900, known as Nordrach-on-Dee (Bashford, 2004: 63; Stell, Shaw, & Storrier, 2003: 328). Previous scholarship has usually assumed that balconies and verandahs for open-air treatment in asylums were used principally for tubercular patients, but in fact the treatment

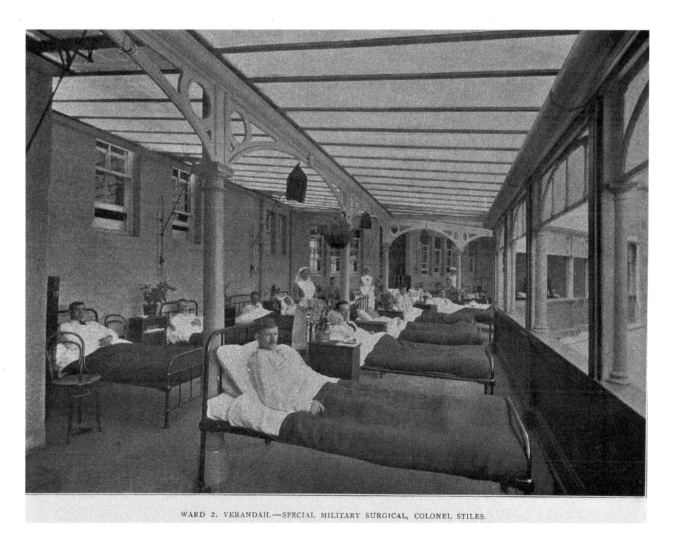

WARD 2. VERANDAH.—SPECIAL MILITARY SURGICAL, COLONEL STILES.

Figure 5-1. Bangour Village Hospital: military patients receiving open-air treatment (hospital building) c1917. Source: Image LHB44/6/3. Courtesy of Lothian Health Services Archive.

was often used for acute insanity (Darragh, 2011:270-271; Ross, 2014:299).[2] A connection between tuberculosis and insanity was postulated in the second half of the nineteenth century, the Scottish psychiatrist Thomas Clouston going so far as to propose a new medical condition called 'phthisical insanity' in 1863. Clouston noted that the frequency of TB was much greater among the insane and attributed this to depressed nutrition of the tissues, leading to a 'general reduction of the bodies of the insane to that state in which they form fertile seed-beds for the tubercle bacillus' (Clouston, 2005 [1892]:482). It is logical therefore, that treatments seen as suitable for the depleted tissues of the tubercular were also used for the insane, and rest in the open-air was used as a treatment for insanity itself from the early years of the twentieth century. The reports of the Scottish Lunacy Commissioners suggest that rest in bed in the open air under the shelter of a verandah was first used as a treatment for acute insanity in Glasgow, at both the Royal and District asylums, in 1904 (SLC 1905:xxx-xxxi).

While Commissioners initially advocated that verandahs be used for the open-air treatment of TB among asylum patients, the use of verandahs as a health measure gradually widened in the period leading up to the First World War. It was often suggested that exposure to the open-air in verandahs could also be used to *prevent* TB and eventually that it was 'calmative and restorative both in bodily and mental illness', so that weak and bed-bound patients of all types were thought to benefit from it (SLC 1910: 99). By the eve of the First World War Commissioners announced that the general benefit of open-air bed treatment in verandahs was 'universally acknowledged', as it could prevent TB, allay mental excitement and improve bodily nutrition (SLC 1914: xxxi). The addition of verandahs to asylums was, therefore, a routine recommendation of Commissioners during the early twentieth century.

Charles Easterbrook, the medical superintendent of Ayr District Asylum, if not the originator of open-air bed treatment for the insane, was the doctor who wrote most extensively about it in Scotland.[3] He proposed treating his patients in bed in the open air on verandahs attached to wards from 1903 when he incorporated such structures into the design of the new asylum at Ayr (opened 1906) (Easterbrook, 1907) (Figure 5-2). Easterbrook found

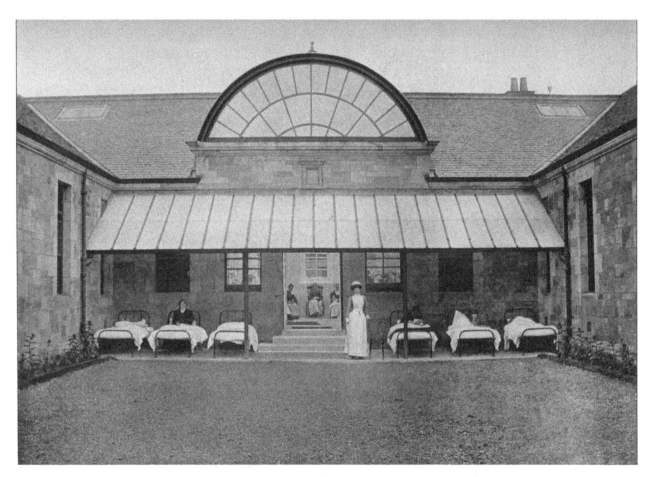

Figure 5-2. Ayr District Asylum: treatment of active insanity by open-air rest under verandahs, 1907. Source: Easterbrook, C (1907) The sanatorium treatment of active insanity by rest in bed in the open air. *Journal of Mental Science,* **53(224), pp723-750. Image reproduced courtesy of Cambridge University Press.**

[2] An exception is Halliday, 2003: 202-209. However, Halliday characterises open-air treatment as a means of controlling patients and a treatment that is self-evidently ineffective, being less concerned with the contemporary belief in its efficacy as a therapy for mental illness.

[3] The LAB deputation to Alt Scherbitz, found open-air treatment taking place there in 1900, and Germany may have been the origin of this kind of treatment (Report of a Lancashire deputation, 1900: 31).

open-air bed treatment most useful for acute cases, casting doubt on the usefulness of *exercise* in the outdoors for the treatment of the acute phases of insanity which he saw as an exhaustion of the nervous system, that would be further fatigued by muscle work. The rest element of open-air bed treatment was considered important to induce calm, reduce restlessness and improve nutrition including weight gain. The beneficial action of open air was said to induce health and contentment and Easterbrook advocated keeping patients outside from 7 am to 7.30pm during the spring and summer, even taking meals outdoors. Patients were routinely kept outdoors from at least 8.30am to 5pm all year round. Improvement was said to take between one and four weeks to achieve.

Easterbrook also stressed that in order 'to prevent the good effects of the exposure to the open air during the day from being counteracted during the night', bedrooms and dormitories should have sufficient air space and ample ventilation. Easterbrook stressed that being outdoors allowed a more rapid subsidence of mental and nervous symptoms when contrasted with indoor rest, patients becoming 'less restless, more manageable and more contented', with improvements in sleep, condition of skin, appetite and digestion. He suggested that fresh air,

'has an undoubted soothing and soporific influence on the nervous centres, and the cooler outdoor atmosphere stimulates general bodily metabolism and appetite, both of which effects render the open air of special value in the treatment of active insanity. But in the treatment of the insane and, indeed, of the sick in general, by exposure to the fresh air of the open, we cannot overlook the concomitant operation of such beneficent influences as the soothing action of soft breezes playing over the features, the comforting effect of the pleasant sounds and prospects of Nature and her surroundings, as commonly associated with the life in the open, the cheerful influence of sunshine, the health-giving action of the ozone and oxygen and possibly other gases of the atmosphere, and the more obscure influences of light, sound, electricity, heat and cold or temperature, humidity, atmospheric pressure and the like' (Easterbrook, 1907).

5.2. Ireland

As we have seen, legislation between 1817 and 1821 initiated the construction of twenty-four district asylums in Ireland, which were constructed in three main phases, from 1825-35, from 1852-55, and from 1865-9 with only three built after 1870, Antrim, Portrane and Purdysburn. The vast majority of asylums were situated a mile or less from the nearest urban centre, within easy walking distance (Cork and Omagh were slightly further, at a mile and a half). The two great exceptions to this, come during the late phase of asylum building after 1900 and are Portrane, which was a new asylum for Dublin, and Purdysburn (Figure 5-3). Even giving credit for rapid urban expansion during this era in Belfast, the new asylum at Purdysburn

was situated at a considerable distance from the city centre where it was not easily accessible by rail or foot and was beyond the reach of the tram system, in a marked shift from the previous norm.

5.2.1. Belfast District Lunatic Asylum (Purdysburn)

While most other asylums in Ireland follow the pattern of nineteenth-century 'fringe belt' development (Whitehand, 2001), in which hospitals, schools and other institutional buildings were constructed on large plots at a short distance from the town centre where land was cheaper and more freely available, Purdysburn is situated so far from the city that the intervening land has only been developed for housing in the last few decades. The siting of Purdysburn, relative to earlier asylum sites, suggests the intensification over time of ideology informing the spatial segregation of the insane poor together with an increasing and deepening consciousness of urban spaces as detrimental to physical and mental health associated with the prominence of degenerationism as an ideology. Purdysburn Villa Colony, constructed between 1902 and 1913, made tangible the desire to provide a place of light, air and hygiene for the mentally ill, in contrast to the dirt, fumes and darkness of the city and it is notable that, just as Belfast was Ireland's only fully industrialised city, it was also the site of its only agricultural colony for the insane.

In the Victorian and Edwardian periods, Belfast underwent an unprecedented period of industrial expansion

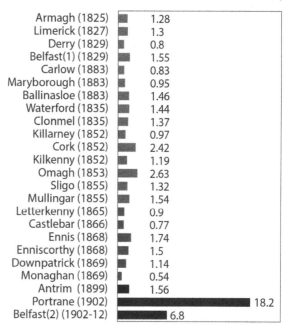

Distance from Town Centre (km)

Armagh (1825)	1.28
Limerick (1827)	1.3
Derry (1829)	0.8
Belfast(1) (1829)	1.55
Carlow (1883)	0.83
Maryborough (1883)	0.95
Ballinasloe (1883)	1.46
Waterford (1835)	1.44
Clonmel (1835)	1.37
Killarney (1852)	0.97
Cork (1852)	2.42
Kilkenny (1852)	1.19
Omagh (1853)	2.63
Sligo (1855)	1.32
Mullingar (1855)	1.54
Letterkenny (1865)	0.9
Castlebar (1866)	0.77
Ennis (1868)	1.74
Enniscorthy (1868)	1.5
Downpatrick (1869)	1.14
Monaghan (1869)	0.54
Antrim (1899)	1.56
Portrane (1902)	18.2
Belfast(2) (1902-12)	6.8

Figure 5-3. District Lunatic Asylums in Ireland and their distances from nearest urban centre. Source: Asylum opening dates obtained from Reuber, M (1994) *State and private lunatic asylums in Ireland: Medics, fools and maniacs (1600-1900)*. Unpublished thesis submitted for the degree of doctor of medicine, University of Cologne. Linear distances determined using google maps.

accompanied by population growth, driven by the linen, shipbuilding and engineering industries. The city (achieving this status in 1888) expanded from a population of 75,000 people in 1841 to 387,000 in 1911, a five-fold increase. Although this expansion was undoubtedly accompanied by considerable feelings of civic pride, expressed and engendered by the ostentatious new buildings constructed in the city (such as the city hall constructed between 1898 and 1906), significant concerns remained about the city's infrastructure and material fabric and their relationship to public health (Dictionary of Irish Architects).

It is generally held that the housing conditions in Belfast were better than in other areas of Britain and Ireland at the end of the nineteenth century and this is thought to be because Belfast's industrial growth came at a relatively late period, when building regulations were already curbing the worst excesses of a previous era (Aalen, 1987: 189). Belfast was in a much better state with regard to housing at the end of the century than Dublin, with only 46 per cent of tenements being of four rooms or less (as opposed to 79 per cent in Dublin) and 1 per cent of tenements being of one room (as opposed to 37 per cent in Dublin) (McManus, 2011:260). Nonetheless, Belfast's rapid growth meant that overcrowding and insanitary conditions were common and there was a perception that numbers of the extremely poor were living in terrible conditions in their own city. A contemporary newspaper report talks of feelings of 'disgust, horror, dread and anger' in relation to Belfast slums (Aalen, 1987: 189; 'In the Belfast slums,' 1907). An 1898 report on the sanitary condition of Belfast records that the city surveyor's department 'has had a great deal to do in the way of destruction, by sweeping away slums and opening out congested areas, and there is no reason to suppose this work is yet at an end'(Lockwood, 1898).

The colony asylum at Purdysburn was situated on an estate which, following a series of purchases, eventually amounted to c500 acres with working farm, dairy and arable fields, another factor that pushed it well into Belfast's rural hinterland, in contrast to the original walled asylum of 1829 which extended to only c45 acres (BDLA Report 1921). It was also at a far higher, and healthier elevation, roughly between 80 and 105 metres, whereas the earlier Grosvenor Road asylum was at an elevation of only 20m. The increased acreage per patient, almost doubling in the transfer to Purdysburn, represented a qualitative change in the embedding of the asylum within a rural/ agricultural landscape in which access to the outdoors was intended to form a much more central part in the environment in which mentally ill patients would live, work and be treated. The Purdysburn site was lauded by the medical superintendent, William Graham, as a refuge from noise and excitement and a means of providing 'plenty of fresh air, exercise and salubrious surroundings', together with a greater degree of freedom for patients (BDLA Annual Report 1898). The Purdysburn estate, when first purchased in 1895, extended to only 295 acres and when part of this, 65 acres, was sequestered for an infectious diseases hospital, there

was consternation about the loss to the insane of land that should have been for their 'employment and recreation' (*Weekly Irish Times* 13th January 1912). The concern that insufficient land remained was addressed by the purchase of additional acreage in 1901, 1904 and 1910, the estate reaching 500 acres in extent by the 1920s (Belfast Corporation, 1929). The provision of a large amount of land for the asylum was not always supported by wider society and a 1909 local government enquiry in Belfast held the asylum authorities to account in this respect. Supporters of the colony system said that a large acreage was necessary 'having regard to modern ideas'. Later supporters claimed that outdoor employment assisted the 'breaking up of morbid mental conceptions, the dissipation of delusions and the withdrawal of attention from ... brooding and self-analysis' (*Belfast Telegraph*, 23rd February 1909; *Irish Times*, 6th August 1910).

The asylum site was situated well into higher land to the south of Belfast at an elevation of between roughly 80 and 105 metres, with the buildings taking advantage of the uneven topography to increase access to health-giving country air (Figure 5-4). The asylum as built differed considerably from the proposed layout (Figure 4-3). The proposed design saw villas arranged around a central open green space, rather as in the typical cottage home design built for orphans in the 1870s and considered below. As built, the hospital and the villas for male patients were situated at the highest, and what would have been considered the healthiest, points of the site, where they were most exposed to the full ventilating powers of the wind. It should be noted, however, that the hospital is exposed to wind in all directions, whereas the male living accommodation receives a degree of shelter from a hill to the northeast. The female accommodation is situated at a markedly lower elevation, suggesting that the ventilating power of the wind was not seen as such a priority for female patients, or perhaps that they were seen as more vulnerable to draughts and cold. This tallies with the finding that female patients were less likely to be required to work in the open air, although outdoor work in the fresh air was frequently cited as of the highest importance for male patients. Unlike the typical male patient, women tended to be associated with a largely interior, domestic sphere where their role as guardians of the home was an important indicator of their return to health (Hide, 2014:102-117).

An analysis of the villa buildings of Purdysburn colony demonstrates how they exemplify good practice with relation to ventilation and therefore provided a healthful environment for patients from a physical, moral and mental point of view. The villas at first sight do not differ greatly, except in scale, from bourgeois domestic houses of the period, and certainly there are no complex ventilation or heating systems of the kind that were sometimes introduced into hospitals.[4] The villa buildings illustrate what was

---

[4] Notably the plenum system at the Royal Victoria Hospital, Belfast of 1903. (Banham, 1984:75-83)

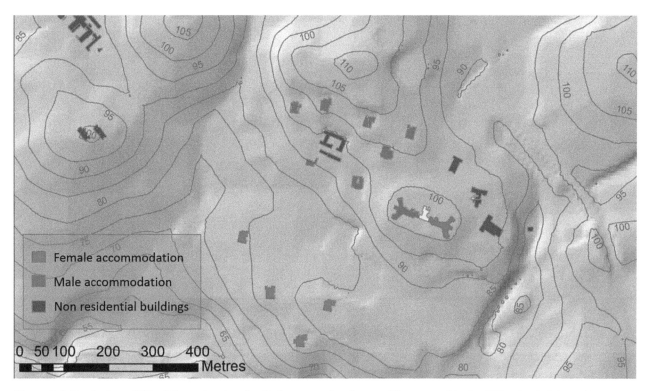

Figure 5-4. Purdysburn Villa Colony showing detailed topography. Source: Map created in ArcGIS using height and buildings data from Land and Property Services with the permission of the Controller of Her Majesty's Stationery Office © Crown copyright and database rights MOU203.

then thought of as a hygienic *domestic* environment and suggest that the 'levelling up' of the lifestyles and daily practices of the poor to more closely resemble bourgeois living conditions was an important part of the therapeutic intention of the villa design (BDLA Report 1911).

The 'bird's eye view' of the asylum at Figure 5-5 was published in an Annual Report in 1921, nine years after the main phase of asylum building was completed. The picture emphasises, by its perspective, the huge spatial expanse of the asylum estate with buildings dispersed and broken up into individual residences that resemble a suburban housing estate, rather than the monolithic structures of a traditional asylum, enabling maximum access on all sides to light and air. The almost idyllic pastoral scene of farmland interspersed with hedges and mature trees, gives no hint of the nearby city from which most of the patients would have come, and we are invited to assume that the air is fresh and healthful. The buildings are visibly situated on the high points of the rolling landscape where they would be most likely to benefit from the movement of air.

The prevailing wind direction in Britain and Ireland is south westerly, with wind having a westerly component for 50 per cent of the time (wind conditions being still or having an easterly component the remainder of the time) (The climate of Northern Ireland, 1983). The villa buildings are orientated roughly north to south, making them easy to ventilate by natural means through the opening of windows on both sides of the building. This allows air to enter on the windward side and exit on the

leeward side having brought with it the vitiated air within the room itself. The central dayrooms and dormitories on ground and first floor allow for maximum benefit from cross-ventilation, the breeze being able to sweep across the room and out the other side. In rooms, such as storerooms, which were not occupied by patients, there is generally only one window, cross-ventilation not being prioritised. The WCs were extremely well-ventilated, with large windows in both outer walls achieving a measure of cross-ventilation, the lack of partitions also assisting with this. However, the rooms ventilated most easily by the prevailing wind were the living and sleeping rooms rather than the WCs, the windows of which face north and east, suggesting that the respiration of patients was a greater concern than emanations from the sewage pipes.

However, a sanitary annexe, which was imposed on five out of the first eight villas to be built, against the medical superintendent's wishes, isolated the WCs on both ground and first floors to a greater degree than in the original design and had better cross-ventilation. The sanitary annexe was a standard feature of hospital design and suggests that the management committee remained fearful of the potential for disease to issue from 'sewer gases' while Graham was more concerned about the destruction to the architectural symmetry of the building that the annexe entailed, which he felt destroyed the homelike character of the villas (BDLA Minutes, 1902: 332).

The ceilings of the rooms themselves were high (12 feet on ground and first floors, 10 feet in attics - Fieldwork measurements), in both living and sleeping areas, allowing

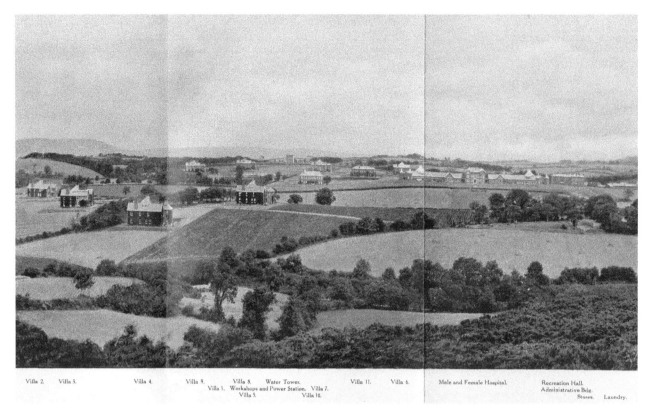

Villa 2.   Villa 3.   Villa 4.   Villa 9.   Villa 8.   Water Tower.   Villa 11.   Villa 6.   Male and Female Hospital.   Recreation Hall.
                                          Villa 1.   Workshops and Power Station.   Villa 7.   Administrative Bldg.
                                                  Villa 5.   Villa 10.   Stores.   Laundry.

Figure 5-5. Purdysburn Villa Colony: bird's-eye view (detail). Source: BDLA Annual Report, 1921.

for a greater cubic area of air within the rooms and a reservoir of fresh air for the patients below, as the warmed, vitiated air rose. Villa fireplaces were not only a means of heating the asylum but also provided ventilation through sucking foul air out of the chimney and drawing fresh air into the room by convection.[5] Each room was fitted with at least one fireplace and associated flue. The exaggerated height of the external chimneys of villas 2-9, reminiscent of tall Tudor chimneystacks, while being a fashionable feature at this period, also demonstrably expels the vitiated products of human respiration from within the asylum rooms at a height substantially above the level of the building, where it could not cause harm. Villa rooms were further ventilated by means of brass gratings fitted in the upper section of the chimney breast which would take up warm air as it rose within the rooms (Figure 5-6, 5-7). No villa had a cellar or basement, as these had begun to seem unhealthy and undesirable,[6] but all the villas were built on a concrete foundation which would have prevented the rise of infected ground air and/or damp into the building. Further ventilation grilles were placed in the outer walls of the space between foundation and ground floor in order to allow noxious fumes and damp to escape

from this danger area close to the ground and grilles were also placed on the outer wall at eaves level to ventilate the wall cavity. The drawings at Figures 5-6 and 5-7 illustrate the architect's concern for the proper ventilation of asylum spaces, showing the flues leading from the grilles within the rooms and the fireplaces. Ventilation grilles within the rooms have their own separate flues leading out to the chimneys expelling foul air at as high a level as possible.

All the buildings at Purdysburn that provided accommodation for patients were fitted with verandahs, including the hospital, all the villas and even the workshops. The standard villa design for chronic patients featured verandahs facing both east and west, so as to benefit from rising and setting sun at times when these working patients would be in the villa. The chronic and observation villas featured a single verandah each, facing southwards, where these more unwell patients, usually not working, could receive the benefit of the outdoors and a sheltered position during the day.

5.3. Scotland

In Scotland, as in Ireland, asylums tended to be located ever further outside urban centres with time (the graph at Figure 5-8 likely underestimates this tendency, as several district asylums which served rural communities were located far from urban centres and are plotted to the nearest settlement). No asylum building (the one striking exception being Perth District Asylum) was located more than 5 km from the nearest urban settlement from which it drew patients, until the 1880s. Following this, Scottish asylums

_____

[5] A popular American magazine commented in 1886, we would be 'healthier and happier if we heated ourselves with open fires [rather than stoves], and in the course of generations would have appreciably and measurably more perfect forms, more active brains, clearer minds and better morals' Robbins E Y (1886) 'How to warm our houses' *Popular Science Monthly* Iss 30, p.239 (quoted in Townsend (1989))
[6] Dr Benjamin Richardson's influential 1876 pamphlet 'Hygeia: a city of health' prescribed that every house should be built on a 'solid bed of concrete' and that cellars should be dispensed with to be replaced by a ventilating space (Richardson, 1876).

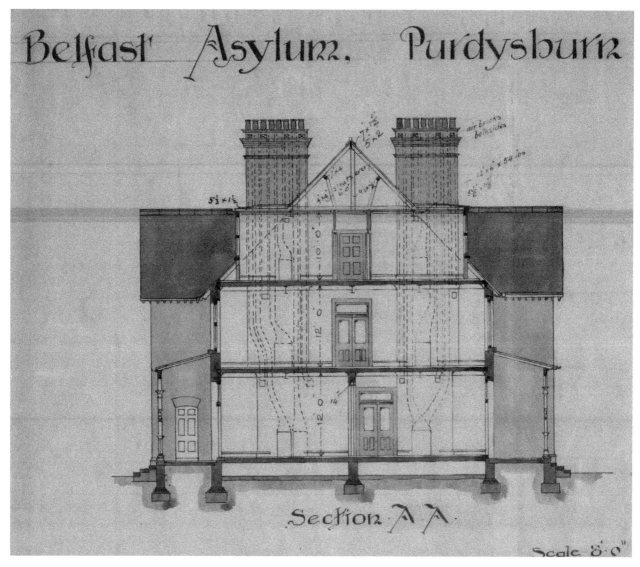

Figure 5-6. Purdysburn Villa Colony: section of villas 8 and 9 showing flues, fireplaces and ventilation grilles. Source: Author's photograph of original architect's plans held by Estates Department, Knockbracken Healthcare Park.

that served urban catchments tended to be located further and further into rural areas. There may have been a variety of reasons for this tendency, as previous scholarship has suggested, a desire to sequester the degenerate and inhibit their reproduction combined with a fall in the price of agricultural land which rendered rural estates better value than land nearer to urban centres (Radford, 1991; Radford & Park, 1995; Jackson 2000:63). However, it is also clear that associated with the move to more rural locations was the dramatic increase in the acreage of asylum sites from the 1880s onwards (Figure 4-9). Before 1880 the average acreage of an asylum site in Scotland was 40, between 1880 and 1910 the size of sites purchased increased more than tenfold to 462 (although initial site acreage must be viewed with some caution, as land was sometimes sold off after obtaining the water rights or leased to local farmers).

Certainly, a move to the country allowed larger sites to be purchased more cheaply, but Scottish Lunacy Commissioners were foremost in advocating larger areas of land for patients. In 1857 their recommendation was

an acre for every four patients, while by 1904, this had increased to one and half acres per male patient, suggesting that a substantial amount of land, providing work and recreation for patients, and guaranteeing a healthy rural environment, became a requirement in the late nineteenth and early twentieth centuries and this affected the location of asylums (Ross 2014: 189-217). However, it was not only acreage that was a concern. The following analysis will suggest that elevation was an additional important factor, with all the sites studied being constructed at elevations well above the earlier accommodation they replaced or supplemented.

5.3.1. Edinburgh District Lunatic Asylum (Bangour)

Edinburgh District Asylum (Bangour Village) was constructed on a 950 acre agricultural site, 23 km to the west of Edinburgh between 1902 and 1906, following increasing pressure of numbers at Edinburgh Royal Lunatic Asylum and the creation of a separate lunacy district for Edinburgh City in 1897. The site chosen was

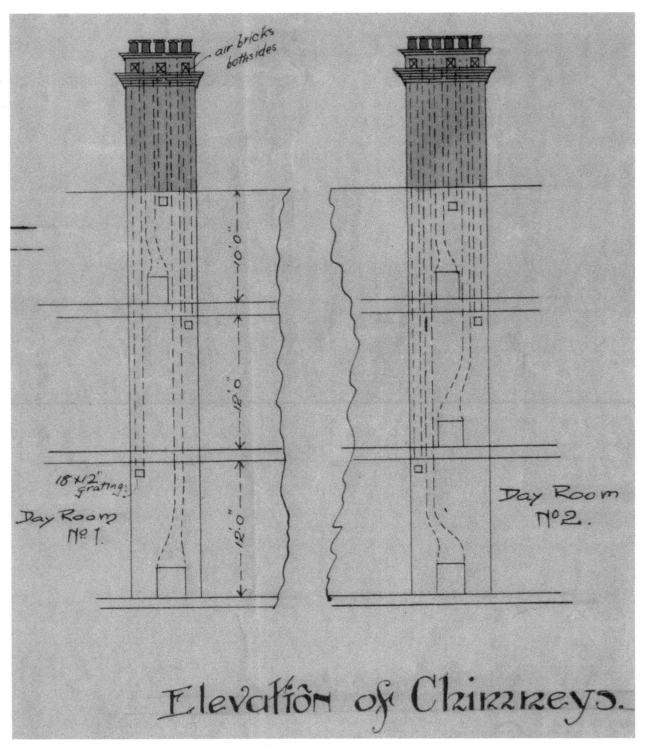

Figure 5-7. Purdysburn Villa Colony: section of villa chimneys showing flues, fireplaces and ventilation grilles. Source: Author's photograph of original architect's plans held by Estates Department, Knockbracken Healthcare Park.

on the eastern slopes of an outcrop of hilly land to the west of Edinburgh, and although not the closest high land (which lay to the south), it is one of the closest areas of high elevation. All the asylum buildings were situated at an elevation between 140 and 180 metres, in contrast to Edinburgh Royal Asylum which was at an elevation of c85 metres. The detailed topographical map shows that the buildings at Bangour Village were, similarly to those at Purdysburn, positioned with regard to elevation and access to ventilation (Figure 5-10). In a similar way to

Purdysburn, the hospital is the most exposed of the asylum buildings. It is orientated north to south and receives comparatively little shelter from surrounding topography, giving it increased access to ventilation. The male villas are situated on similarly high ground and are orientated northwest to southeast, giving some protection from direct wind, protection also being offered by the ridge to the rear of the buildings. However, these male villas are situated with greater access to ventilating breezes than the female villas, which are on lower ground, together with the communal

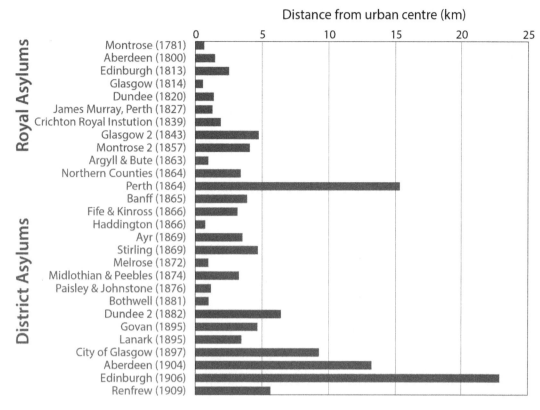

Figure 5-8. Distance of Scottish asylums from nearest urban centre. Source: Linear distances determined using google maps.

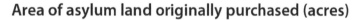

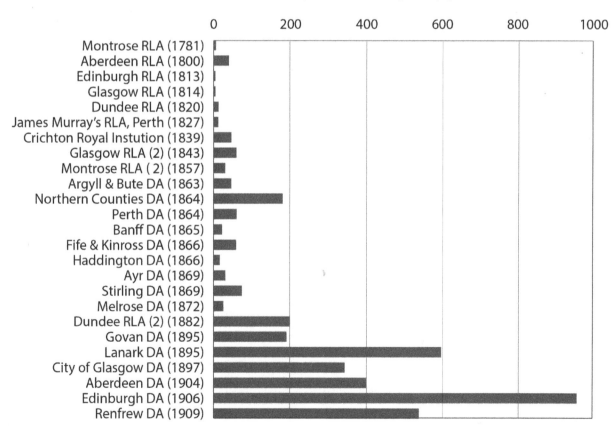

Figure 5-9. Acreage of Scottish asylum sites plotted against year of opening of asylum. Source: Darragh, A (2011) *Prison or Palace? Haven or hell?* Unpublished PhD thesis, University of St Andrews. Three sites have been omitted where data was not given by Darragh, acreage has been added for Renfrew from RDLB Minutes 6th September 1902

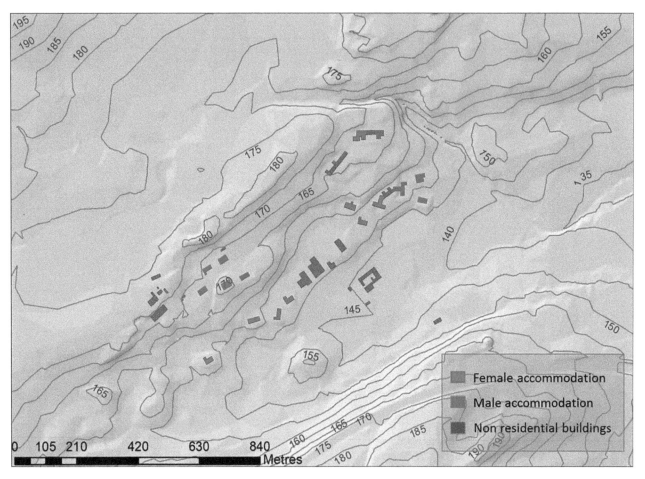

Figure 5-10. Bangour Village Asylum showing positions of principal (surviving) buildings in relation to detailed topography. Source: map created in ArcGIS using height and buildings data from OS OpenData © Crown copyright and database right 2016.

buildings and administration and admission wards. The very lowest ground on the site, near the main road, was avoided for building purposes, and may have been seen as less healthy. A bird's eye view of the original plan for the asylum (Figure 3-12) shows that considerable changes were made with regard to siting as the plans progressed. The original plan shows that all the asylum buildings including the hospital were originally to be sited on the medium height land (between 145 and 160 metres), where the female villas and the power station were eventually built, and that it was not intended to use the higher land to the rear. The original plan presented a layout that much more closely resembled an idealised suburban housing estate with dispersed villas arranged at regular intervals around a central green, not unlike pioneering cottage home institutions that had been introduced for pauper children in England in the 1870s, and that also often used the epithet 'village' (Figure 5-11). However, the regularity and order of the original design may have perhaps seemed a little mechanistic, and ultimately the decision to take advantage of higher points of land in siting the buildings leads to a random, organic quality in the layout which was admired by commentators. For example, a writer sent by *The British Architect* commented,

'...the eye is met by what appears to be a series of villa residences, some of larger and others of smaller

dimensions, scattered one almost might fancy, at random on the sunny southern slope of undulating pasture land. Here and there a coppice or belt of trees gives further variety to the scenery which, in diversity of contour, is typical of the Scottish midlands. There is nothing to suggest restraint, everything to attract by pleasing variety. No two houses are alike either in their exterior form or interior arrangement and decoration. The keynote of the settlement is variety of environment.' (*The British Architect*, 5th October 1906)

South-facing verandahs were added to the male villas at Bangour in 1904 and all accommodation for patients built subsequent to that date, featured verandahs. The hospital featured south-facing, west-facing and east-facing verandahs, allowing patients to obtain the benefit of sun and air at all times in the day. South-facing verandahs were double-height, giving more patient accommodation towards the milder south (Figures 3-18, 3-19). The good health of asylum patients in the early years of the asylum's opening was attributed to 'the use of the spacious, well-ventilated wards of the hospital and from the more extended use of open air in the treatment of disease in general'. Open-air bed treatment was found to be 'calmative and restorative and of advantage in many directions' (Bangour Village Annual Report 1909).

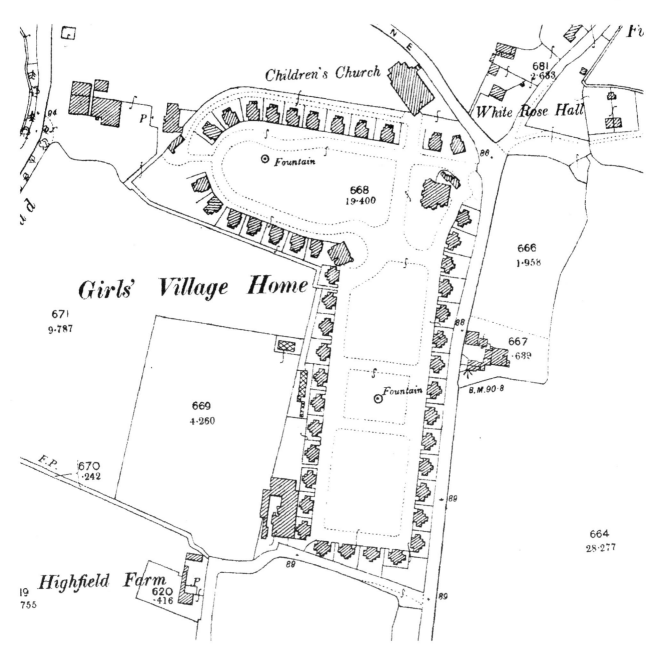

Figure 5-11. Dr Barnardo's Village Home for Orphan, Neglected and Destitute Girls at Barkingside (opened 1873). Source: 1:2 500 County Series 1st Revision [TIFF geospatial data], Scale 1:2500, Tiles: esse-tq4489-2, Updated: 30 November 2010, Historic, Using: EDINA Historic Digimap Service, <https://digimap.edina.ac.uk>, Downloaded: 2021-05-18 12:31:07.163. © Crown Copyright and Landmark Information Group Limited 2021. All rights reserved. 1897.

The asylum as built (Figures 3-14, 3-15) departed considerably from the original plan by moving the hospital and male accommodation to higher and healthier ground. This not only gave male villas greater access to ventilation, as at Purdysburn, but also increased the distance of males from females, without, however, placing any kind of physical barrier between sexes as was customary in asylum accommodation. The female villas follow the original plan in terms of using different orientations, adding to the 'variety' and 'individuality' which was sought for in the asylum design and was also a noted characteristic of the layout of the colony villas at Alt Scherbitz (this differs markedly from the Barnardo's village home which emphasizes regularity and order in villa positioning). However, the female villas are all situated with their

long facades facing north to northwest and south to southeast, allowing for a south-facing frontage and some protection from prevailing winds. The fact that the villas are positioned on higher ground, however, suggests that ventilation was also a concern. Villa 21, for instance, was situated at some distance from the other female villas, in a departure from the proposed plan, but its positioning takes advantage of slightly higher land further to the west of the site, and avoids a slight dip in the land adjacent to the other villas. Variation in the orientation of individual buildings has been retained, as has the congregation of a majority of the buildings along a central area of mid-height, retaining open spaces between clusters of buildings in a possible attempt to create a 'village green' style settlement. Figure 3-15, a bird's eye view by the architect, depicts the final

205

result as an entirely successful evocation of the village ideal, with buildings dotted around a rural landscape that is spacious and open, to a far greater degree than would usually have been possible, due to economic constraints, in middle-class suburban developments. The image at Figure 3-15 was first reproduced in the *Illustrated London News* in 1906, under the headline 'A Garden City for Lunatics'. The *ILN* claimed that the Lunacy Board for Edinburgh had 'erected an asylum for their insane poor on the garden-city principle', the first complete example in Great Britain and an experiment that would be 'watched with much interest' (*ILN*, 13th October 1906: 508). As far as can be determined, however, the comparison with a garden city was not made by the asylum builders or the architect, despite the obvious analogies with Howard's ideal of planned settlements incorporating spacious plots and open, green spaces as a response to overcrowding and bad air in the urban slums. The design for Bangour had been produced by the end of July 1898, before the October publication of *To-morrow: a Peaceful path to real reform*, containing Howard's ideas for the layout and financing of a network of garden cities (*Morning Post* 6th October 1898; *Edinburgh Evening News* 28th July 1898). However, although there is no obvious similarity with Howard's designs in terms of the layout at Bangour, we will consider below how Howard was motivated in his creation of the garden city concept by some of the same concerns that were significant for asylum builders of the period. It was far from unthinkable

to associate an institution for the poor with the concept of the garden city. Although the Barnardo's Home for girls at Barkingside (Figure 5-11) was first built in the 1870s, well before Howard's ideas gained currency, it was renamed the 'Girls' Garden City' in 1903 (*Cambridge Daily News* 24th November 1903, *The Sketch*, 20th July 1904).

5.3.2. Renfrew District Lunatic Asylum (Dykebar)

Renfrew District Asylum (Dykebar) was constructed between 1904 and 1909 following the establishment of a new lunacy district in Renfrewshire. During the period leading up to the commencement of building works, the medical advisor to the Lunacy B0ard committee, Dr Oswald, asked for a relief map to be made of the site, so that the positions of proposed buildings could be seen in relation to the topography, indicating the level of importance that attached to building situation (RDLB Minutes 19th June 1903). As the topographic map shows, Dykebar asylum was constructed on a plateau of land with villas and hospital being positioned on higher points of the landscape and surrounded by a ring of small hills (Figure 5-12). It is exceptional in this study, as the site chosen (between 30 and 40 metres) is not at a higher elevation than previous asylum provision in the county, being at roughly the same elevation as Riccartsbar and Craw Road asylums outside Paisley (38m) and considerably lower than the Greenock Parochial asylum in the hilly north

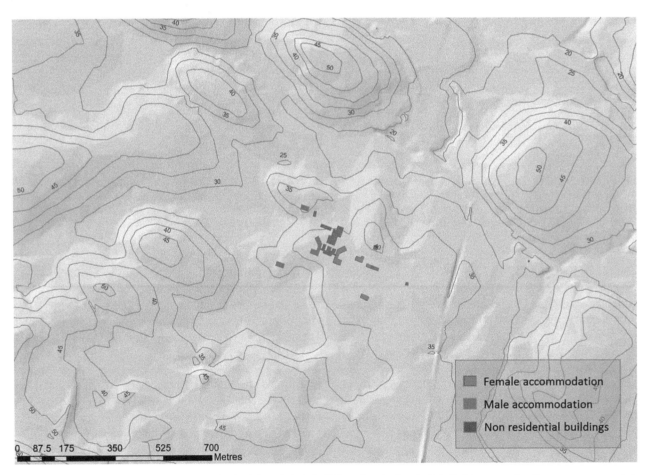

Figure 5-12. Dykebar Asylum showing principal (surviving) buildings in relation to detailed topography. Source: map created in ArcGIS using height and buildings data from OS OpenData © Crown copyright and database right 2016.

west of the county (112m). However, the site is at a higher level relative to urban areas around Glasgow, Renfrew and Paisley. There is no clear difference in positioning between female and male villas, but the female chronic villa is situated close to the laundry while the male chronic villa is positioned close to the farm, the workplace for these categories of patient (Figure 5-13). Male and female closed villas for more severely ill patients are situated at a distance from the other asylum buildings. The administration block with its hospital wings is placed at the heart of the site. Instructions for attendants at Renfrew gave special mention to ventilation and enjoined that staff were to 'give constant attention to the ventilation of their wards, day-rooms, dormitories, closets, staircases etc and to see that the air is kept free from pollution and as nearly as possible at a temperature of 58 degrees [14 degrees Celsius]. The windows are always to be kept open when the state of the weather makes it practicable to do so' (NRS MC14/4 *General Rules and Instructions for Nurses and Attendants*, 1912). The first annual report from Renfrew remarked that TB had been kept at bay by healthy surroundings and open-air treatment, and staff had benefitted in health terms from moving between villas in the fresh air rather than using corridors (RDLB Annual Report 1907). Ventilation in villas was 'natural' i.e. by the use of open windows but electric fans were also used in the living accommodation, laundry and kitchen and the asylum was praised by Commissioners for having 'carefully ventilated' wards (RDLB Annual Report, 1911). Field observation has determined that, relative to

other sites, there is a greater emphasis on ventilation in building design, and this may have been a compensatory measure given the relatively low elevation of the site. All windows in the hospital wings had exterior ventilation grilles going through to internal radiators, the rising of the warm air drawing fresh air in, without creating draughts and there were also ventilation turrets on the ridge line of the roof. The admission block showed an even greater concern with building ventilation with, in addition to ventilation grilles behind radiators, also adjustable vents at intervals, drawing fresh air inside at ground level and at ceiling level for the removal of vitiated air. These could be closed internally with a key, if necessary, and provided a further means of removing vitiated air, most likely to flues that vented through the chimneys. All the villas feature ventilation grilles under windows, on the ground and unusually, on the first floor as well. All villas additionally have a ventilation turret at roof level, the only villas for chronic patients in this study to demonstrate this feature. All villas also had south-facing verandahs sheltered from the west and east by the wings of the building. The admissions block features verandahs almost the full length of its south-facing elevation (Figure 5-14) and the hospital blocks featured south-west and south-east facing verandahs which were used for open-air treatment of patients (RDLB Minutes, 31st May 1907). Unlike the other colony asylums in this study, however, which made much of their lack of walls and fences, Renfrew was enclosed with an iron fence around the perimeter (RDLB Minutes, 31st May 1907).

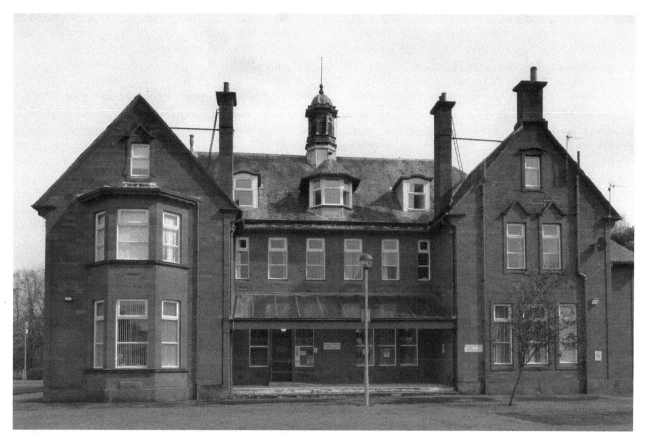

Figure 5-13. Renfrew District Asylum: laundry villa showing ventilation turret Source: Author's photograph.

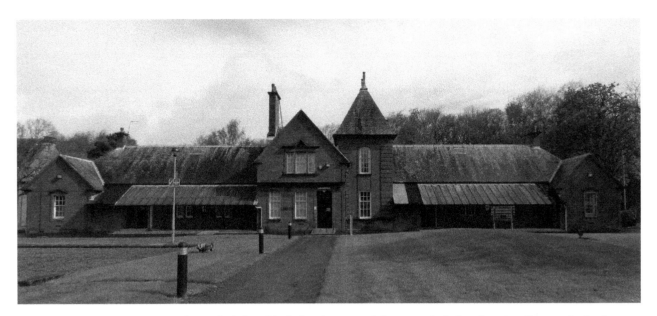

Figure 5-14. Renfrew District Asylum: admissions block showing verandahs on south-facing elevation. Source: Author's photograph.

5.3.3. Aberdeen District Lunatic Asylum (Kingseat)

The nature of the decision-making process with regard to the planning of Kingseat is unclear, as early records are no longer extant. What is known is that the asylum builders, the architect and many of those influential in public health in Aberdeen were exposed to the ideas of Ebenezer Howard as set out in his 1898 work, *To-morrow: a peaceful path to real reform*. The *Aberdeen People's Journal* reviewed *To-morrow* in an extensive two-part piece, a matter of weeks after the establishment of the Garden City Association in 1899 (*Aberdeen People's Journal* 29th July 1899 and 12th August 1899). The paper reprinted extracts from the book, urging readers to buy it and noting that the Garden City Association was 'progressing in numbers and influence'.[7]

Likely to have been much more directly influential, however, was the Annual Congress of the Royal Institute of Public Health which took place in Aberdeen on 2nd to 7th August 1900, attracting 800 delegates from all over Britain and Ireland. The Congress was attended by the architect of Kingseat, Alexander Marshall Mackenzie, by prominent members, including the chair, of the ACDLB and by William Reid, the Medical Superintendent of Aberdeen Royal Asylum. By the time the Congress took place, the garden city concept had acquired considerable momentum, prompting 'a good deal of discussion' in popular, as well as more specialist, circles and it is highly likely that Howard's scheme was a topic of informal discussion among delegates *(Yorkshire Post,* 4th January 1900). A section of the Congress was devoted entirely to 'Architecture and Engineering', much of this concerned with hospital construction and domestic, particularly working class, housing. Banister F Fletcher, architect, gave

a lecture speculating on the place of public health in the architecture of the coming century and justifying attention to the environment in bio-social terms, and although he does not cite Howard directly, the percolating influence of Howard's ideas is apparent, as Fletcher appropriates the term 'garden cities' and suggests that well-designed streets and beautiful buildings 'help to a healthy condition of mind'. He advocates planned settlements which provide 'the latest sanitary improvements both in the planning of the cottages and in the abundance of light and air and tasteful surroundings' and comments on the economics of removing factories and workers to the countryside where rents are low and health benefits high (*RIPH Transactions*, 1901: 422-432).

By 15th August 1900, plans for the new asylum at Aberdeen had been prepared by Alexander Marshall Mackenzie (*Aberdeen People's Journal,* 15th August 1900). The earliest surviving architect's plan of the site dates from some years later, 1906, the year that the asylum was deemed completed and all the villas were brought into use and apparent parallels can be traced between this plan and Howard's diagram No 3 (Figure 5-15 and Figure 5-16). The essential form of the layout in both cases is a south-west quadrant circle sector, with main axial paths converging on the public/administrative centre of the site and curved paths arranged concentrically. The plan of Kingseat is tilted out of true north giving the main axes a similar angle to Howard's Boulevard Columbus and Boulevard Newton. The drawing is coloured in a way which emphasises the 'zoning' that was also one of Howard's main contributions to town planning. A small green area corresponding to Howard's central garden is situated between stores and laundry and the recreation ground follows the placement of Howard's Central Park. The administrative building (correlating to Howard's Town Hall) is situated in front of the recreation ground/Central Park, while the main patient accommodation is arranged either side of what may be

---

[7] The *Aberdeen People's Journal* does not record any visits to Aberdeen by Howard, who made his first visit to Scotland to promote garden city ideals in February 1902 (*Edinburgh Evening News*, 6th February 1902).

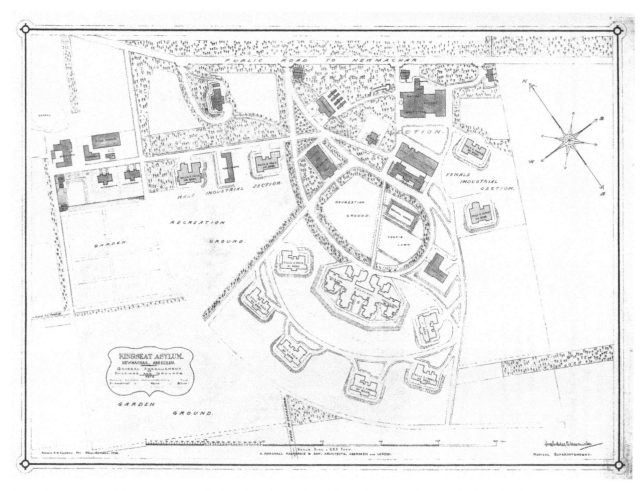

Figure 5-15. Kingseat Asylum: architect's drawing of layout, dated 1906. Source: Jenkins & Marr (1997) *Kingseat Village Proposals.* **Unpublished report for Grampian Healthcare NHS Trust.**

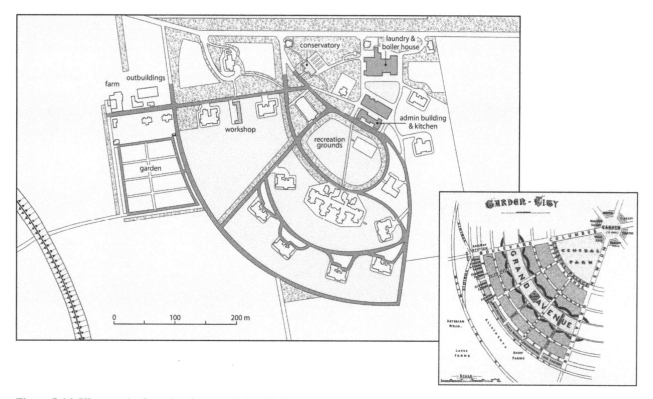

Figure 5-16. Kingseat Asylum showing parallels with Howard's Diagram No 3 Source: plan of Kingseat redrawn from architect's drawing by L Mulqueeny of Queen's University, Belfast; Diagram No 3 reproduced from Howard, E (1898) *To morrow: a peaceful path to real reform* **London: Swan Sonnenschein & Co Ltd.**

termed the 'Grand Avenue' of the site, with the paths leading to patient villas from either side approximating the 'crescent' form of Howard's housing enclaves. The farm buildings are located at the edge of the site, together with the garden/allotments, as in Howard's plan, and the main line railway is located just to the west of the site, curving towards the asylum in a form strikingly similar to Howard's diagram No 2. A conservatory for cultivating flowers is located with a similar orientation to Howard's 'Crystal Palace', albeit on a smaller scale.

Kingseat was built on high land to the north of Aberdeen at an elevation of 105-120 metres, a considerably increased elevation over the Aberdeen Royal Asylum which was at a height of 33m. The general topography of the site is a slope protected by a hill to the north-east. The ground is fairly level, although sloping away to the south, and therefore ideal for replicating the rather regimented design of Howard's garden city (Figure 5-17). Kingseat therefore differs from the other asylums in this study in presenting a slightly more ordered and symmetrical layout, although individual villas are orientated in a variety of ways within this layout. In fact, the buildings which occupy the higher ground at Kingseat are those which parallel the buildings at the apex of Howard's diagram number 3, the administration building and the recreation hall, rather than, as might be expected, the hospital (the difference in

elevation between hospital and administration building is c10m/30ft) (Figure 5-18). This perhaps suggests that replicating the diagram with some exactitude was a high priority for the asylum builders. The most significant departure from Howard's layout is the positioning of the laundry and boiler house with its associated chimney at the apex of the site's triangular formation. Howard would certainly have placed this 'industrial' building beyond the outer ring of the site where it could easily be supplied by the railway in an efficient manner. *To-morrow* contains an elaborate plan for the provision of electricity by means of developing water power pumped by windmills, thus producing 'smokeless' cities, the result of which would be 'health, brightness, cleanliness and beauty' (Howard, 1898: 165). Howard's primary motivation for removing factories to the edge of towns was, therefore, not the smoke or odours they would produce but the ease of connection with the transport network. However, in practice, this idea did not work either for Kingseat or for Letchworth Garden City, Howard's first experiment in bringing his garden city principles to fruition. At Letchworth, when the hydro-electric scheme was dismissed, Howard was advised that the encircling of towns with industrial estates was 'not suitable in a country where the prevailing wind is from the south-west' and therefore factories should be sited in the north-east corner of any settlement (Beevers, 1988: 101). The motivation for siting the boiler house and

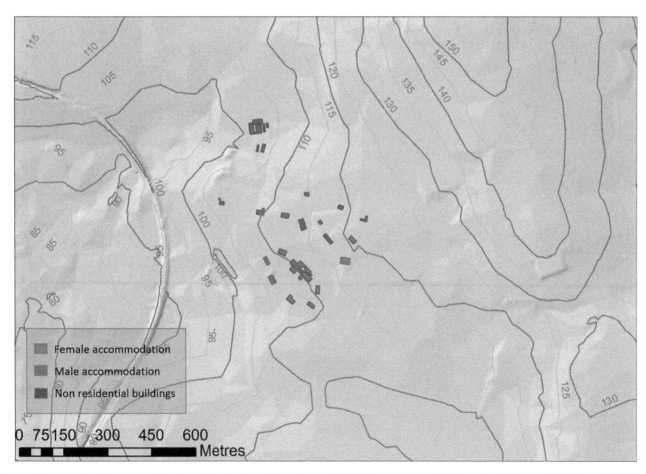

Figure 5-17. Kingseat Asylum showing principal (surviving) buildings and detailed topography. Source: Map created in ArcGIS using height and buildings data from OS OpenData © Crown copyright and database right 2016.

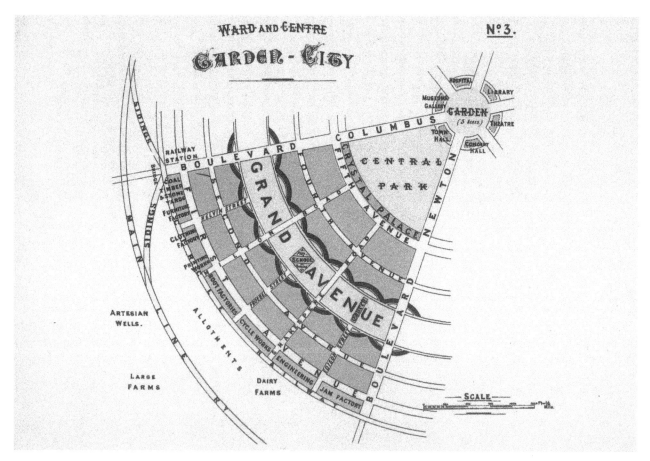

Figure 5-18. Howard's Diagram No 3. Source: reproduced from Howard, E (1898) *To-morrow: a peaceful path to real reform* **London: Swan Sonnenschein & Co Ltd.**

laundry in the north-east corner of Kingseat, ostensibly the administrative/public centre of the site, appears to have been similar—smoke and odours would be carried away from the patient accommodation, whereas siting nearer the railway would carry the smoke over the site.

The original plan for the asylum featured an underground tramway carrying meals from the general kitchen to dining rooms in the individual villas 'but this system was dropped on the score of too great first cost' (*Aberdeen Weekly Journal,* 5th December 1900). This idea may be an echo of Howard's proposal for an 'underground railroad' to connect peripheral towns with Central City. Underground trolleys to carry food were part of the American 'Kirkbride' asylum design, but although asylums such as the Essex County asylum at Claybury were built with walkthrough tunnels for pipework, underground food delivery does not appear to have been a feature of British or Irish asylum construction (*Report of a Lancashire deputation,* 1900:29; Godbey, 2000: 35).

The same year (1906) that the plan at Figure 5-15 appeared, Kingseat was first referred to as a garden city in the Aberdeen press, which enthused that it was 'as unlike a lunatic asylum as one could possibly imagine any place to be. No high wall, in fact, no fence of any kind, surrounds Kingseat, its outward appearance, with its finely laid out grounds, bowling greens, cricket and football pitches &c,

being more like a modern garden city' (GA GRHB8/6/2 Scrapbook of newspaper cuttings). An extensive search of the early archives relating to Ebenezer Howard and the establishment of Letchworth Garden City has given no indication, however, that either he or the Garden City Association were aware of Kingseat.[8] It is clear, however, that Howard saw the garden city as a potential response to what was perceived by contemporaries as a crisis in the growing numbers of insane. At a meeting in 1902 to discuss the prevention and cure of insanity, Howard suggested that garden cities would 'act indirectly as a preventive' to insanity and other diseases (*Reading Mercury,* 27th December 1902).

5.4. England

5.4.1. Sixth Lancashire County Asylum (Whalley)

In 1901, Lancashire was a highly industrialised and densely populated county, with 13 per cent of the population of England and Wales inhabiting only three

---

[8] The early records of the GCA are incomplete, comprising the minutes of AGMs (from 1901), some early pamphlets and the publication *The Garden City* (1904-1908). Howard's surviving early writings and correspondence likewise contain no allusion to Kingseat, although one of the earliest drafts of his ideas suggests that the 'city of health' would need to attract an institution (namely a home for waifs and strays) in order to bring in capital, population and markets (DE/Ho/F1/5 City of Health and how to build it c1890-1891).

per cent of the area. The cotton industry dominated, and was a major driver in the doubling of the population in the second half of the nineteenth century (*200 years of the census in Lancashire*, 2001). The provision of sufficient asylum space for this burgeoning population was a continual problem, and Lancashire and Yorkshire were second only to London in terms of the number of asylums constructed, Lancashire building six by 1915. In 1904, a positive decision was made to build a colony asylum as Lancashire's sixth asylum and plans were produced, but these were then dropped. It was decided, in 1905, to build an asylum along more traditional lines, similar to those built at Caterham, Leavesden and Banstead, and consisting of rows of pavilions behind one another connected by corridors, with administration buildings running down the centre.

Because of the construction of Whalley as a series of blocks connected by corridors, arranged in a linear, symmetrical fashion, it was not possible for the blocks to take advantage of irregularities in topography, and, indeed the layout required a large area of flat land. When the site for Whalley was purchased in 1902, the asylum authorities intended to build a colony asylum, but the decision to drop this idea, and build a more traditional asylum instead, was only possible because the site was level, and it is conceivable that the site was chosen with this flexibility in mind. However, at the time, strong objections were raised to the purchase of Whalley because it was low-lying and had clay soil and, by implication, bad air. It was thought that the low site, (60m/200ft) 'would be found to be conducive to phthisis and other tubercular diseases among the patients, who were generally in an enfeebled state of bodily as well as mental health' (*Lancashire Daily Post*, 8th June 1905). However, no pre-WW1 Lancashire asylum was built at an elevation of over 100 metres and despite the evident belief that a higher elevation would be healthier for patients, later asylums in Lancashire were built at lower elevations than earlier ones, very likely because of their increasingly large size (Table 7).

Whalley is situated in a river valley with higher land all around (Figure 5-19), and the pavilion blocks are orientated slightly towards the south-west, where forward-facing dayrooms could obtain the benefit of sunlight from the south. In the original plans for Whalley only the blocks

Table 7. Lancashire asylums, elevations in metres (elevations obtained from http://en-gb.topographic-map.com/).

Asylum (opening date)	Elevation (m)	No of patients built for
Lancaster (1816)	75	150
Rainhill (1851)	77	400
Prestwich (1851)	96	500
Whittingham (1873)	82	1,000
Winwick (1902)	35	2,050
Whalley (1915)	60	1,260

for 'sick' patients are shown with south-facing verandahs, which were for 'fresh air treatment', although it is not clear whether this treatment was used only for patients who were physically unwell. Other patient accommodation did not originally feature verandahs, although some were added in later years. The design of the asylum, with parallel rows of pavilions connected by corridors was very similar to a plan used at Leavesden (1871), Caterham (1871) and Banstead (1877) (Taylor, 1991:39). However, the Leavesden plan was much criticised at the time and the plan at Whalley was slightly modified to decrease pavilion sizes and increase access to light, air and views. Acute and sick wards at Whalley were smaller than those at Leavesden with 100 rather than 160 patients (*The Builder*, 25th July 1868). Pavilions were placed somewhat further apart (on average around 20 metres further apart than those at Leavesden (distances calculated using measurement tools for historic maps at digimap.com). Although this arrangement did not provide the access to light, air and views that was provided by the generally more favoured 'compact arrow' design where pavilions were stepped back in echelon, it was a slight improvement over the Leavesden model.

5.5. Germany

5.5.1. Alt Scherbitz

The asylum of Alt Scherbitz was founded in 1876, at first making use of buildings already existing on the site. The first phase of construction took place between 1876 and 1878 (the medical section) and colony villas were added in the 1880s and 1890s. It was originally planned to accommodate 450 patients but by the mid 1890s, patient numbers had grown to 960 (*JMS* 1894 (40) 487-499; Sonntag, 1993: 11-12)). Alt Scherbitz was constructed on a plateau cut through by a river valley. The continental terrain here is at a high level (c120m/400ft), even the river valley which is the lowest land in the area being at a high elevation when compared with sites in Britain and Ireland. However, the land in this area is flat, offering no significant topographical features other than the valley cut through by the river Elster (100 metres/330 feet). The level nature of the site that was chosen, suggested that finding an asylum site which was at a higher elevation than the surrounding area where natural ventilation would be maximised was perhaps not the foremost priority for the German authorities. However, the medical section of the asylum, constructed first, occupies the higher land on the site, whereas the colony villas for working patients occupy ground sloping down to the river valley. Almost all villa buildings have some sort of verandah on the ground floor, often with a balcony over, serving the first floor. Colony villas generally feature a verandah but as all colony villas were slightly differently orientated these face a variety of different directions. However, most face either west or south. The Lancashire Asylums Board, when visiting Alt Scherbitz, noted an 'ingenious arrangement' for wheeling a patient in bed out of doors onto a balcony or verandah, by means of detachable wheels, which was probably part of an open-air treatment regime (*Report of a Lancashire deputation*, 1900: 31).

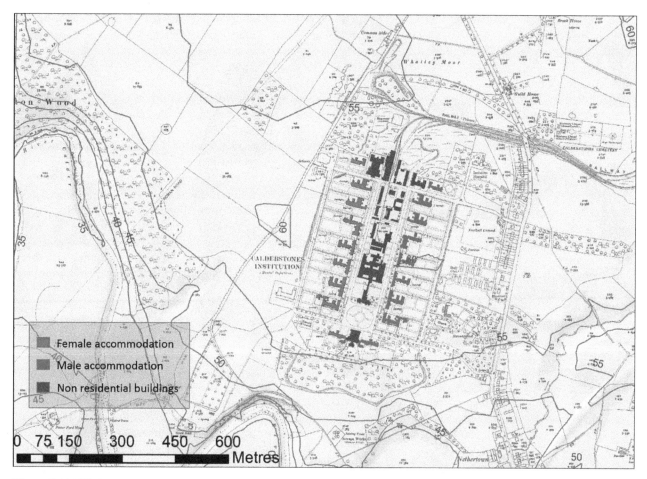

Figure 5-19. Whalley Asylum showing detailed topography. Source: Map created in ArcGIS using OS OpenData overlaid by OS County Series (1932) 1:2500 TIFF geospatial data from EDINA Historic Digimap Service (original site largely demolished) © Crown copyright and database right 2016.

5.6. Discussion and conclusion

It is clear from the foregoing that the colony asylum provided advantages with relation to the siting of buildings that could not be offered by the traditional asylum layout. In Scotland and Ireland, sites were chosen which were of mid height in relation to surrounding topography, that is, they were situated between the highest and lowest ground in the vicinity, often with an area of higher ground affording shelter to the north (e.g. Kingseat, Bangour, Purdysburn). Most of the sites (Kingseat being an exception) were built on sites with varied, rolling topography, and individual buildings took advantage of small hills or areas of higher ground. The opportunity to site buildings in relation to the topography lead to healthier situations and greater access to ventilation. This is seen clearly at Purdysburn and Bangour Village where the hospital and male villas were placed on the highest land. The villas and hospital at Renfrew were also situated on the higher land, rather than the surrounding valleys and it is only at Kingseat, where other factors were a consideration, that the hospital does not occupy the higher land on the site. The symmetrical layout of Whalley, with blocks connected by corridors, meant that it had to be situated on a large expanse of level and low-lying land, which was deemed at the time to be less healthy. Although Whalley was actually at a higher elevation than

one of the Scottish sites, Renfrew, it was a virtually flat site in a river valley, surrounded by higher ground. We can therefore see that the absolute elevation of a site may have been less important than its relative elevation with regard to nearby settlements, and that the rolling character of a site with hills and valleys, was sometimes seen to offer an advantage. In the case of Bangour and Purdysburn, the original layout of the asylum was much modified in order to take advantage of topographical features, and therefore hygiene and ventilation can be assumed to have been a priority for the asylum builders. The altering of asylum layouts to take advantage of topography did not necessarily render them less domestic or village-like in aspect. In fact, this may have been a factor that increased the perception of 'variety' and 'individuality' in layout, that was noted by commentators. Alt Scherbitz is unlikely to have been the inspiration for layouts which took advantage of topography in this way, as it was built on largely level ground which is likely to have been less well ventilated.

Fresh air was of paramount importance, being seen to have an impact on moral, mental and physical health, to the extent that even patients who were unfit to be out of bed, or who were in the 'active' stage of their insanity were exposed to fresh air beneath the many verandahs provided on each site. However, the prioritisation of fresh air and hygiene is only one of the considerations that has been at play in designing the layout of colony asylums in Scotland and Ireland, and other factors must be drawn in to account for differences in asylum provision between Scotland and England. A distinct Scottish asylum culture in which moral, mental and physical health was more strongly linked to the qualities of environments, appears to be responsible for differences in Scottish and English approaches to institutionalising the insane. Scottish asylum authorities were alarmed by the tendency to asylum growth, overcrowding and disease in England and elsewhere. It is suggested here that Ebenezer Howard's garden city, which sought to address the dangers of degeneration, overcrowding, and disease represented by the urban slums, is a possible source for the layout of the asylum at Kingseat. Kingseat strongly resembles Howard's garden city template, a resemblance which has not been identified in the years since its construction (Richardson, 1991; Halliday, 2003: 307-310; Darragh, 2011: 16-17; Ross, 2014: 214, 224). If inspired by Howard, the asylum (opened in 1904) may have been the earliest complete expression of Howard's vision, comfortably predating Letchworth, which is usually known as the First Garden City (ACDLB Minutes 19th June 1904).[9] An idealised community combining the advantages of town and country may have had much to commend it to asylum authorities who were addressing problems related to health, both physical and mental, similar to those that the garden city sought to confront. It is plausible for asylum authorities to have been attracted to the utopian elements of Howard's vision as they related to health and to have attempted to access them through the close reproduction of his diagrammatic forms, but other potential sources of inspiration for the asylum at Kingseat may also have been influential. By the time of the publication of *To-morrow: a peaceful path to real reform* in early October 1898 Ebenezer Howard had presented his vision in public on numerous occasions and had arrived at a conception of the garden city which was informed by a variety of concerns, chiefly aesthetic, sanitary and socio-economic. Although a large portion of the book was devoted to discussion of the economics of funding his network of cities through the recovery of the 'unearned increment' resulting from rising land prices through 'rate-rent', far more influential for future planned settlements was Howard's spatial and aesthetic concept of the city, with low density housing situated within garden plots, the city itself characterised by plentiful open, green spaces, rationally planned so that public buildings, housing, shopping and factories occupied clear zones in an environment of the highest quality (Hall & Ward, 2014:29-35).

Asylum builders of the late Victorian/Edwardian period were facing, in many ways, similar problems to those who sought to combat urban overcrowding and disease through planning and housing reform. A recurrent theme is the low mood and lack of energy of slum inhabitants, entailing a symbiotic relationship with their environment that was detrimental to mental as well as physical health. The tendency of the poor to mental ill health was triggered or exacerbated by poor environment and their poor environment was in turn caused by their degenerate practices. Mental, physical and moral health were irrevocably connected within these discourses, which were informed by the medical understanding of mental illness as broadly somatic in origin (Scull, 1993: 325). While poor environments were responsible for causing disease, environmental improvements could lift up the poor from their degraded physical and mental condition. By the time that the colony asylums in

Scotland were being constructed, asylum authorities were also facing the endemic problems brought about by the asylum system itself. As the numbers of insane grew ever higher, existing asylum buildings which had been constructed as models of healthy and hygienic environments were extended and new asylums proliferated. Early public asylums were built for less than 300 patients, whereas by the late decades of the nineteenth century some new English asylums were built for 2,000 and more (Taylor, 1991: 133-155). This engendered some of the very same problems that were thought to be the consequence of overcrowding in urban slums. English Lunacy Commissioner reports of the late nineteenth century are increasingly concerned with outbreaks of disease in asylum buildings, posing a threat not only to the patients themselves but to the communities within which the asylums were situated. A survey of Lunacy Commissioners' reports suggests that outbreaks of zymotic disease, 'asylum dysentery' and other contagious infections were a particular source of concern from the 1890s onwards. For example the Commissioners' report for 1896 complains of 'an unusually large number of cases of colitis, dysentery or dysenteric diarrhoea and typhoid fever … which, in some instances, assumed an epidemic character' (ELC Report, 1896: 20). The same report also refers continually to overcrowding and the pressure for accommodation at county and borough asylums which was seen as an important contributor to deaths from phthisis and pneumonia.

It was not only overcrowding and disease that made the old-style asylums appear increasingly unattractive. Previous research has suggested that there was a strong antipathy within Scottish asylum culture to the 'aggregation' of large numbers of patients, and that large, 'barrack' style English asylums were pointed to as examples of the kind of monotonous architecture that was to be avoided. From the mid-nineteenth century onwards it was suggested that an ideal asylum might resemble 'a large English homestead, or some large industrial community', 'a farming or industrial colony', or might be composed of 'separate houses, in which the patients are distributed

---

[9] Although Letchworth is often dated to 1903, no building work was commenced until the summer of 1904. The First Garden City Company Ltd was registered on 1st September 1903 and Parker and Unwin's layout for Letchworth Garden City was issued as 'the company's plan' on 11th February 1904, following a survey of the site in the winter of 1903 (Miller, 1990, 54-56). Development of the estate began a few months later, when infrastructure such as roads, waterworks and sewerage were constructed, fifty plots were let and the first houses were started (Purdom, 1913, 45-6).

according to their dispositions and the features and stages of their disease'. Scottish authorities praised Alt Scherbitz for avoiding the 'monotonous uniformity' of large asylum buildings, implying that 'barracks' architecture rendered the inhabitants dull and passive. Although the barrack style of asylum was also criticised in England, there appears to have been greater resistance than in Scotland to the 'villa system' as an alternative, because of difficulties with 'administration, supervision and cost of maintenance' (Taylor, 2007: 276). Indeed, after the opening of Kingseat its first medical superintendent concurred with some of these criticisms, saying that a village asylum required a larger staff and was 'perhaps less easy to supervise' (ACDLB Annual Report 1907).

The signifier for Howard of health in his garden city is fresh, pure (and smoke-free) air, a consequence not only of the rural situation but a product of its spatial organisation, with roads 'so wide and spacious that sunlight and air may freely circulate', removing deleterious 'vitiated' air produced by the overcrowding of people (Howard, 1898:32). It is no surprise, therefore, that when a garden city for Scotland (at Rosyth) first began to be seriously proposed in 1903, the influential Edinburgh psychiatrist, Thomas Clouston was prominent among those pushing for the adoption of Howard's principles north of the border, stating that 'there was not a doctor in Scotland who would not welcome the scheme' (*Manchester Guardian*, 2nd March 1904).[10]

The 'garden city' at Kingseat, and the colony asylums in Scotland and Ireland should be seen as idealised environments which sought to overcome the besetting issues of working class housing, the darkness, odours, lack of ventilation, the overcrowded conditions and dirt which affected patients physically and hence morally and mentally. The correlation of the garden city with health was no doubt appealing to asylum builders, seeking to avoid the endemic problems of disease and overcrowding, presented by the former monolithic style of building. The division of the asylum into a series of separate villas spread out across a rural site was important in preventing the spread of infectious illnesses. The clean air of the countryside was vital for restoring health that had deteriorated in the slum living conditions of the city. However, reformist asylum builders had routinely constructed their buildings in beautiful, elevating (and elevated) surroundings within the 'fringe belt' of cities and towns and surrounded by acres of open space. Overcrowding could be, and often

was, dealt with simply by extending the accommodation already on offer, by constructing additional wings or pavilions connected by corridors onto existing buildings. Alternatively, there were many models of the 'colonisation' of institutional space available to the Aberdeen asylum builders including the example that they cite most freely, the colony asylum at Alt Scherbitz.

If we are to accept that the garden city is the model that has been followed at Kingseat, this is likely to have been motivated by additional factors. The garden city gave form not only to the marriage of town and country, and to the unity of urban development with health but also to the wedding of social conformity with liberty and individual freedom with co-operative living. Ebenezer Howard's garden city presented a utopian 'marriage' of a series of opposed concepts, the separation of which troubled the early twentieth century asylum builder as much as his colleague, the social reformer. Howard sought to bring the benefits of society, intellectual stimulation, amusements, and plentiful work into the healthy clean air and sunlight of the country. He sought to promote individual freedom within a framework of social cooperation that would benefit all while providing the minimum of restraint and to release the vitality of the inhabitants by allowing them to benefit from the fruits of their labours and to express their individuality.

In the same way, asylum builders in Aberdeen were concerned with the insane poor who were frequently understood at this period as a herd-like mass whose vitality and individuality were compromised, through bad heredity and/or bad environment. The uniformity and repetitiveness that characterised asylum architecture and furnishings was easily seen as correlating with a loss of individuality and a consequent loss of vitality and energy that were detrimental to physical and mental health and replicated the repetitiveness and monotony of urban housing and environments. The village asylum made use of the physical arrangement of buildings and spaces to emphasise patient individuality, a theme which will be returned to in chapter 8. The following chapter will concentrate on an under-researched aspect of asylum construction, the provision of natural light through windows and glazing.

---

[10] Clouston was physician super-intendent of Edinburgh Royal Asylum from 1873, the first official lecturer in mental diseases at the University of Edinburgh between 1879 and 1908, president of the Medico-Psychological Association, editor of the *Journal of Mental Science* and writer of numerous publications on mental illness including *Clinical Lectures on Mental Diseases* which went through six editions. Clouston has some claim to be thought of as the most influential psychiatrist in Scotland at this period (Beveridge, 1991). Howard and Clouston may well have met in 1902 or 1903, when Howard travelled to Scotland to promote the garden city, and they certainly met in 1908, when Clouston was present at a meeting to constitute the Edinburgh and East of Scotland branch of the Garden City Association at which Howard spoke (*The Scotsman*, 25th November 1908).

Light and the colony asylum[1]

6.1. Introduction

'Pinel it was—eternal honour to him—who, with wisdom, and courage, and humanity, first struck from the limbs of the insane the heavy chains that galled them, destroyed the scourges that tortured them, led them forth into the light of day, and gave them an opportunity of regaining their right minds.' *Inaugural Address on The History and Progress of Psychological Medicine by J Crichton Browne, Senior President of the Royal Medical Society, Edinburgh (reported in the* Journal of Mental Science *1861 (7): 19-31)*

The narrative above, which paints a vivid picture of the early alienist Philippe Pinel liberating the insane, freeing them from their chains and leading them from their dark prison-like cells into an environment characterised by light, freedom, cleanliness, and therapeutic care can lay some claim to be the founding myth of the asylum movement in Europe (Bynum & Porter 1993:1358-1368; Foucault 1965:242-243). As state institutional provision for the insane poor spread across the continent from the first half of the nineteenth century, their humane treatment within the modern asylum was explicitly contrasted by asylum doctors with unenlightened institutions of the eighteenth and early nineteenth centuries that held patients in dark and airless 'cells'. Discursive practices informing the establishment of asylums for the insane poor in Britain and Ireland constituted the asylum as an enlightenment project in a sense that is often very immediate and entirely literal. The insane were being led out of the darkness, from dark dungeons into dayrooms flooded with light, in the same way that the medical understanding of madness and its treatment was moving from the darkness of ignorance to the light of knowledge. An understanding of the cultural context in which asylums came to be built raises some interesting questions for the archaeology of these institutions. If the provision of natural light forms part of the mythos of the asylum, can we 'read' this in the buildings themselves? In what other ways did natural light resonate for the nineteenth and twentieth century asylum builders and how can this inform our interpretation of asylum architecture?

The contemporary requirement for light in asylum and hospital buildings has been noted by historians, architectural historians and archaeologists who have made use of both the evidence of the buildings themselves and contemporary sources (Taylor 1991: 28-29; Yanni 2007: 33; Piddock 2007: 58). Among archaeological approaches,

Susan Piddock (2007: 58,61,76) notes that nineteenth-century asylums in Britain, South Australia, and Tasmania were influenced by contemporary prescriptions in terms of light provision. Asylum buildings were often arranged and orientated to benefit from natural light for considerations of health. The construction of separate pavilions and the lowering of walls were ways of maximising access to light. Eleanor Casella (2001:110) suggests that the typical provision of large windows in nineteenth-century institutional designs can be explained by the need to provide 'free light for work spaces', and both economic and therapeutic themes are echoed by Katherine Fennelly (2014: 417-425) who points to the importance of light in choosing asylum sites in Britain and Ireland, suggesting that asylum authorities had an 'awareness of the benefits of natural light, whether for economic (cost-saving) motives or as a form of treatment'. Charlotte Newman, (2010: 97-98, 276, 284) writing on English workhouses, finds that the more light-filled rooms within the workhouse structure were associated with accommodation for 'deserving' cases such as the sick and elderly, but again concludes that the provision of large windows was largely a money-saving measure. Other writers focus on the provision of windows as a means of providing therapeutic views for patients in asylums, underplaying the additional purpose of windows as providers of internal lighting (Edginton 1994: 580; Hickman 2009: 431).

While practical considerations should not be underestimated, the resonances that attach to 'light' and to which previous scholars have alluded, require further exploration. The significance of light as historically situated cultural discourse and its meaning as a therapeutic agent and symbol of paternalistic care have not been fully elaborated. As a result, the provision of light within asylum and other institutional buildings remains under-recorded and its overall importance for the understanding of the material culture of asylums has been unfairly minimised. Light in the second half of the nineteenth century assumed an importance in medical discourses that was linked to multiple layers of meaning, layers which are amenable to excavation from within the mental health literature and are indispensable to our reading of institutional buildings themselves.

Understanding how light has been managed in the design and construction of a building is problematic because windows perform more than one function. They can admit light (or not, if shielded by blinds and curtains), but they can also be opened to admit air, their size and shape can be dictated by architectural style or by a perceived need to balance an architectural composition. Their form may be influenced by expediencies, such as the availability of materials or financial constraints and they may also

---

[1] Parts of this chapter have been reprinted with permission from Springer, from Allmond, G. 'Light and darkness in an Edwardian institution for the insane poor - illuminating the material practices of the asylum age.' International Journal of Historical Archaeology, 20 (1), pp.1-22

facilitate observation, allowing people to see and be seen, and provide views of surrounding landscape. The light-admitting properties of windows cannot be isolated from these other considerations, but we can start to understand this particular quality by addressing ourselves to contemporary discursive practices. This assists us in assessing the likely significance of light as a phenomenon in the building of asylums and hospitals at this period. Having noted the prominence of light within medical discourses, we are able to assess the meaning of large and numerous windows as not merely architectural fashion or economic expediency but constituted by discursive practices. Similarly, having analysed the attention to light in these buildings we are able in some sense to quantify the significance of discourses surrounding light, by tentatively formulating an answer to the questions, 'How important was light in the building of the asylum?' and 'How was light important in the asylum?'.

6.2. Light and its discourses

Recent scholarship relating to light has analysed aspects such as developments in artificial lighting in the Victorian period (Otter, 2008), the 'sunshine movement' of the 1920s and 30s (Carter, 2003; Freund, 2012) and early modernist architecture (e.g. Overy 2008) and these writers have explored discourses of natural light that emerged during the late Victorian and Edwardian period and their relationship to health. However, a detailed analysis of the medical discourses on natural light that informed the asylum movement and its material culture has not been carried out. For the purposes of this study, a search of the *Journal of Mental Science (JMS)* (1855-1914) yielded approximately 1500 references to natural light in this period and provided the primary categories set out below, with additional material extracted from the contemporary texts outlined, the majority of which were cited or reviewed within the *JMS*.

1. *The light of knowledge dispels the darkness of ignorance.* The cultural ground against which medical discourses of light are set, within the pages of the *JMS,* derives from the enlightenment conceit of knowledge dissipating the darkness of ignorance and it is this metaphorical usage of light which is the most frequently seen. However, the position of mental health professionals within these discourses is a vulnerable one. Light is occasionally 'thrown' on a field (madness) which is painted as a vast unknown, a mysterious and troubling adversary, the 'dark depths of our science' *(JMS* 1897 (43): 387-391) and there is a discursive implication that the victory of light is partial and contingent. Alienists writing in the *JMS* at this period, continually display an awareness that their understanding of mental illness is in its infancy and the light which they are able to throw on the subject is surrounded by darkness at every turn.

2. *Light exposes wrongdoing to the gaze of the proper authorities.* Among the frequent references to matters 'brought into the light,' are a number that discuss maltreatment or neglect of patients either within or outside the asylum. In these cases the 'light' correlates with moral opprobrium and proper supervision while

darkness has concealed either the wrongdoing of asylum staff or the unfit and often morally suspect living conditions of the poor. As in the founding myth of Pinel leading the unfortunate insane out of the dungeons of the asylum, the darkness that characterises abusive treatment of patients is sometimes literal as well as figurative, with patients being removed from dark cells in workhouses or domestic settings *(JMS* 1855 (2): 114-120). Within the asylum, light permits observation, a mutual gaze between patients and staff and is a disciplinary requirement (Foucault, 1977). Nightingale (1863:92) proposed that the plans of hospital buildings should be simple because complication of plan interfered with light and hence 'facility of supervision,' 'discipline,' 'protection' and 'polic[ing]'. However, in Nightingale's, largely military, hospitals there is an implication that it is nurses (largely female) who require protection from patients (largely male), rather than the reverse. Discourses of light suggest that the supervisory gaze protects the vulnerable whether these are patients or staff, by imposing norms of acceptable behaviour and should not exclusively be seen as a means by which the authorities exercised control over patients.

3. *Light is cheerful.* Consistent reference is made to 'cheerfulness' as a quality associated with light *(JMS* 1856 (2): 376, (5): 161) so that asylum accommodation that is light, is also cheerful. Light is one aspect of the therapeutic influence of environment, which is expected to operate on the mentally ill by elevating mood. Forbes Winslow elaborates on the effect of light on mental health, calling the solar beam essential for 'serenity and integrity of the mind' and comparing the 'bright, ruddy, happy faces and buoyant spirits of those who reside in the country...and upon whom the sun is generally shining' with the 'pale phlegmatic faces. and nervous depression' of the urban labouring poor (Winslow 1867: 4-5). The light and fresh air of rural areas is explicitly contrasted with the darkness and dirt of the city, the countryside being constituted as healthful, mentally as well as physically, in opposition to the gloom and dirt of the city. Conversely, light eliminates the dark corners and shadows that are troubling to disturbed minds. Dr. T W McDowall suggests that 'light often dissipates nocturnal hallucinations' because abnormal sensory impressions are more distinct than normal ones in the dark *(JMS* 1886 (32): 112) while Bibby (1895: 97-98) cautions against ornamental work in the design of the asylum that is 'grotesque' or casts 'undesirable shadows' so that there may be 'as little as possible for the disordered mind of the patient to dwell upon'. The mentally ill are understood as making errors of perception which cause them to wrongly interpret, and fixate upon, the shapes and shadows of darkness.

4. *Light provides the vitality that is necessary for healthy physical and mental development.* In this respect of requiring light for healthy development, a continual correlation is made between human beings and plants. Florence Nightingale observes that people turn to the sun as plants do, her influential *Notes on Nursing* adding that, 'Put the pale withering plant and human being into

the sun, and, if not too far gone, each will recover health and spirit' (Nightingale 1860:49). The idea of light as stimulating is related to a pervasive understanding in medical and wider discourses of the period that human beings and plants shared a similar physical response to their environment. A popular American work on hygiene, summarises the thinking of this period, pointing out that light is essential to the development of plants and animals, who both become blanched and stunted without it (Hammond 1863: 206-210). Human beings could not develop properly in the dark and would become thin, deformed and etiolated. Etiolation, a term usually applied to plants grown in the dark, and which become spindly, pale and weak is here used to describe human beings who were characterised by watery blood, pale skin, rapid pulse, underweight, lack of energy and susceptibility to illness. Light is described as a 'most healthful stimulant, both to the nervous and physical systems...The delirium and weakness which are by no means seldom met with in convalescents kept in darkness, disappear like magic when the rays of the sun are allowed to enter the chamber' (Hammond 1863: 206-210). Forbes Winslow elaborates on this, suggesting that etiolation in human beings could also be '*moral* and *mental*' leading to intellectual deterioration and crime as well as bodily deformity, disease and death (Winslow 1867: 4). Winslow postulated that human beings diminished in strength and energy without light because of the effect of lack of light on the 'vital fluid' of the blood in diminishing the numbers of red-blood cells (1867: 155). Some classes of the insane, such as the 'idiot' were characterised as lacking in vital force and, correspondingly, having no 'light' in their eyes *(JMS* 1861 (7): 243). Nightingale and others repeat the belief that cretinism, a condition which was categorised with mental illness at this period, could be caused by lack of sunlight, probably also on the basis that it was perceived as a lack of vitality (Nightingale 1860:49; *JMS* 1873 (19): 171.

5. *Light is stimulating and can cause adverse effects in those who are susceptible.* Because of its stimulating qualities, care had to be taken in the exposure of some patients to light, because bright light 'frightens one, rejoices another and agitates all' (Esquirol, quoted in Bucknill & Tuke 1879: 79) and therefore rest in darkened rooms was often recommended for manic patients. However, the beneficial properties of light were felt to be, by some, so overwhelming that Kirkbride, for example, advises that the admission of light into asylum spaces 'ought not to be excluded for even the most excited cases' (Kirkbride 1854: 29). Light was to be avoided at times when stimulation was not required or desirable and Forbes Winslow recommends that light is excluded entirely from the bedrooms of the insane 'in order to tranquilise them and cause sleep' (Winslow 1867: 151).

6. *Light is a purifying agent that kills disease and promotes healing.* In the 1850s light was already being described as 'amongst the foremost sanitary requirements' for asylum buildings *(JMS* 1856 (2): 273). Florence Nightingale continued with this theme, stating that light

has a 'purifying effect' upon the air of a room, removing odours and disease-causing agents, and therefore the sun must reach rooms both in the hospital and in the home at some point in each day. She further states that 'a dark house is always an unhealthy house' and that want of light 'promotes scrofula' (a form of tuberculosis) among children (Nightingale 1860: 16, 1863: 18-20). Forbes Winslow (1867: 162) goes further in claiming that light chemically purifies the blood of those who are unwell and Nightingale concurs that people 'lose their health in a dark house and if they get ill they cannot get well again in it' (Nightingale 1860: 16). Wounds were thought to heal more quickly in field hospitals because of the benefit of exposure to light and air (Parkes 1887: 761). It was not until 1895 that the news of Robert Koch's finding that the 'tubercle bacille' was destroyed by direct sunlight was discussed in the pages of the *JMS* (1895 (41): 230) (the discovery was made in 1890), but although the idea of light as a specific curative for tuberculosis gained ground, Koch's discovery emerged during a period when the disease-fighting benefits of light were already a familiar part of medical discourses. Light was, by this time, a significant element of hospital design having become fully embedded in discourses of mental and physical health. The antibiotic properties of light were important to hospital designers from the late nineteenth century and buildings were to be orientated towards the sunlight with areas of shadow to be avoided (Kisacky 2000: 315; Galton 1893: 15).

7. *Light, together with air, cleanliness, exercise and diet, is part of the hygienic regime of the asylum.* The provision of light formed part of discourses relating to hygiene which saw an 'intimate connection' between bodily and mental functions. Preventing physical decay or degeneration through hygiene could stop even a hereditary taint of mental illness from taking hold *(JMS* 1861 (7): 319). Critics of the 'hygienist' orthodoxy in asylum medicine claimed that the influences of food, air, water and light were 'dubious and unregulated' and that medical superintendents should make more use of drugs in their treatments *(JMS* 1866 (12): 312). Others were content to acknowledge the benefits of light, while noting the lack of 'positive facts' concerning its effects (Parkes 1883: 95). The Medical Superintendents of asylums were sometimes criticised for neglecting their 'duties as physicians' i.e., to investigate the pathology of madness or develop new therapies, in favour of 'architecture, farming and questions of hygiene &c,' but this accusation was resisted with the argument that 'bad architectural arrangements' and 'neglect of sanitary precautions' was harmful to health, both physical and mental, and was likely to prolong a patient's illness *(JMS* 1874 (20): 327-351). Burdett (1891: 187) specified that asylums must be run by doctors because, as well as drugs, the Medical Superintendent needed to be an expert in 'hygienic treatment' including light and atmosphere, furnishing and decoration, diet and clothing and occupations and amusements.

8. *Light is a requirement for a well-built and humane asylum.* The asylum movement represented itself as

an enlightenment project that had swept away the misguided and often brutal treatment of the insane in the past, replacing it with the humane regime of the modern asylum. Key to this narrative, as continually replayed in the pages of the *Journal of Mental Science*, was the understanding that the insane were, before the era of the public asylum, kept in dark, prison-like cells and physically restrained and/or beaten (e.g. *JMS* 1873 (19): 329). The light-filled rooms of the asylum were therefore a literal and metaphorical counterpoint to the inhumane treatment of the past. Asylums in Britain, Ireland and around the world were discursively policed and lauded or condemned to a large degree on the basis of how light or dark were their dormitories and dayrooms. Light was explicitly correlated with 'freedom' *(JMS* 1867 (12): 603-606) and the provision of facilities that were 'home-like' rather than 'prison-like'.

The discursive elaboration of light as a requirement for asylums existed alongside sets of prescriptions for asylums and other hospitals in terms of the provision of windows, among which was the influential work of Florence Nightingale. Nightingale (1863: 19) dictated that hospital pavilions should be orientated north to south so that the sun could shine in one side or the other from sunrise to sunset, with a window to at least every two beds so that as 'great a surface as possible should receive direct sunlight'. The window-space should be one-third of the wall space and the windows should reach from 2-3 ft (0.6-0.9 m) from the floor to 1 ft (0.3 m) below the ceiling, not only to admit light but also to allow a view. Ceilings 15-16 ft (4.5-4.8 m) high would allow for sufficiently tall windows while the pavilions should be as low as possible; 'two stories are better than three; and one is preferable to two', and the distance between them should be at least twice the height of the walls so that the buildings would not interfere with the light and ventilation from each other. Patients should be arranged along walls with windows so as to obtain maximum benefit from the light, and passages and corridors should be light and airy. The walls should always be light-coloured to make the room light, whitewash should be used and the plans should show the 'utmost simplicity' in order to avoid 'skulking places', for disease-causing agents. Nightingale's specifications were hugely influential from the 1860s onwards and demonstrate that a concern with light informed the construction of hospitals and other public health institutions as well as asylums (Livingstone, 2003: 64-65).

6.3. Darkness in the Victorian slums

Contemporary discursive practices constituted asylums as a necessary and beneficial response to the unenlightened treatment of the insane which was practised outside the asylum movement. But medical discourses leave much that is unsaid, but yet is implied, within the understanding of light and it is clear from an examination of the wider cultural context that important discourses around light and darkness developed in this period, which positioned the extremely poor in places of darkness from which an active

reform movement, including the asylum movement, was poised to deliver them.

The visceral descriptions by social explorers of the smell, dirt, damp, the claustrophobic lack of light, air and space characterised slum inhabitants as desensitised, apathetic and animal-like, unable to resist the temptations of vice and alcohol, and therefore to be pitied, not unlike descriptions of the insane in their pre-enlightenment dungeons. Compassion mixes in these accounts with anxiety as the spectre is raised of 'dark and noisome' haunts which are concealed away from the main thoroughfares in which squalid poverty lurks, threatening to spill out and contaminate other social strata (O'Hanlon 1853: 1).

In his *Walks among the Poor of Belfast* the Rev W M O'Hanlon emphasises a continual theme of this genre; the association of darkness with what is often called a 'promiscuous' lack of segregation. Adults and children, related and strangers are to be found huddled together 'without the slightest regard to decency and order' (O'Hanlon 1853: 17). Darkness obscures boundaries between persons and categories and under cover of darkness, incestuous relationships are allowed to take place. Darkness is associated with crime and vice of all kinds but particularly sexual transgression, such as prostitution and the ensuing syphilitic disease, a prime cause of insanity. The association with physical disease and death, 'social and mental putridity and malaria' threatens to poison the community and 'moral-sanitary reform' is called for, in order to save society as a whole (O'Hanlon 1853: 49).

This theme is returned to by General William Booth of the Salvation Army, 'In Darkest England and the Way Out' (1890). At this key period of colonial expansion which was characterised by the 'saturation of British culture' (Ledger and Luckhurst 2000: 133) with the images, symbols and rhetoric of Empire, the urban slums are compared in racist/ imperialist discourse with the tropical forests of Africa 'where a ray of sun never penetrates' and where human beings are deformed physically and mentally by the foul air and lack of light, becoming 'dwarfed into pygmies and brutalised into cannibals.' The dark regions of the city are compared to malarial swamps which are liable to spread disease and immorality. The struggle to reform the slums, in parallel with the struggle to cure the insane, is seen as a civilising one, waged against a formless mass of the dehumanised who are to be led from darkness to light, literally and figuratively, from dirt, darkness, immorality and insanity to order and hygiene.

6.4. Natural light provision in Scottish, Irish and English asylums

Instructions for the guidance of asylum architects, produced by the relevant authorities in each jurisdiction (England and Wales, Ireland, Scotland) specified that asylum buildings should have free access to sun and air (England and Wales, Scotland) and that asylum windows should be 'large', but state no specific dimensions, other than in some cases stating that windows should be low enough for patients to see out of them (*Sixteenth report from the Board of Public Works, Ireland*, 1848: 236; *SLC Report (Scotland)*, 1859: 115-119; *Commissioners in Lunacy (England)*, 1870). However, domestic building regulations in most geographical areas of Britain and Ireland at the turn into the twentieth century specified that windows must measure 'the equivalent of $^1/_{10}$ of the floor area of the room', and this standard has been used in the following analysis of asylum window size in order to provide a comparative measure for gauging the extent of natural light provision within asylum buildings (Muthesius 1979 [1904]: 23). Window area is given as a proportion of floor area for each room in a selected villa at each site, usually a villa for chronic, long-stay patients.

Table 8. Purdysburn – percentage window to floor area in villas 2-5 (dimensions obtained from plans and field measurements).

Room	Floor area (m²) (dimensions in ft)	Number of windows (standard size 3.18m²)	%age window to floor area
Ground Floor			
Dayroom 1	46.36 (20 x 25)	2 (and glazed door)	20
Dayroom 2	46.36 (20 x 25)	2 (and glazed door)	20
Dayroom 3	53.92 (29 x 20)	5	30
Reading Room	27.88 (20 x 15)	2	23
First Floor			
Dormitory 1	27.88 (20 x 15)	3	34
Dormitory 2	27.88 (20 x 15)	3	34
Dormitory 3	92.64 (25 x 40)	6	21
Dormitory 4	92.96 (50 x 20)	5	17
Attic Floor			
Dormitory 5	26.8 (24 x 12)	1 (non-standard)	31
Dormitory 6	44.6 (16 x 30)	1 (non-standard)	19

Table 9. Kingseat - percentage window to floor area in villa 4 (dimensions obtained from plans and field measurements).

Room	Floor area (m²) (dimensions in ft)	Window area (m²)	%age window to floor area
Ground Floor			
Dayroom 1	65.09 (35x20)	2.25 x 4 = 9	14
Dayroom 2	46.36 (25x20)	2.5 x 1 2.25 x 3 = 9.25	20
Dining Room	59.48 (32x20)	2.5 x 1 2.25 x 3 = 9.25	16
Downstairs Dormitory	46.36 (25x20)	2.5 x 1 2.25 x 3 = 9.25	20
First Floor			
Dormitory 1	46.36 (25x20)	1.98 x 1 1.44 x 1 1.76 x 2 = 6.94	15
Dormitory 2	46.36 (25x20)	1.98 x 1 1.26 x 1 1.44 x 1 1.76 x 2 = 8.2	18
Dormitory 3	46.36 (25x20)	1.98 x 1 1.44 x 1 1.76 x 2 = 6.94	15
Dormitory 4	46.36 (25x20)	1.98 x 1 1.26 x 1 1.44 x 1 1.76 x 2 = 8.2	18

Table 10. Bangour Village - percentage window to floor area in villa 18 (dimensions obtained from plans and field measurements).

Room	Floor area (m²) (dimensions in ft)	Window area (m²)	%age window to floor area
Ground Floor			
Dining Room	73.6 (42 ft 9 in x 18 ft 6 in (excluding bay))	2.06 x 4 2.34 x 5 = 19.94	27
Day Room	133.48 (45 ft 11 in x 24 ft + 18 ft 6 in x 18 ft (excluding bay))	2.06 x 4 2.34 x 5 1.99 x 3 = 25.91	19
First Floor			
Dormitory 1	73.6 (42 ft 9 in x 18 ft 6 in)	2.06 x 5 1.43 x 4 = 16.02	22
Dormitory 2	61.93 (37 x 18)	2.06 x 4 = 8.24	13
Second Floor			
Dormitory 3	73.6 (42 ft 9 in x 18 ft 6 in)	2.06 x 5 1.43 x 4 = 16.02	22
Dormitory 4	61.93 (37 x 18)	2.06 x 4 = 8.24	13
Dormitory 5	33.49 (18 x 20)	1.43 x 4 = 5.72	17

Table 11. Whalley – percentage window to floor area in chronic villa (dimensions obtained from plans and archive photographs).

Room	Floor area (m²) (dimensions in ft)	Window area (m²)	%age window to floor area
Ground Floor			
Day Room	286.2 (85 ft x 36 ft 3 in)	3.2 x 17 2.32 x 2 3.03 x 1 = 62.07	22
Dormitory	144.38 (37 x 42)	3.2 x7 2.32 x 1 = 24.72	17
First Floor			
Day Room	286.2 (85 ft x 36 ft 3 in)	3.2 x 17 2.32 x 2 3.03 x 1 = 62.07	22
Dormitory	144.38 (37 x 42)	3.2 x7 2.32 x 1 = 24.72	17
Second Floor			
Dormitory 1	164.31 (48 ft 9¼ in x 36.3)	2.55 x 11 1.85 x 2 2.42 x 1 = 34.17	21
Dormitory 2	247.85 (73 ft 7¾ in x 36.3)	2.55 x 14 = 35.7	14

Alt Scherbitz, the explicit model for the majority of the asylums in this study, averages 20 per cent for the ratio of window to floor space across patient accommodation, with dormitories slightly less well-lit than dayrooms. Bangour Village and Preston, which is slightly less sunny on average than Edinburgh, had a ratio of 19 per cent overall, roughly twice the minimum specified for domestic housing in the British Isles at this period.[2] The ratio at Kingseat, near Aberdeen was somewhat lower at 17 per cent overall, despite the fact that it is approximately as sunny as Edinburgh. This is less than the other asylums in the study (although still well above the domestic requirement), and may perhaps be accounted for by the slightly cooler temperatures in the north of Scotland, which may have made larger windows more problematic due to the potential heat loss. Two asylums were much better lit than Alt Scherbitz—Purdysburn and Renfrew—although the exact ratio of window to floor area cannot be calculated for Renfrew as no original plans survive giving room dimensions. However, the villas at Renfrew are of a similar size to those at Purdysburn, and the average window height

---

[2] Climate data for Scottish and English cities was obtained from the Met Office (https://www.metoffice.gov.uk/public/weather/climate) and for Leipzig from Deutsche Wetterdienst (www.dwd.de). The raw data has not been provided here as data for 1900-1914 may differ. For the purposes of this thesis, it has been assumed that *relative* temperature and sunshine hours have, however, not altered greatly.

Table 12. Alt Scherbitz – percentage window to floor area in male villa G (dimensions obtained from plans and field photographs).

Room	Floor area (m²)	Window area (m²) (standard size 3m²)	%age window to floor area
Ground Floor			
Dayroom 1	6 x 4 (24)	3 x 2 (6)	25
Dayroom 2	8.7 x 6.2 (53.94)	3 x 3 (9)	17
Dayroom 3	6 x 4 (24)	3 x 2 (6)	25
Dayroom 4	7.5 x 6.3 (47.25)	3 x 3 (9)	19
Dayroom 5	7.5 x 6.3 (47.25)	3 x 3 (9)	19
First Floor			
Dormitory 1	17 x 6 (102)	3 x 7 (21)	21
Dormitory 2	7.8 x 13 (101.4)	3 x 6 (18)	18
Dormitory 3	6.2 x 8.5 (52.7)	3 x 3 (9)	17

at Renfrew is 9 feet 2 inches. Although window widths are variable, a survey suggests that the Renfrew villas were lit at least as well as those at Purdysburn, which has a window to floor area ratio averaging 25 per cent. Glasgow and Belfast are very similar in terms of temperature and yearly sunshine hours and are both significantly less sunny than nearby cities. It appears, therefore, that there may be some correlation between comparatively low sunshine hours and larger windows, with perhaps also a correlation with colder average temperatures and smaller windows. (It is difficult to speculate about window size at Alt Scherbitz as comparisons have not been made within Germany. German attitudes to light in asylum buildings were not explored in this research, although window/floor ratios were similar to Edinburgh and Preston. While Edinburgh and Preston window sizes may have reflected a tension between admitting more light and not letting out heat, the issue at Alt Scherbitz is likely to have been managing light admission in a much sunnier climate.) In the following analysis, Purdysburn has been used as case study, both because of the large ratio of window to floor area, but also because there is excellent survival of plans, photographs and interiors (also showing internal glazing).

6.5. Light at Purdysburn

The eight standard villas that provided accommodation for most patients on the Purdysburn site, are orientated in the same direction, roughly north to south with the majority of the villas inclining towards NNE-SSW (Figure 4-5). The main entrance to each villa is on the north elevation, with verandahs to west and east when the villas were originally built (the verandahs are now missing or closed in) (Figure 6-1). The villas are orientated in the way prescribed by Nightingale for hospital pavilions, although the arrangement of the space into internal rooms, on a domestic model, has somewhat reduced the numbers of windows when compared to a rectangular hospital ward. The villas are three storeys high, higher than Nightingale specified, but early villas (Figure 4-5, numbers 2, 3, 4 and 5) are separated by at least twice the height of the walls, as

she recommended. Villas 8 and 9 are closer together than this but approach each other on only one elevation, the remaining elevations being fully exposed to light and air. The western elevation, in each case, is privileged in terms of numbers of windows, having three to each gable on the ground floor, while the eastern elevation has two to each gable. The buildings are orientated to take advantage of sunlight when it is available and the increased brightness in the direction of the sun on days of broken cloud, the most frequent sky conditions in cloudy climates (the distribution of luminance in a fully overcast sky is symmetrical about the zenith and independent of the position of the sun) (Hopkinson *et al.* 1966: 23).

The windows at Purdysburn are immediately striking as tall and as occupying a large proportion of the wall area, particularly on the ground floor of the building (Figures 6-2, 6-3). Of a standard size, (other than the dormers, the windows to the WC and to the stairwell) the majority are 8ft 3in (2.51 m) in height rising to 8ft 7in (2.61 m) and 4 ft (1.22 m) in width. Sets of three windows across the ground floor gables of the western elevations provide almost a wall of glass in these pre-modernist buildings.

Every room was lit far in excess of the domestic requirement, at least twice as much (with the exception of two of the dormitories). The best lit rooms are the WCs on the ground and first floors. However, the attention to windows here can be assumed to be at least partly the result of a perceived need for cross-ventilation (i.e. windows are provided in at least two walls in order to allow air to enter in one side and exit through the other). The largest dayroom (3), the scullery and visitor's and attendant's rooms, the special cases room and three of the six dormitories have more than three times the window provision required for domestic houses. The remaining living and sleeping rooms have twice or more the required provision (apart from Dormitory 4 at 17 per cent). Cross-lighting, where rooms are lit from more than one direction, occurs in the main dayroom (3) and WCs on the ground floor, and three of the first-floor

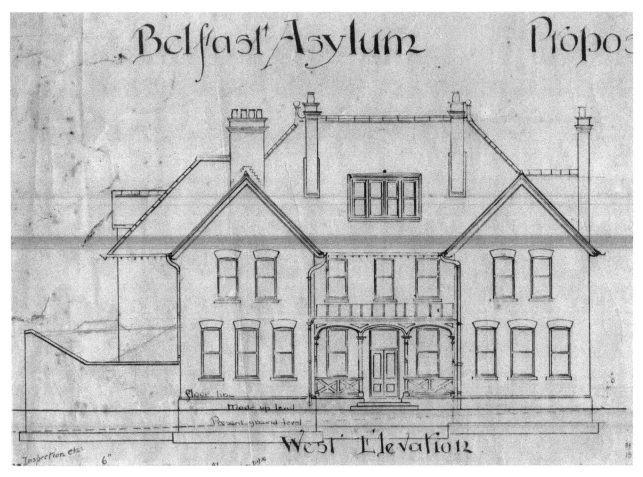

Figure 6-1. Purdysburn Villa Colony: standard villa western elevation, showing original verandah. Source: Architect's drawing, Estates Department, Knockbracken Healthcare Park.

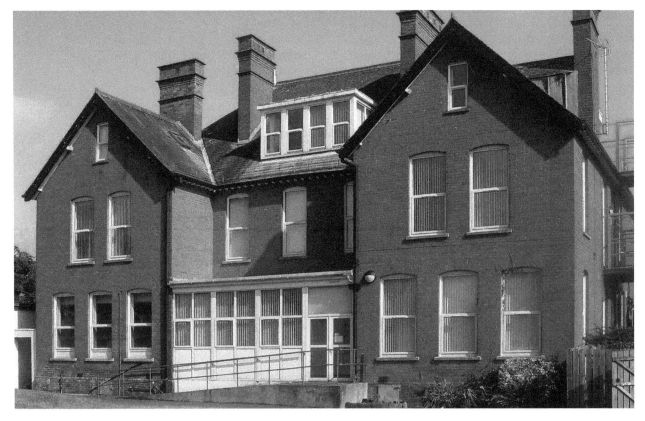

Figure 6-2. Purdysburn Villa Colony showing mid-afternoon light (3.30 pm, mid-September) falling on western elevation of standard villa. Source: Author's photograph.

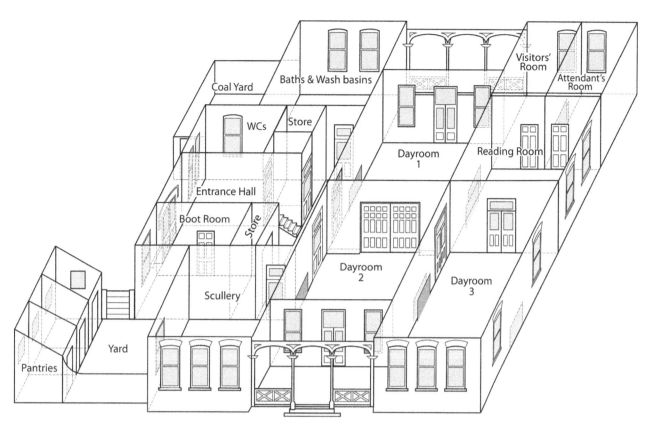

Figure 6-3. Purdysburn Villa Colony: perspective drawing of ground floor of standard villa. Source: redrawn from original plans held by Estates Department, Knockbracken Healthcare Park, supplemented by fieldwork. Not to scale.

dormitories (1, 2 and 4).[3] Nightingale's more stringent recommendations for hospital wards, that windows should form at least one third of the external wall space are generally met by the rooms at the perimeter of the villa, while the central dayrooms fall somewhat short of this requirement with about a fifth of wall space glazed. However, because the internal walls are glazed only at door openings, the rooms are not as well-lit as a typical hospital pavilion. This apparent compromise in light provision could be seen in terms of the discursive requirement to produce a 'home-like' or domestic space in the asylum with internal divisions corresponding to the layout of a domestic house. It can also be surmised that light provision, while critical for mental health, could be somewhat reduced relative to the provision made for those who were physically diseased or injured.

6.6. Interior movement of light

Moving into the interior of the building, the height of the ceilings, again far in excess of what was required domestically at this period (building regulations specified 8.5 ft (2.59 m)) are 12 ft. (3.66 m) on ground and first floors and 10 ft (3.05 m) at attic level. Apart from aiding the circulation of air within the building, this

allowed for taller windows and increased light provision, windows beginning at 2.5 ft. (0.76 m) from the floor and terminating approximately 1 ft. (0.30 m) from the ceiling. This fits with Nightingale's prescription for the windows in hospital pavilions and allowed for patients to be able to see out of the windows while seated or in bed in the dormitories, but the ceilings are lower than her recommendation for hospital wards (15 ft/4.57 m), giving a more domestic scale. The main entrance doors on the north side of the building are half-glazed, admitting light to the hall and stairwell but in general the hallways and stairways are poorly lit compared to living areas (Figure 6-3). The majority of internal doors are half-glazed and have transom lights over, doors into the dayrooms from the verandahs being double doors, as are the doors into the reading room and between dayrooms 2 and 3. Solid doors with transom lights over are fitted at the entrance and exit to the scullery and solid doors without transom lights to the bootroom and storerooms. The doors to the visitors' room and attendant's room may have contained small glazed panes, to facilitate observation. These can still be seen in some of the villas and appear to be original. On the first floor, doors to the main dormitories are half-glazed and fitted with transom lights over, while doors to attendants' and special cases rooms are solid (again perhaps formerly with small observation panes) without transom lights (Figure 6-4). Doorways on the ground and first floors are on average, 7 ft. (2.1 m) high, with transom lights 2.5 ft. (0.7 m) in height and 3 ft. (0.9 m) in width. On the attic floor which was used for patient and staff accommodation as well as storage, doors to storage spaces

---

[3] The *Belfast Newsletter* of 21st October 1929 in a report on Purdysburn states that, 'Cross lighting is a feature of the villa apartments. In every room the light comes in on both sides, for light is now being regarded as an all-important factor in mental and physical healing'. However, as the standard villa design was drawn up in 1902, the importance of light can be presumed to date from much earlier.

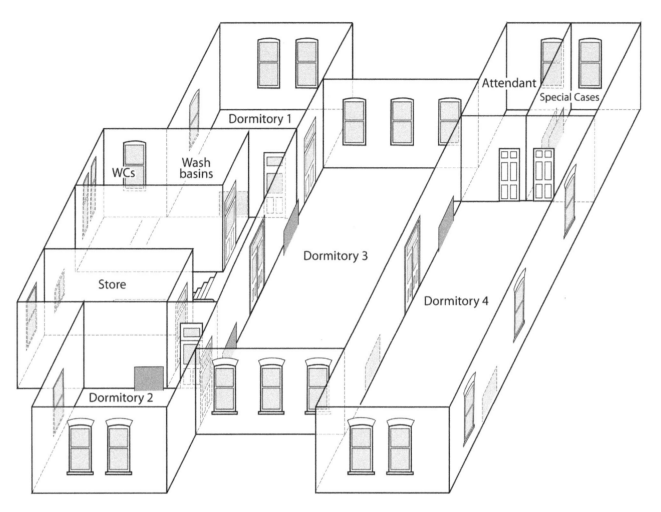

Figure 6-4. Purdysburn Villa Colony: perspective drawing of first floor of standard villa. Source: redrawn from original plans held by Estates Department, Knockbracken Healthcare Park, supplemented by fieldwork. Not to scale.

are solid, without transom lights (Figure 6-5). The main dormitories appear to have been fitted with half-glazed doors although subsequent changes make this difficult to determine, while the staff rooms have solid doors but are also fitted with 'borrowed lights' that distribute light from the windows into the passageway. None of the villas was constructed with cellars, although they are built over an air space fitted with terracotta ventilation grilles (PRONI LA/7/29/CB/22 Builder's Specification, 1902).

The contemporary photograph, portraying the interior of dayroom 3 (Fig 6-6) can be interpreted as a deliberate discursive construction of the asylum as a place of light. The image has been captured facing towards the large windows and their full height has been brought into the picture, emphasising the light flooding through them. The windows are partially open, showing that fresh air is moving into the room but they are not hung with curtains, although blinds appear to be fitted. At this period, heavy curtains were a feature of domestic interiors and the absence of curtains here can be understood as allowing more light to enter the room, as well as eliminating furnishings that would trap dust and dirt. The blinds would have assisted the staff and patients to manage over-stimulating glare. The presence of potted plants near the windows and

flower vases on the mantel shelves discursively signals the healthy properties of this interior, the vigorous growth of the plants demonstrating that the environment is one of strength and vitality for the patients who can be likened to plants in their response to light. Reflective surfaces within the room render the light more visible, such as the polished linoleum on the floor, and the mirrors over the fireplaces which reflect, not only light, but the windows themselves. Walls and ceilings are pale-coloured which further reflects light around the room. Light also falls prominently on, and is reflected from, the tables running down the centre of the room and the books which lie upon them. The type of reading material provided in the asylum is not recorded but it is known that books were intended as a distraction from morbid or misguided thoughts and the light falling on the books in this photograph acts to emphasise discursively the provisions made by an enlightened asylum regime. The patients themselves are absent from this picture, their absence signalling that they are fit and active and about their healthful employment during the day, rather than sedentary. The photograph presents the asylum as a light environment with all that entailed in terms of health, hygiene and enlightened care and would have been read as fulfilling and most likely exceeding requirements for a public asylum for the insane poor.

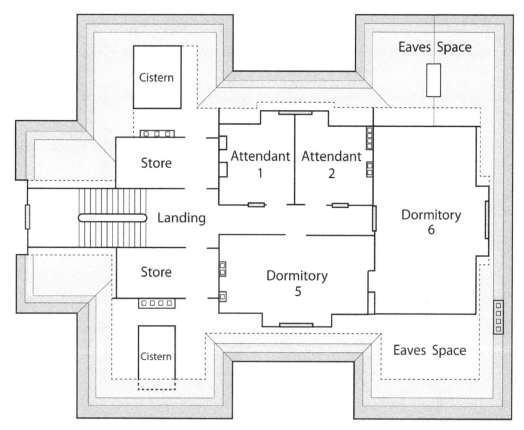

Figure 6-5. Purdysburn Villa Colony: plan of attic floor. Source: redrawn from original plans held by Estates Department, Knockbracken Healthcare Park.

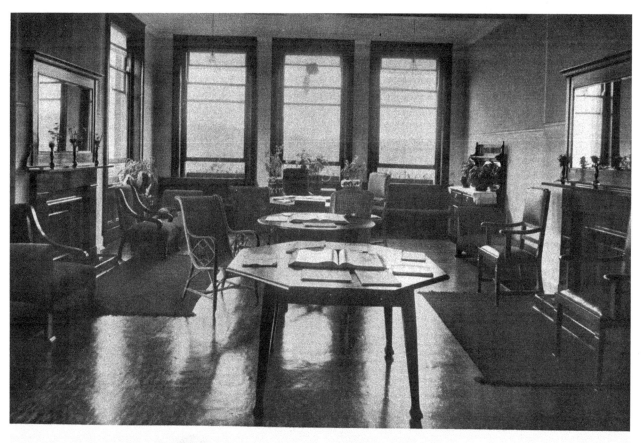

A VILLA DAYROOM.

Figure 6-6. Purdyburn Villa Colony: villa dayroom interior. Source: BDLA Annual Report 1921.

Light is enacted within the material practice of the building itself with the orientation of the main dayroom (3) towards south and west meaning that it would have been light-filled all day long and was no doubt used by patients who were not able or willing to be out at work during the day. However, for the majority of patients day-time work, perhaps on the farm (for men) or in the laundry (for women) was considered an essential part of the therapeutic regime, the labour of patients being indispensable for the smooth running of the asylum. The orientation of the central dayrooms (1 and 2) with verandahs facing west and east reflects this regime. Dayroom 1, facing east, could be used for breakfasting, when it was filled with the rays of the rising sun, Dayroom 2, facing west, for dining when it would benefit from the setting sun, but outside these times, these would have been among the least well-lit rooms. Dayrooms 1 and 2 were divided with sliding doors that could open to form a large space, lit from either direction, as necessary. The verandahs (no original verandah survives) were originally fitted with glass roofs, allowing light to enter into the dayrooms beyond. The plans of the rooms take the simplest form possible, their rectangular shape eliminating dark and shadowy corners, perhaps not only for the sake of hygiene and ease of supervision but also to reduce the possibility of morbid or manic fancies among the patients.

Areas where cleanliness and elimination of disease-causing agents were particularly important are also well-lit, particularly the scullery and WCs. The scullery/kitchen faces west, receiving its greatest usage during the preparation of the evening meal, with the cleansing and food-preparation functions arranged under or near to the windows and the cooking range opposite the window at the back of the room. The bathroom and 'lavatory' (as the washing area was called at this period), faces eastwards where it would be lit in the early part of the day, this room most likely receiving much of its use during the morning period, the wash-hand basins being situated under the windows. Neither WCs nor baths were partitioned, suggesting that light and vision extended into the most intimate parts of the patients' lives. The visiting room and staff room are well lit by windows, but the absence of transom lights over the doors suggests spaces that are more private and perhaps only in temporary use. The darkest area of the ground floor is the corridor, although it is clear that efforts have been made to increase the natural light reaching this area by means of transom lights and glazed doors leading into the rooms off the corridor. Dark corridors were seen as less than desirable, Nightingale (1863: 56) specifying that they 'must be light and airy', while Burdett (1891:100) called dark corridors at Darenth asylum their 'greatest blemish'. The extent of corridors in the villa buildings has been reduced to a minimum, in comparison with both contemporary asylums and pavilion hospitals.

Although many specialised asylum fixtures and fittings were available at this date, none appears to have been used on the windows at Purdysburn, although moulded wood stops were to be fitted to top and bottom sashes 'to allow

them being open 5 in.' (PRONI LA/7/29/CB/22 Builder's Specification, 1902). The restricted opening would have prevented patients falling or jumping from windows, while allowing them to be used for ventilation, but would not have distinguished the windows from ordinary domestic examples.

The ratios of window to floor space in the first floor dormitories are slightly reduced in comparison with the ground floor dayrooms reflecting the fact that patients were not likely to be in these rooms except at night-time and that light could be an impediment to rest and sleep. However, the dormitories are nonetheless almost as well-lit as the ground floor rooms, which would have assisted the 'sunning' of the rooms during the day in order to eliminate disease-causing agents. It can be assumed that the 'special cases' room on this floor was used for patients deemed disruptive or requiring close supervision. The provision of a standard window correlates this space conceptually with a domestic space rather than a prison cell with high barred windows and indeed Burdett's (1891:9) instructions for 'single rooms' specify that these rooms must resemble cells as little as possible, the gauge of this being that the patient should be able to see out of the window. This room, which would have been used for the most disruptive patients and therefore might be expected to be somewhat carceral in nature, is constitutive of the enlightened nature of the treatment in this asylum and by implication of the enlightenment of the asylum project as a whole. Seemingly, the provision of light was so powerful a marker of humane treatment that it was maintained by the President of the Medico-Psychological Association that fastening the door on a patient 'whether for bodily illness, for observation, or for mental excitement' in a room that was well-lit was a valuable strategy, while locking patients in a dark room was worthy of the Lunacy Commissioners' criticism *(JMS* 1874 (20):332-334).

The attic storey is slightly lower in height (at 10 ft; 3.05 m) than the rest of the villa but this is compensated for by wide dormer windows, and the use of borrowed lights to feed light into the corridor, defeating the expectation that this part of the villa would be darker than the lower floors. The borrowed lights, fitted with obscured 'muranese' glass, in the walls of the attendants' quarters, would also have facilitated observation of patients passing along the corridor while maintaining some privacy for the staff. The eaves spaces and cistern rooms were to be whitewashed (PRONI LA/7/29/CB/22 Builder's Specification, 1902), suggesting that these unventilated and badly lit recesses (small rooflights appear to have been fitted over the cistern rooms) were sources of concern as potential repositories for dirt or foul air. Forbes Winslow recommended whitewashing as a means of 'distributing light by artificial means' (Winslow 1867: 198) and whitewash may have been used for its light reflecting as well as antiseptic properties.

The number, size and orientation of the external windows at Purdysburn and their positioning to facilitate the regime of the asylum allowed patients to benefit from more light at times of day when they would be in the villas. Living quarters are better lit than sleeping quarters or uninhabited spaces, and the internal glazed doors and transom lights, the whitewashed eaves spaces, dormers and borrowed lights in the attic spaces and the elimination of dark cellars, all speak of the importance of light in the construction of the asylum. Although a hospital pavilion might have been better served with windows, light has been maximised at Purdysburn, while the villas remain within an architectural idiom of domesticity.

6.7. The winter gardens at Purdysburn

Purdysburn's hospital building with twin integrated winter gardens was designed by prominent English asylum architect George Thomas Hine and built between 1909 and 1912. The building comprises a three-storey central block with single-storey wings on either side, the west wing for males and the east, identical, wing for females. The building is orientated roughly west to east and open verandahs originally ran along the length of both wings, facing southwards where patients could be exposed to air and sunlight during fine weather (Figures 4-14). Classical architectural theory, which correlates constructed forms with the proportions of the human form, allows us to view the low wings either side of the tall central block of the hospital as articulated limbs, curving forwards in a gesture that is embracing/confining. The Winter Gardens are situated in the position of the 'palm of the hand' on both male and female wings of the building with adjoining dorms and annexes forming 'fingers' (Figure 4-15). The three dormitories of each hospital wing all open onto the Winter Garden as does the service annexe for each wing (kitchens) and the sanitary annexe (baths, wash basins and WCs). The Winter Garden, therefore, provided a panoptic hub for each wing of the hospital, with all dormitories visible and accessible from it.

However, while the Winter Garden was certainly intended to provide good visibility into areas occupied by patients, another primary function was its construction as a light-filled space that acted as a funnel feeding light into the Winter Garden itself and the adjoining dormitories.[4]

In the closing decades of the nineteenth century, a winter garden was an indispensable addition to the facilities of hotels, health resorts and spas and was associated with health, leisure, and freedom from the stresses and constraints of modern living (Koppelkamm 1981:45-46). Winter gardens were usually on a grander scale than the domestic conservatory and commonly featured masonry or brick walls with large windows. The earliest winter gardens were built with tiled or slated roofs, in a style that echoed early orangeries, but the early nineteenth century saw a change to glazed roofs arising out of an increasing understanding of the importance of overhead or perpendicular light to the growth of plants. John Claudius Loudon, one of the most prominent horticultural writers of this era (Grant 2013: 25), observed that: 'the summits of all bodies in the free atmosphere receive more light than their sides; and hence the trees in dense forests continue to grow and thrive though they receive little benefit from light, except from that which strikes on the tops of the plants. Hence the great importance of perpendicular light to plants under glass' (Loudon 1845:91).

Although overhead light in summer was thought essential for the ripening of fruit, Loudon considered that a glass roof was also important for a 'greenhouse in which no fruit is ripened but in which the abundance of light is required all the year'. He recommended that such a greenhouse should have, 'perpendicular glass to receive a maximum of light during winter and a sloping roof of glass at an angle of 45°, which is found favourable for the admission of light at every season' (Loudon 1845:91). Loudon's ideal for a greenhouse was based on the understanding that when rays of light hit glass at an angle of between 90° and 40°, more than 85 per cent of the light passes through the glass. However, at angles lower than this, the amount of light transmitted through the glass rapidly begins to fall off until, at a 10° angle, more light is lost than passes through (Lawrence 1963:107-109). Given that the altitude of the sun does not rise above 40° for several months of the year in northern latitudes, the glass surface of a greenhouse or winter garden must approach the vertical on at least some portion of the structure in order to capture a maximum amount of light during the cooler seasons.

The original two-stage lantern roof of the Winter Garden at Purdysburn (roof no longer present) was hexagonal, the lower stage a vertical glazed plinth with windows that opened on three sides and a roof of fixed panes at an approximate pitch of 35-45° (Figure 6-7). This was surmounted by an identical smaller scale lantern of vertical fixed panes and an angled roof, and the whole was finished with a tall iron finial. The roof lantern presents a substantial surface of vertical glass to lower angles of the sun in the early and late hours of the day and through the winter months. The design also captures the overhead sunlight which was deemed so important to the development and health of plants, and a large glass surface is available to catch diffused light from all directions.

An image, taken from a Belfast District Lunatic Asylum annual report, which was captured within a few years of the hospital's opening in 1912, depicts the Winter Garden on the female side of the hospital and shows the room dominated by a large and verdant tropical plant whose great size, dark leaves and vigorous growth give a strong impression of an environment of optimum health (Figure 6-8). The presence of the plant implies that the room is light-filled but the light is also made visible within the lofty room by the pale colours of the floor and walls and the glazed surfaces of the wall tiles. Half-glazed doors, set in a glazed screen, marked the entrances between the

---

[4] According to a former member of staff at Purdysburn the Winter Garden was known as the 'solarium' at one point in its history (Hamilton and Martin, 2013).

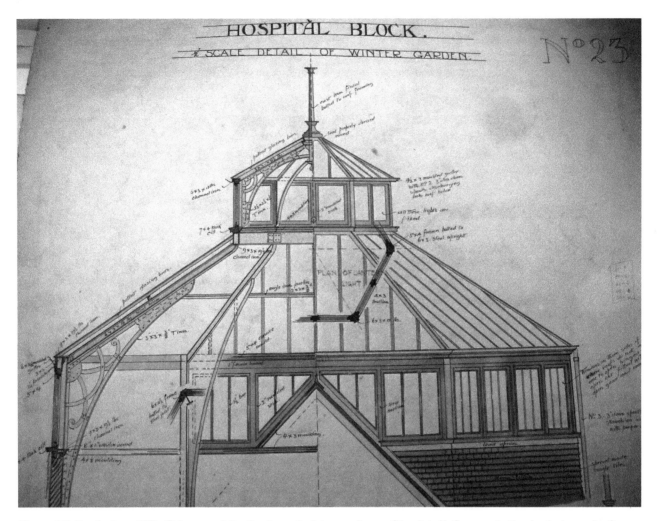

Figure 6-7. Purdysburn Villa Colony: architect's plans of winter garden roof (undated). Source: Author's photograph of original architect's drawings, Estates Department, Knockbracken Healthcare Park.

Winter Garden and the dormitories. The glazed screens are brought into the picture showing how the light from the Winter Garden feeds into the other areas of the hospital. The only visible shadows are those cast by the elegant tables on which books are placed. These cultural objects are balanced with the natural object, the plant, and occupy a discursive position that would have been occupied by statues or works of art in a public winter garden.

The patients are shown enjoying rest and recuperation in a genteel bourgeois context, with the emphasis on humane treatment in an ambience which is suggestive of a hotel or spa rather than the spartan working class homes from which they are likely to have come, and which contemporary discourses reviled as dark, dirty and airless (Mearns 1883: 4-5; Booth 1890: 166). The scene speaks of the beneficial effect this environment is having on the patients. They are sedate and composed, there is no agitation and apparently no noise, all the patients appear to be silent. They are sedentary, but well enough not to be lying in their hospital beds which are seen vacant in the background. This space would be understood by contemporaries as one where the patients could obtain exercise by walking around the room, perhaps stopping to look at the pictures or words laid out on the tables, rather as promenaders would use

a public winter garden, pausing to view the works of art while sheltered from inclement conditions outdoors.

The Winter Garden at Purdysburn asylum was constructed to offer patients the benefit of the therapeutic qualities that light was thought to possess. A Winter Garden, with its cultural associations of health and freedom from the stresses of modern living, was provided for the more fragile patients as a means of allowing them to be 'outdoors' while indoors, and thus avail of the many benefits that exercise in the open air could afford including bathing in the overhead light that the roof lantern was carefully designed to capture, without being exposed to the cold and wet. The design of the roof ensured that the Winter Garden was filled with light, whenever light was in the sky, with its vertical panes angled to catch light in the cooler seasons and the sloping roof able to capture beneficial perpendicular rays and diffused light from all directions.

The explicit meaning of the Winter Garden as light-filled space often overlaps with more indirect and symbolic resonances. A Winter Garden is ostensibly a space for the cultivation and display of tender tropical plants and the plant that was placed at the centre of the room is shown

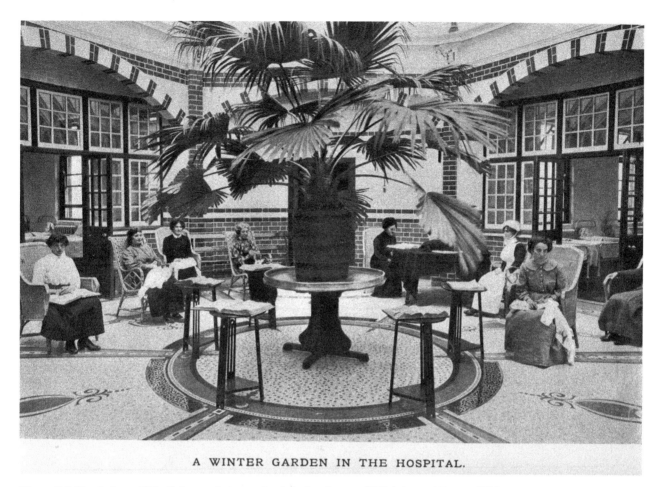

A WINTER GARDEN IN THE HOSPITAL.

Figure 6-8. Purdysburn Villa Colony: winter garden interior. Source: BDLA Annual Report 1922.

as thriving within this environment, with large, strong leaves of a deep colour and exuberant growth reaching above head height. The plant stands in vivid contrast to the blanched and spindly specimens that would be grown in a less healthy and darker environment. The mentally fragile patients are implicitly correlated with tender and fragile tropical plants and the light that benefits plants is perceived as also engendering vitality, energy and vigour in the patients, extending to their weak and disordered minds which could be properly nurtured within the asylum and encouraged to heal. The perceived continuum between physical and mental disease during this period meant that there was often no clear division between treatment for psychiatric disorders and bodily ones. Providing a physically healthy and hygienic environment including well-lit accommodation was part of a regime that was intended to promote recovery in the insane.

6.8. Discussion and conclusion

The discourses of light and mental health that have emerged in the material practices of this asylum are multi-layered and a broad separation can be made into those aspects which are likely to have formed part of the explicit intention of architects, builders and medical superintendent, such as the elimination of disease-causing agents and the promotion of cheerfulness and those that are implied, such as the fear of degeneracy and societal

collapse. However, any such separation is likely to be somewhat arbitrary, for, as we have seen, the figurative and literal lie extremely close in discourses of light, and the symbolic force of light is likely to account for some of the quasi-scientific belief in its medical efficacy.

In giving attention to the admission and movement of light through the buildings the colony asylum is discursively situated within an enlightenment project which has delivered the insane poor both from the barbarous treatment they would have received outside the asylum and from the misguided and brutal regimes of the eighteenth- and early nineteenth-century asylums which imprisoned the insane in dungeons. Additionally, the light of the asylum justified removing the insane from their homes, which were discursively constructed as mentally, morally and physically unhealthy. Light was identified with the superior knowledge and understanding of the medical hierarchy and illuminated their surveillance and control within the building. However, a link can be drawn between the light of observation and that of protection, light protects the patients from abuse even as it facilitates control and discipline. Light was also to be seen as a significant part of therapeutic care in promoting physical and mental health, elevating mood and in banishing the shadows on which hallucinations were built. The asylum environment was a caring one, providing strength and vitality, but also a self-interested one, protecting society from the threat that was spreading from below, of mental disease and degeneration emanating from the darkness of the slums.

Darkness was to be kept at bay within the material practices of the asylum, all recesses were to be eliminated so that light could reach into every corner and kill the disease-causing organisms that lurked there. Situated on rural sites, outside the urban area, with rooms that were spacious and well-ventilated, admitting copious amounts of light, asylum villas take their cue, architecturally, from the homes of the middle classes and a developing cultural orthodoxy of the bourgeois home as light, airy and hygienic and the antithesis of the claustrophobic, filthy and noisome slums, hidden from sight, that render their inhabitants idiotic, animal-like and desensitised. The bourgeois-style colony villas can further be seen as constituting discourses on the nature of legitimate socio-sexual relations, their separation as buildings allowing for the sorting of patients into types and genders, and their well-lit and open, yet divided, internal spaces allowing for categorisation, separation and policing of sexual and social contact, inter and intra patients and staff. The insane poor, like the sane poor, are constituted as lacking the strength, moral and physical, to construct appropriate socio-sexual divisions, one of the most potent measures of their descent into 'darkness' and one that is seen as ultimately threatening to civilisation itself. The bourgeois environment of the asylum emphasises the paternalistic control of the medical establishment and regulates the bodies of the insane poor within light-filled spaces that keep order through promoting health, sanity and sexual continence.

The foregoing discussion has sought to extend our understanding of the cultural context and the values informing explicit decisions that were taken in the construction of asylum buildings, as well as what can be 'read' as implied but was not a part of the agency of medical superintendent, architect or builder. This study seeks to go beyond a concept of 'unchanging rationality' (Burke 2008:2) in which 'light' is perceived as timeless, but is in fact very much informed by our own contextual understandings, and to move towards an understanding of the values held by the society that produced the villa colony asylum. Material practices; the buildings, spaces and ways in which they were inhabited can only be usefully understood in the light of discursive practices; the words, symbols and ideas used by contemporaries to represent light and darkness.

Discourses of mental illness were constituted by medical professionals and not patients, but, although discursive practices are not linked to material practices in any formal or predictive way, the material remains of the asylum confirm an emphasis on light, air and space. Although we would expect an attention to light in the asylum buildings constructed at this period, the exact form this takes is not entailed by medical discourses. The fact that the buildings 'fit' with contemporary discourses on light provides additional evidence of the degree to which we can accept the values of these discourses as significant, because they are materially enacted. The material evidence cannot be written off, in the same way as the potentially self-serving treatises of the medical establishment might be.

We have already noted that reading the provision of light within a building can be a complex matter. If we take the staff accommodation within the asylum as an example, this highlights some of the difficulties. Attendants' rooms within Purdysburn are largely as well lit as the accommodation of patients, but it would be simplistic to conclude from this that the connection of light with mental health cannot be sustained. Light provision within asylums was subject to regulatory and economic considerations which sometimes acted to standardize window sizes within institutions. Furthermore, as we have seen, light is multivalent and carries meanings that are the unconscious reproduction of cultural norms as well as those that are the result of agency of builders and designers. As a consequence, our understanding of the meaning of light at any particular place and time is unlikely to be entirely amenable to linear, correlative strategies. Because of this, a close reading of contemporary sources is essential in order to tease out the ways in which we should understand the buildings we see. Strategies which read light as resonant, evocative, and discursively powerful are more likely to bring us close to contemporary understandings than strategies which attempt to correlate the specific size and shape of windows to singular meanings such as 'health,' 'surveillance' or 'economy.' However, broad tendencies in hospital and asylum architecture should be pursued and further research may profitably be able to examine changes in window sizes and the ratio of window to floor space over time, clarifying differences in the light provision for patients of different types within and between hospital and asylum buildings. The age of asylums, which saw new buildings constructed across Europe and North America in large numbers, has left a rich legacy in terms of numbers of institutions and the time span they cover. This may negate potential difficulties caused by the fact that buildings persist where ideas do not, and that it may have been difficult to practically implement changes in discourses around light in pre-existing buildings.

The next chapter will focus on the ways in which the architecture, spaces and décor of the colony asylum attempted to embody ideals of the 'domestic' and 'home-like'.

7

Domesticity and the colony asylum

This chapter will begin by exploring the historical context to the provision of 'home-like' accommodation in asylums for the insane at the beginning of the twentieth century, by means of a short review of the existing literature. We will then move to a consideration of the contemporary primary material relating to domesticity in the asylum in order to determine what types of meaning coalesced around the idea of 'home-like' in this period. This will be followed by an analysis of selected buildings within each of the sites in this study, examining how each of these conform or depart from the cultural ideals that have been uncovered. Finally, the provision of 'home-like' surroundings in the colony asylum will be related to wider cultural trends such as the cult of domesticity and ideas of liberty and individuality.

7.1. Historical background to domesticity in the asylum

'... of all the ills that beset us, lunacy was the first to be defined as something that should be treated away from home. Acutely conscious of this rupture, psychiatric reformers then explicitly set out to recreate homes.'
(Stevenson, 2000: 8)

Previous scholarship has suggested that the late eighteenth and early nineteenth centuries saw a radical change in the way that the insane were conceived of and treated. Earlier conceptions of the insane as bestial, violent and raving and needing to be tamed through brutal and harsh treatment, such as beatings and physical restraint, gave way to the rejection of physical punishments and attempts to engage the insane person's 'desire for esteem', under the supervision of a patriarchal 'Moral Governor' within a therapeutic, domestic-style environment (Scull, 1983: 245). The archetype for this change in attitude was the York Retreat, which was modelled on a domestic home, both architecturally/spatially and in terms of the regime followed. The asylum itself was built to resemble the country seat of a bourgeois family and the patients were encouraged to develop self-control through working towards privileges, some of which were associated with the spatial arrangement of the building, as patients worked towards the centre of the structure where the patriarchal figure of the 'moral governor' had his quarters. Interiors were broken down into spaces equivalent to those occupied by a bourgeois family, such as dayroom, dining room and library and aspects of restraint, such as locks and walls, were concealed so as to preserve the 'home-like' appearance (Edginton, 1997, 2003).

With the establishment of the public asylum system in Ireland, England and Wales and Scotland from 1821 onwards, the importance of maintaining a domestic/home-like scale and appearance within the asylum continued to be emphasised in the growing literature relating to asylum construction and management (e.g. Browne, 1837; Clouston, 1879; Connolly, 1847). In the early days of the asylum movement, it was unusual to be treated away from home for any kind of illness, and it was only the very poor who were subject to this type of medical provision (Taylor, 1991: 11). Stevenson contends that lunacy was the first disease in which treatment away from home was deemed necessary to a cure (Stevenson, 2000: 8). The early asylum system was built on the premise that the insane could only be treated away from home, the homes of the insane frequently being seen as an 'exciting cause' of insanity, due to domestic conflict and cruelty or to poor environmental conditions (Philo, 2004: 463-4; Yanni, 2007: 54).

However, in the second half of the nineteenth century, institutions such as lunatic asylums were becoming ever larger, and the asylum system in particular began to creak under the strain of vastly increasing numbers of patients, many of whom were long-term, often cognitively impaired rather than mentally ill in the way this would be understood today. The aspiration to keep asylums small-scale and domestic in the accommodation they provided began to suffer, as ever more vast buildings were constructed. Attempts were made to include domestic details in furnishings and to break up the interiors of asylum buildings into smaller, domestic-style spaces (Yanni, 2007: 6). In the second half of the nineteenth century, the suggestion that asylum buildings themselves should be broken down into smaller units, whether cottages, blocks, pavilions or villas, was increasingly put forward, partly because this was seen as more 'homely' than the alternative (Philo, 2004: 649). To some degree this trend was also observable outside the asylum system. By the end of the nineteenth century, the appellation 'home' was used for several types of institution, convalescent homes from the 1860s, cottages homes for orphans from the 1870s and homes for the feeble-minded from the 1890s, as the institutional landscape increased in complexity and made provision for long-term residents. Domestic architectural models were also used for ordinary hospitals, notably the cottage hospital (also from 1860s), which aimed to lessen the suggestion of a public building dedicated to the sick, with even Florence Nightingale proposing that the best convalescent hospital would be composed of a string of cottages (Taylor, 1991: 44, 74-5). A great deal of idealisation of the 'cottage' is discernible in these trends, although at this period the homes of the poor were, in reality, often seen as unhealthy and squalid (Richardson *et al.*, 1998: 45). A consciousness of the effect on minds and spirits of institutional buildings appears to have influenced these attempts at domestic scale and feel, but they can also be viewed as associated with a late Victorian cult of domesticity, in which the home (particularly the middle-class home) had developed into a sanctuary 'sealed off from the sullying sins of the secular world'. The home was increasingly seen as a refuge from society's shortcomings—immorality and materialism—and was managed by women as 'moral supremacists' who were associated with the material fabric of the house as preservers of healthy environments (Adams, 1996: 3-4; Rafferty, 1996: 38-9).

At this period, the aspiration for mental nurses was that they would be trained in domestic ideology and as Hide and Boschma have suggested, as women they were presumed to be responsible for preserving morality within the family and, by implication among patients (Boschma, 2003:84; Hide, 2014:75). It was hoped that middle-class women, or at least women of a certain refinement could be attracted towards mental nursing, and it was often a subject of complaint that such women were not available for this type of work (Boschma, 2003: 92-99). Insofar as insanity was often connected with moral failings and defined as a departure from acceptable social standards, women's role as moral guardians was brought to the fore. The 'home-like' setting of the asylum was an environment in which women could enact bourgeois practices, raising the morally deficient (working-class) patients out of insanity and bringing civilisation to degenerate lower-class behaviours (Boschma, 2003: 141). It has been suggested that the association of women with the home and men with work and outdoors was influential on the type of activities that male and female patients were expected to carry out in the asylum. Women were more likely to work in the laundry or dressmaking or other 'domestic' activities and less likely to be encouraged to go outdoors. Outdoor work was largely the preserve of men, and it has been suggested that women were more stigmatised by institutionalisation because of their greater association with the domestic sphere (Porter & Wright, 2003: 44). This may explain why some asylums ran the male side of the asylum on the model of a barracks and the female side like a residential home (Berrios & Freeman, 1991: 22). The female asylum patient was being consciously restored to her idealised role as guardian of domestic morals and hygiene, while the chief concern associated with male patients was that they should be restored to their families as productive providers, whose major role was outside the domestic sphere. It is also possible that degeneracy was more clearly associated with male patients, who were more prone to GPI (Gittins, 1998: 164).

Previous scholarship has addressed the question of how a home-like environment was provided in the asylum from several points of view. With regard to external architecture, Taylor has analysed the buildings themselves, pointing to the usage of 'traditional domestic-scale details' in hospitals such as verandahs, half-timbering and steep, tiled roofs (Taylor, 1991: 74). Richardson notes the avoidance of the 'grand façade and gigantic institution' in order to give a homely feel at Derby County Asylum (1851) (Richardson *et al.*, 1998: 168). More recent scholarship

has examined asylum interiors, Guyatt contending that in the period between 1880 and 1914, 'homeliness' was more important than questions of sanitation, security or cure in English asylums (Guyatt, 2004: 48). Using photographic evidence, Guyatt shows that, even in Claybury public asylum, a high standard of internal furnishing was provided (although Claybury was heavily criticised for its lavishness by London County Council). Guyatt sees the asylum as a 'hybrid' space, private in the sense of only being accessible to a minority, but public in the sense of housing 'large, unrelated and transitory populations'. She notes that the asylum dining room with its proliferation of bentwood chairs, plants and pictures resembled most closely, not a domestic space, but a late Victorian restaurant. Contemporaries sometimes made comparisons with hotels, clubs and hospitals, as well as domestic homes (Guyatt, 2004: 50-54). Asylum interiors mirrored changing trends in domestic interiors, heavy furniture and dark colours giving way in the later nineteenth century to lighter styles and colours, with medical superintendents, as the asylum managers, becoming heavily involved in decorating decisions. However, most of the interiors that Guyatt considers are those in private asylums, complicating her assertion that asylum authorities were increasingly concerned with greater domesticity, as she acknowledges that paying customers may well have expected a high standard of internal furnishing. As the sole example of a public asylum for non-paying customers, it is not clear how typical Claybury was of asylum accommodation in England. Guyatt suggests that the main reason that more attention was given to domesticity at this period was because, for many patients, the asylum would indeed become their lifelong home. Additionally, the medical establishment understood physical surroundings to have a 'beneficial influence' on patients, increasing their self-control and improving their behaviour, although she also asserts that public asylums were restricted to a version of domesticity that was appropriate to the station in life of the patients (Guyatt, 2004: 58-62).

Jane Hamlett is the leading scholar of domesticity in public asylums in the Victorian and Edwardian period and she posits that some patients were indeed helped to feel 'at home' in the asylum by their environment. Hamlett de-emphasises the ways in which a domestic environment was used as a method of control and suggests instead that asylum authorities wished to differentiate asylum spaces from those of prisons, placing a high value on the emotional importance of a home-like environment (Hamlett, Hoskins and Preston, 2013:21). Hamlett credits the establishment of the Lunacy Commission and their cycles of inspection with the imposition of an asylum standard that required domestic furnishings of a standard equivalent to a middle-class home. This coincided with a trend towards increasing middle-class consumption of consumer goods, rising middle-class incomes and a belief in the power of objects and surroundings to exert moral influence within wider society. Domestic interiors and the objects they contained could be used to inspire correct behaviour, such as occupying the chairs and seats 'in a proper manner' and using eating utensils in a way which chimed with social norms (Hamlett, 2015: 20). However, Hamlett emphasises that 'cheerfulness' was constantly invoked in relation to interiors and that 'the material world was thus granted emotional power, to raise up patients and improve their condition', and should not therefore be understood merely as a means of control (Hamlett, 2015: 21-22). Hamlett, in contrast to Guyatt, perceives a tension towards the end of the century between domesticity and hygiene as guiding principles within the asylum, paralleling an increased concern with hygiene in the domestic home. For example, rather than domestic finishes such as wallpaper, in later asylum interiors there was an emphasis on glazed brick and paint.

In the following section, we will consider the meaning of 'domestic', 'home' and 'home-like' as these terms were applied to asylums in the late nineteenth/early twentieth century.

7.2. Contemporary primary evidence relating to domesticity

The following discussion, is based on an analysis of some of the primary published sources relating to insanity in the period 1880-1914, principally the *Journal of Mental Science* and the annual reports of the Scottish Lunacy Commissioners. Using the search terms, 'home', 'domestic' and 'home-like', it was possible to establish some of the associations that these terms had for asylum culture, and more particularly, Scottish asylum culture in the late nineteenth/early twentieth century.

It is clear that by the end of the century some of the conception of an asylum as an extended family circle that began with *The Retreat* at the beginning of the century had been retained, especially for the smaller (and often private) asylums in which there was a close paternalistic relationship between the superintendent and the patients (*Journal of Mental Science* 1885, 31 (134): 272-275). By this period, the term 'asylum' had come to have considerable negative associations and the word 'home' was sometimes suggested and used as an alternative, but the interest in providing a home-like environment extended far beyond the use of the term and entailed a close interest in how buildings were divided and laid out and how they were decorated and furnished. The clearest and most frequent association of 'home' and 'home-like' in the primary published literature surveyed is with 'comfort'. This appears to signify principally physical comfort, but there is also an implication that the 'comforts of home' are related to kind and gentle treatment. In this respect the asylum is seen as the antithesis of the workhouse and the prison. Many categories of insane were seen as particularly physically, as well as mentally weak. For instance the feeble-minded were said to all labour under more or less constitutional weakness and therefore required comfortable, home-like surroundings more than the general population (*JMS,* 1910, 56 (233), 253-261).

However, some critics doubted whether an asylum could ever be truly home-like. Irish medical superintendent Connolly Norman commented that,

'When can an asylum be home-like to the poor? It needs to be handsome if it is not to present the unutterably dreary and demoralising desolation of an Irish workhouse ward, than which no more melancholy form of habitation has been occupied by man since the days of the cave-dwellers. But the handsomer and brighter you get the great precincts of an asylum, the further you are from home. Home surroundings have an educative, a supporting, a calming effect….the rigid discipline, the unvarying routine, the monotonous and uninteresting life of an asylum can do harm' (Norman, 1904: 61).

The contemporary medical establishment recognised a tension between domestic and institutional, and also often acknowledged that this was a tension that was difficult to resolve, because the nature of an institution required a certain grandeur that was antithetical to the idea of home—large spaces and high ceilings being opposed to the cosiness and confinement that represented domesticity in the popular mind. Scottish Lunacy Commissioners frequently talk of the homes of rural Scottish peasants, though dark, cramped and unhygienic, as representing an ideal of simplicity and domesticity which is difficult to replicate in the asylum setting. However, the peasant home is also subject to much implicit and explicit criticism, principally for 'squalor' and lack of cleanliness and it is clear that there was some uneasiness about placing patients in humble, yet homely settings. While it was admitted that the 'standard of taste' in some Scottish rural dwellings 'may be very different from our own', the cottages could still provide 'much enjoyment of life' because of their qualities of homeliness (SLC 1880: 133). While middle class aesthetic taste was seen as one of the signifiers of home, working class homeliness, which was an option for some patients through the Scottish system of boarding out, was still admitted to have a certain appeal, and allowed the patients to come into contact with sane individuals and to have a greater degree of liberty, which were both seen as important. However, it was clear that although home comforts had been increasing among the poorer classes, the standard of home environment provided by them could not equal that of a properly equipped asylum, which could more nearly replicate a desirable bourgeois home.

A significant characteristic of 'home' was that it should not contain too many people, and the more patients, the more institutional a setting was bound to be (Brodie, 1881: 25). The disaggregation of patients into smaller blocks, cottages and villas and the grouping of these into 'villages' was therefore praised as more 'home-like'. The congregating of patients into large groups was seen as antithetical to home and the English asylum superintendent Steen commented that, 'it is most disastrous to the home feeling to have gangs of patients from the different wards merging into one huge herd in the dining hall' (Steen, 1900). In some, usually private asylums, the provision of single rooms for patients, was seen as more home-like (*JMS*, 1884, 30 (129): 17-19). However, single rooms rarely provided more than a small proportion of accommodation in public asylums for the insane poor, and were generally used temporarily for patients suffering attacks of acute mental illness or who needed special supervision. Small wards were, however, seen as more desirable than large ones for the same reasons (Wallis, 1894: 335-344).

A further attribute of 'home' was the absence of what is often referred to as 'irksome discipline', suggesting that 'home' in this period is seen as a welcome relief from rigid routine and regulation, and that there were some attempts to free the asylum from these kinds of considerations. Irksome discipline was seen as leading to increased irritability among the patients and a need for more staff (SLC 1884: 111). Mentioned as particularly 'irksome' are the routine, the lack of personal freedom and the lack of privacy, including the removal of an individual's personal clothes and possessions. The liberty of home life was of particular concern to Scottish Lunacy Commissioners who stated that liberty, particularly passing through a building and in and out of it freely, and also the ability to choose freely the company of others, was more home-like, added to the comfort of the patients and benefitted their mental condition (SLC 1882: xvii, xxxviii, 62). Home life and its associated liberty was seen to increase the physical and mental well-being of patients and gave them 'a full opportunity of realising and developing their individuality' which was seen as an important factor in rendering the patients productive (SLC 1895: xl).

Domestic life was considered as having the potential to elevate morally the condition of patients, in an era when mental illness was seen as connected to physical and moral health. An English medical officer, describing the ways in which epileptic colonies could be organised to replicate family life, quotes the French philosopher Renan,

'The professor cannot teach that purity and refinement of conscience which is the basis of all solid morality, that bloom of sentiment which some day will be the great charm of the man, that mental subtlety with its almost imperceptible shades—where then can the child and young man learn all these? ... These things are learned in the atmosphere in which we live, from our social environment; they are learned in domestic life and nowhere else.' (Renan quoted in Ewart, 1892)

The idea that refinement and subtlety are the products of family life, suggests that the bourgeois domestic domain and a bourgeois psychic identity—with its supposed sensitivity and intellect—is being held up as an ideal for the socially excluded, and a means by which their mental condition can be improved. At Lanark District Asylum the Commissioners noted with approval that 'at tea time the same women preside at their respective tables and help the tea from their own teapots'. This particular replication of bourgeois practices was said to have 'a refining effect on

the patients' behaviour' (*SLC* 1896: 80; Ross 2014: 269-273).

The fourth International Home Relief Congress in Edinburgh in 1904 suggested that the 'influences of home life' should supersede the assistance given to 'social weaklings in the prison-, convent-, or barrack-like 'institutions' of the past'('The International Home Relief Congress', 1904). This was a period, therefore, where the institution was beginning to seem harmful to 'social weaklings' including the insane, and the environment, practices and personnel of family life were often considered to be elevating and healing. The desire for home was seen as both natural and instinctual and having a persistent force even in those with severe and chronic mental disease. The advocate for colony asylums in Lancashire, social campaigner John Milson Rhodes, wanted asylums to be, 'less like a combination of factory and weaving shed and more like a home', because this would lead to greater happiness among the patients. He quoted the American neurologist W P Spratling,

'the home instinct, the love of home associations, and the desire for pleasant and sympathetic companionship, are the last of the natural desires to die in a people who suffer from mental enfeeblement or decay through chronic and far-reaching diseases' (Rhodes, 1905: 687-688).

Home as a social construction, produced by the rising middle classes, was therefore cast as something 'natural' and 'instinctual' that was fundamental to the nature of being human, and it was therefore this that should be reached for in trying to revive the lost humanity and social functioning of mentally ill or diseased people.

A number of artefacts were strongly associated in Scottish Lunacy Commissioners' reports with providing more homely surroundings in asylum interiors. 'Objects of interest', which included plants, flowers, books and other reading material or pictures were prominent among these, but also important was the painting and papering of walls, window treatments and the provision of comfortable furniture. A direct relationship was drawn between furnishings and decoration and the manageability and productivity of patients. For example, the Commissioners commented of Dumfries District Asylum,

'The entrance hall has been much improved by opening it up and substituting coloured tiles for the stone pavement ... Painting and papering have been done on an extensive scale ... windows have been furnished with valances; coloured tablecloths have been introduced; chairs have taken the place of benches; carpeting and pictures have been increased; and unnecessary doors have been removed. By these and other such means the brightness and cheerfulness of the corridors, dayrooms and dormitories have been increased, and a more homelike aspect given to them, with the result, which always attends such changes, of adding to the tranquillity and contentment of the patients, and making them better able and more willing to engage in active, useful work.' (*SLC* 1882: 66)

The furnishings and decorations of accommodation for the insane were often examined in minute detail by the Commissioners who made very precise recommendations. For instance, the Commissioners suggested that a rug, about 11 feet square, should be placed opposite each fire place in the Dundee West Poorhouse lunatic ward, to add to the brightness and cheerfulness of the rooms and give it a more 'homelike and comfortable aspect ... because pleasant surroundings have an important practical effect in making the patients more easily managed and more contented' (*SLC* 1888: 92).

In conclusion, the 'home-like' quality of provision for the insane poor was seen as vital to their mental and physical well-being. It was also important in increasing their contentment and manageability as asylum inmates and developing their individuality which were all important factors in encouraging asylum patients to take part in productive work and hence resume their place as useful members of society. The domesticity of the asylum aimed to replicate the elevating forms and practices of bourgeois life which had the capacity to elevate the mental and moral condition of patients. Bourgeois home life was constructed as 'natural' and 'instinctual', and was to replace the bestial and asocial tendencies of mentally ill patients which had led to their exclusion from normal social circles.

The following section will look at the architecture, interiors and spatial organisation of the asylums in the study, in order to determine what was prioritised in the attempt to make asylums more home-like.

7.3. External architecture

For the purposes of this section, a selection of villas from each site will be examined in detail for their external architectural features and attributes. In addition, primary sources—principally Annual Reports and Lunacy Board Minutes—will be mined for clarifying information about the domestic character of the buildings that were constructed.

7.3.1. Alt Scherbitz, Germany

For the purposes of this section, it is not proposed to analyse Alt-Scherbitz for its approximation to contemporary German norms of domesticity in terms of external architecture. Instead this section will treat Alt-Scherbitz as an influence on the design of the Scottish and Irish sites and will examine how contemporary visitors to the Prussian asylum viewed the external design of the buildings, in terms of British and Irish conceptions of the home-like and domestic. George Miller Beard, who wrote the first account of Alt Scherbitz to be published in English, described it as consisting of 'six or eight cottages, a small distance from each other, each cottage

being about the size of a moderate country home—all plain brick buildings, pleasing in appearance outside and comfortable in reality inside'. The asylum was further publicised among the international psychiatric community in 1889 on the publication of *The Insane in Foreign Countries* by William P Letchworth who was President of the New York State Board of Charities. Letchworth noted that the buildings were 'unpretentious brick structures, with outer porches' that were entirely separate without corridor connection and 'resemble private dwellings'. He felt that they demonstrated the 'feasibility of substituting inexpensive, comfortable structures, something like ordinary dwellings, for the generally prevailing massive palatial edifices built on the congregate plan for the insane' (Letchworth, 1889: 288).

A later visit by Sir John Sibbald found that the buildings were approximated 'as far as possible to the character of ordinary private dwellings, as regards their size, their style of architecture ... and their grouping' (Sibbald, 1897: 20). Sibbald describes the colony houses of Alt Scherbitz as 'indistinguishable from private houses' with no wall surrounding the asylum and 'ordinary well-kept villa gardens' surrounded by wooden palings, due to be replaced by hedges, with higher palings surrounding the closed villas (Sibbald, 1897: 24). The architecture was 'of the simplest character. There is nothing grand or imposing about any of them, but they are all pleasant to look at, and many of them are picturesque. No attempt has been made to secure uniformity of design, on the contrary, uniformity appears to have been avoided ... the style of architecture of both sections of the institution is generally that of the plain villa with overhanging eaves, or of the Swiss chalet. Simple balconies and verandahs are frequent, and the walls are, in all cases, more or less adorned with climbing plants' (Sibbald, 1897: 25).

Sibbald also noted that tree planting ensured that only a few houses could be seen at a time so that, 'no inmate can be oppressed, as an inmate of an institution consisting of one huge pile of buildings often is, with the feeling that he has lost his individuality, and is only an insignificant unit in a great aggregation' (Sibbald, 1897: 25). He commended Alt Scherbitz for the absence of connecting corridors and pointed out that corridors added greatly to the expense of an asylum and also meant that the buildings could not be freely distributed on the site. Worst of all, that they gave the buildings 'somewhat of a prison character'. According to Sibbald, 67 per cent of the patients in Alt-Scherbitz were in open houses where the doors were unlocked during the day and could be opened with an ordinary handle (Sibbald, 1897: 27-33). Rhodes also concurred that the houses of Alt-Scherbitz 'closely resemble ordinary good villa residences'. The ivy and other creepers on the houses was said to give 'a very pleasant and homely look to the buildings' (Rhodes & McDougall, 1897: 7-15).

The Edinburgh deputation which visited Alt-Scherbitz in 1897 found that the asylum tried to assimilate 'the conditions of life of the patients to those of sane people in an ordinary rural community'. They were impressed by the lack of walls, railings, gates or porter's lodge so that the asylum was not separated in any way from the outside world. The administration house was said to be 'entirely of the character and appearance of a private dwelling house' and the impression of the closed part of the asylum was 'of a thriving suburb of London or some English town'. 'Trees, creepers, flowers, are everywhere cultivated in profusion and given an indescribable home-like appearance to the whole settlement'. The villas were of a 'comfortable, domestic appearance,' but 'although architecturally of the same type, have none of that dead uniformity of design which produces monotony ... monotonous uniformity has been avoided, whether it be in the design of the villas or the pattern of the tea-cups'. All the mechanisms of restraint, such as window locks were not made visible to the patients. The colony part of the asylum was said to even more resemble an ordinary village community because the buildings were 'scattered' and 'irregular' ... The most striking feature of the place is *the absence of the appearance of an institution'* (*Report of Deputation from the Edinburgh District Lunacy Board* 1897: 14-28).

The Lancashire deputation found that the administration building, although small, had 'nothing mean or insignificant in its appearance' but was 'elegant and tasteful'. They conclude that 'the idea of a *home* is, in fact, at the bottom of the village colony system' by which they mean that 'those whose tastes, habits, interests and occupations are similar might be enabled to associate and live together apart from others'. The division of patients was also thought to increase the individual interest of attendants in their patients and the individual interest of the patients in themselves. It was thought important to stem the loss of individuality which leads to 'loss of initiative and mental energy, in short, of mind' by appealing to the personal initiative of patients. This could only be done by more normal living conditions and intimate and close contact with sane attendants. Variety was expected to have a good effect on the medical staff as well as patients, as they visited a variety of houses and communities rather than the daily ward round in an asylum. 'Large unsympathetic wards and corridors' were felt to depress the spirits and were not cheerful like the arrangements in a colony (*Report of a Lancashire deputation, 1*900: 27-35, 63).

Although the villas built in Scotland and Ireland are very variable in styles and layout, it appears that the villas at Purdysburn and at Dykebar in particular, may have been influenced by the style and layout of villa G at Alt-Scherbitz (Figure 7-1). The basic form of double-fronted

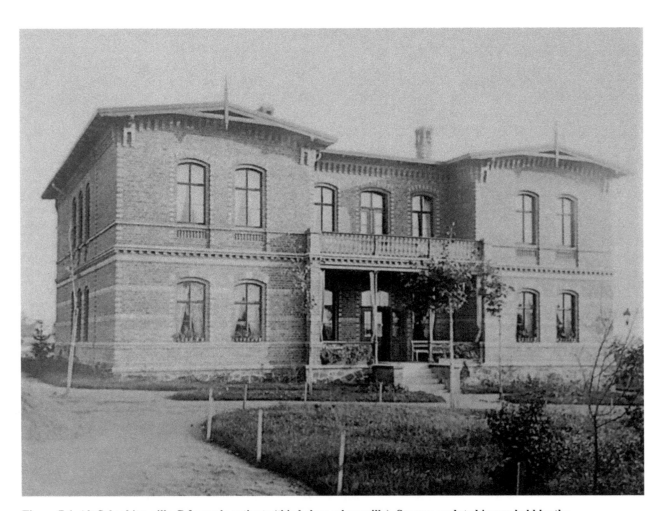

Figure 7-1. Alt Scherbitz: villa G for male patients (third class colony villa). Source: undated image held by the Traditionskabinett at Sächsisches Krankenhaus, Alt Scherbitz.

villa with gabled end bays and recessed central bays spanned by a verandah represented by villa G is replicated by design one at Purdysburn and by the two villa designs at Dykebar, although the decorative details in each case are very different.

7.3.2. Aberdeen District Asylum (Kingseat)

Designs for Kingseat asylum villas were prepared by the local architect Alexander Marshall Mackenzie in August 1900 and the asylum was constructed between 1901 and 1904, making it the first complete general asylum of the colony type to be opened in Britain or Ireland. The architect stated that his aim was to have 'some degree of quality in architecture without a single vestige of ornament' (*Aberdeen Journal* 14th January 1901). Early commentary on Kingseat stated that the village asylum was 'more efficient and more adaptable' and made the patients happier than 'under the old, more expensive and more cumbersome method of erecting palatial, prison-like buildings' (Macpherson, 1905: 490). Kingseat, unlike Bangour which suffered from lengthy disputes almost amounting to scandal in relation to cost, was built relatively cheaply at £253 per bed. The asylum was praised for looking less like an institution than the traditional asylum, and was noted to be 'cheerful and homelike ... without

architectural pretensions', and harmonising with its surroundings ('The First British Village Asylum', 1906).

Alexander Marshall Mackenzie (1848-1933) produced a wide variety of designs, many for domestic houses and manses but also for a number of larger buildings such as schools, hospitals and churches. Many examples of Mackenzie's domestic work still survive in Aberdeen and some of these share characteristics with his work at Kingseat. Figures 7-2 and 7-3 show two of his domestic designs and his design for Villa 5 at Kingseat is shown at Figure 7-4, exhibiting the use of stonework, timber framing and gables of varying sizes. Two main architectural styles are perceptible in the design of the asylum. A style the architect called 'old English', was used for the recreation hall and villa 5 and features overhanging eaves and timber panelling above a more traditionally Scottish stone building. A second style identified as 'late Scottish renaissance' was a revival borrowing from seventeenth-century Scottish dwelling houses, many of which were recorded in the influential five-volume work, *The Castellated and Domestic Architecture of Scotland,* published between 1887 and 1892 (Macgibbon and Ross, 1887-1892). The Scottish Renaissance is illustrated in this work by dwelling houses that use a quasi-symmetrical arrangement of windows and doors, and the positioning

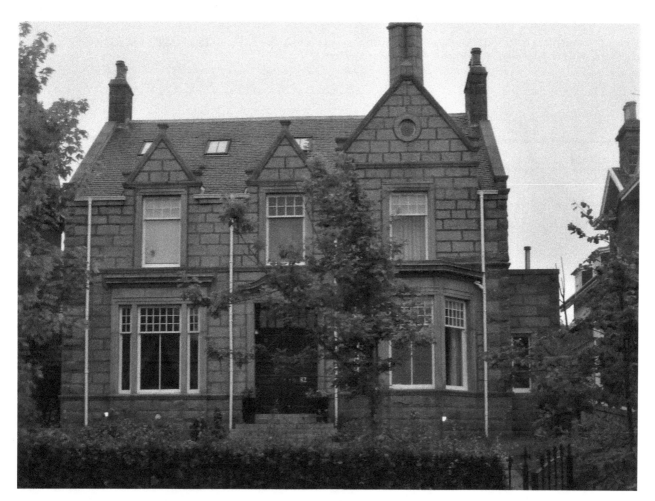

Figure 7-2. Designs of A Marshall Mackenzie in Aberdeen: domestic house at 82 Queen's Road (1898). Source: Author's photograph; dates and locations, Dictionary of Scottish Architects.

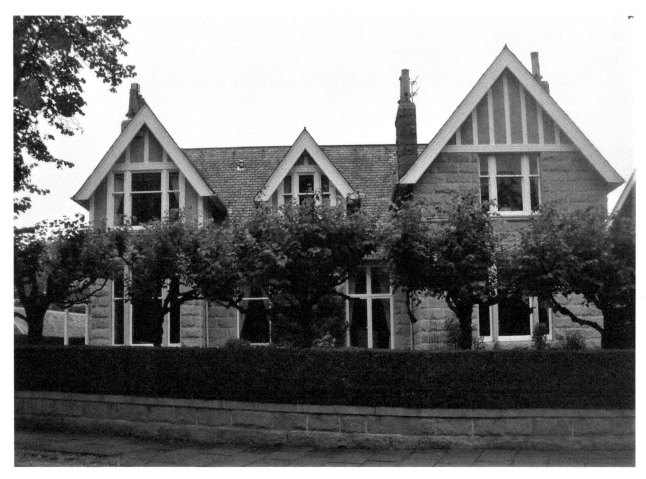

Figure 7-3. Designs of A Marshall Mackenzie in Aberdeen: domestic house at 31 Forest Road (1899). Source: Author's photograph; dates and locations, Dictionary of Scottish Architects.

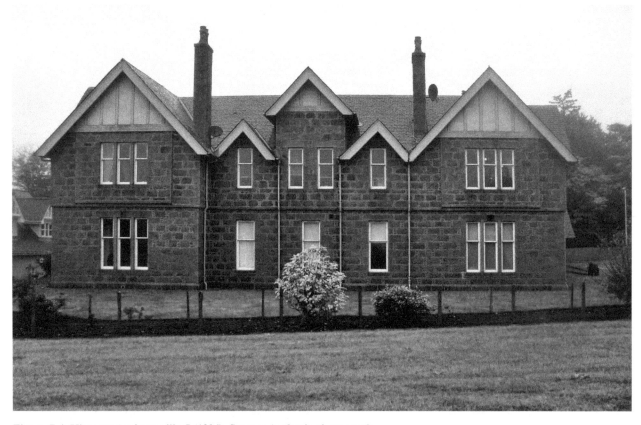

Figure 7-4. Kingseat Asylum: villa 5 (1904). Source: Author's photograph.

of gables to approximate classical features. The designs retain a vernacular character, however. The symmetricality is rarely perfect and the oversized chimneys and sweeping roofs of an earlier era persist (Figure 7-5). The Kingseat buildings are designated a 'late' form of this style, in that the turrets, bartizans and crowsteps of the Scottish gothic are entirely absent. The highly decorative window and door architraves present in some historical dwelling houses of this style are not replicated at Kingseat and architectural ornamentation is kept to a minimum, with quoins unemphasised and no window sills or architraves to window or door openings.

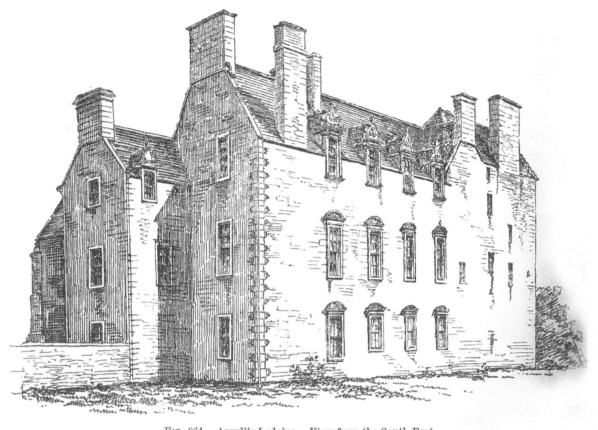

FIG. 864.—Argyll's Lodging. View from the South-East.

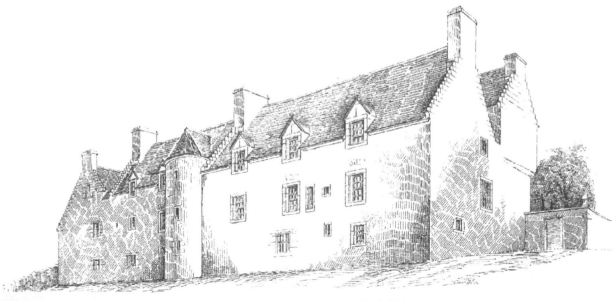

FIG. 973.—Fountainhall. View from the North-West.

Figure 7-5. Examples of Scottish Renaissance architecture. Source: David Macgibbon and Thomas Ross, *The castellated and domestic architecture of Scotland from the twelfth to the eighteenth century*. Volume II (top: p424; bottom: p552) (Edinburgh, 1887-1892).

However, the buildings are all constructed of local pink granite (this is said to have been quarried on the estate (Blanc, 1908: 328) (a quarry is marked on the site plan, NW of the farm steading), roughly hewn and laid in courses on a prominent plinth, with galleting between the stones providing one of the few modest decorative flourishes. Entranceways and window openings have been altered in the renovations of the building, so the original appearance is, in most cases, uncertain, except for those buildings recorded photographically in Annual Reports. There were five villas for males and five for females divided into two sections, 'industrial' or 'colony' and 'medical'.[1] Two of the three villas in each side of the medical section were villas for acute and incurable patients requiring close supervision which were 'closed', i.e. doors were locked during the day, all villas being locked during the night. The third villa was an 'observation villa', for incurable patients requiring less supervision. The six medical villas were situated within easy reach of the hospital building, with male villas grouped to the west and female villas to the east. The 'closed' male and female villas are situated close to each other, while the 'observation' villas (number 3) are either side of the hospital and less accessible to each other. Female industrial villas are situated near the laundry and kitchens where many of the women would have worked. Male industrial villas are likewise situated near the farm and workshops, the traditional male places of work. There is a clear spatial division between industrial and medical sections and between male and female open villas, although there are no physical barriers as there would have been at more traditional institutions. The architect wanted to build all the villas (two on each side) in the industrial colony in the 'old English' or 'woodwork' style with projecting eaves and gables. He though this design looked 'exceedingly well' but the idea was rejected by the Board on the grounds of expense and ultimately only one villa on each side was built in 'old English style' (ACDLB Minutes 14th January 1902, 27th January 1902).

Villas 1-3 (Figures 7-6, 7-7, 7-8) are of a similar style but each of the three villas uses a different arrangement of wall-head dormers and gables to achieve variety, although villas one to three on the male side are exactly replicated on the female side. Decorative details are at a minimum, the designs using only the broad forms of dormer and gables to decorative effect, in the case of villa two, this arrangement is more informal and asymmetrical. However, this very plain style is common in Aberdeen domestic housing, and, as we have seen, may well have evoked the domestic more readily than more elaborate styles at this period. None of these villas appears to have had an entrance on the main elevation, the buildings being entered by doors on the rear elevation.

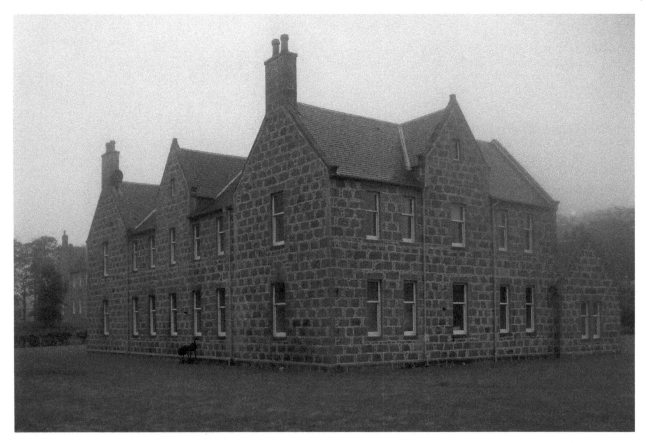

Figure 7-6. Kingseat Asylum: villa 1 (medical section). Source: Author's photograph.

[1] Richardson incorrectly states that the colony section of Kingseat comprised six villas (Richardson, 1991:75)

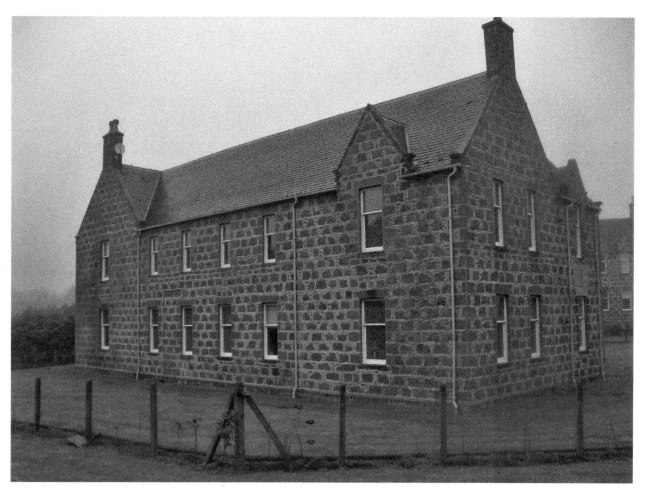

Figure 7-7. Kingseat Asylum: villa 2 (medical section). Source: Author's photograph.

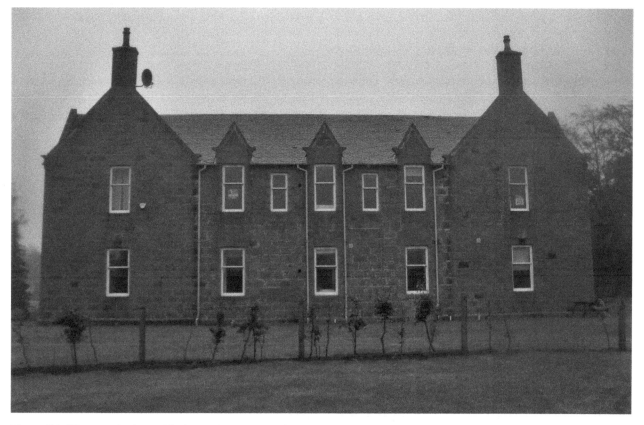

Figure 7-8. Kingseat Asylum: villa 3 (medical section). Source: Author's photograph.

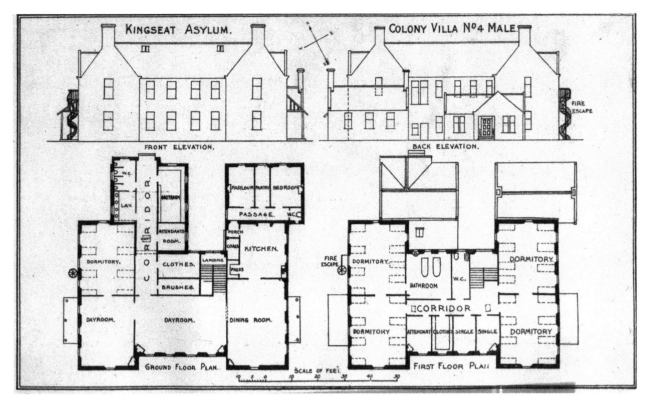

Figure 7-9. Kingseat Asylum: villa 4 (male) elevations and plans. Source: Kingseat Annual Report, 1904/5 GRHB8/6/1. Courtesy of NHS Grampian Archives.

Villa four (male) (Figure 7-9, 7-10) was for farm and garden workers, convalescent and chronic patients who were supervised by one attendant and one nurse. The main six-bay elevation (80 feet (24.4m) in width) is symmetrical and consists of a central four-bay section with gabled cross-wings each side. The detailing is very simple and this is one of the simplest designs on the site, without even a pedimented dormer to lift the design and having the feel of a country farm house. The main elevation does not signal its importance in any way, there are no entrances on this elevation; it is only the unusual width of the building (24 metres) that perhaps detracts from its domestic character. Side elevations are identical and are six bay with a twinned gabled roof over the central four bays. They have been altered since construction but would originally have had access from the first floor on the left-hand side to the fire escape. The elevation drawings also show that there was originally a small verandah on the west and east sides of the building. (The verandahs are shown on the 1906 plan on male villa four but not on female villa four. However, a contemporary photograph shows that female villa four did in fact feature verandahs.) The rear elevation has now been altered but originally consisted of a central five-bay section with gabled cross-wings to each side and a single-storey 'cottage' abutting each gable. The left-hand cottage consisted of accommodation for the attendants but this 'cottage' was only present on the male villa four, the female villa four did not have attendant accommodation, the nurses who looked after the villa retiring to the nearby nurses' home at night.

Villa five (male) was originally designated for tradesmen and skilled artisans and could house 32 patients who were supervised by two nurses. Villa five (female) housed 34 patients, supervised by two nurses and was the dwelling for kitchen and laundry workers. These were open or 'parole' villas and the patients who lived here were designated 'chronic' and worked on the grounds and in the workshops. Supervision at night was by night patrol rather than by staff who lived in.

Villa five is the most architecturally sophisticated of all the patient villas (Figures 3-11, 7-4). It is asymmetrical but when viewed from the front gives an impression of symmetry. The main elevation of this building is the south elevation and there do not appear to have been any verandahs, perhaps in the assumption that patients in the colony would spend a great deal of time outdoors anyway.[2] The main elevation consists of two gabled crosswings, the left hand protruding slightly, with a central section of three wallhead dormers, the central dormer of extended height with a small square window illuminating the attic space within. Variation in window size and shape is used for decorative effect, with narrow windows grouped into threes on the gable ends and wider single windows on the central bays. The side and central gables are marked with painted, timbered panels, in a style the architect referred to as 'old English'. The upper floor is separated from the lower floor by a corbelled course giving a very subtle jettying effect. This effect is emphasised by a further corbelled course below the upper window on the gables which results in a flat raised panel around the

---

[2] The relative lack of verandahs at Kingseat was lamented after its construction, and more substantial verandahs were subsequently added to some of the villas (Kingseat Annual Report 1908)

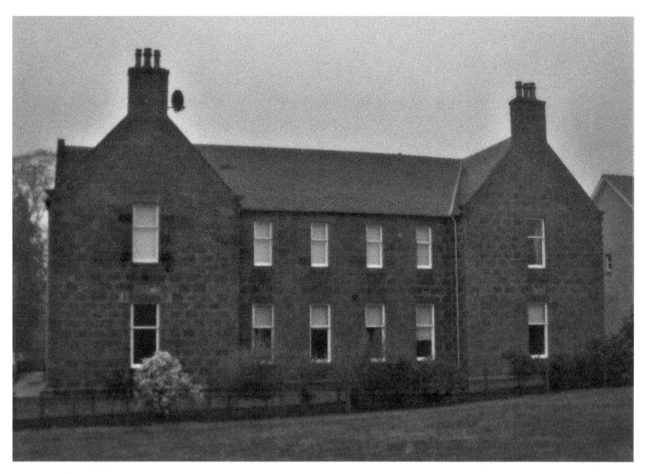

Figure 7-10. Kingseat Asylum: villa 4 (male). Source: Author's photograph.

upper windows, giving a suggestion of oriel window. The west and east elevations are arranged as paired gables with mock-timber panelling matching the main elevation. The rear elevation consists of the two gabled crosswings and a further off-centre gable which is echoed with a narrow 'stair tower', the upper storey of which is emphasised by two courses of corbelling and a tripartite window. The stair tower and the side gables are timber panelled at the top. Abutting the left gable is a single-storey 'cottage' which probably once formed the staff accommodation at the villa, as its previous internal divisions echo those of the staff accommodation in villa four.

We have seen that all the villas on the Kingseat site were of slightly differing styles (although male and female villas were identical), that were largely of a very simple, unornamented character resonating with modest domestic architecture of the period and alluding to Scottish Renaissance styles of the past. The more elaborate and decorative example is described as 'old English' which is perhaps a further allusion to the garden city layout that appears to have been an inspiration for Marshall Mackenzie in designing the asylum, but is also very similar to domestic designs he produced elsewhere in Aberdeen. Entrances are problematic, as the main elevations in all cases are not the location of the villa entrance. These are usually located at the rear of the villa and are not given any kind of decorative prominence.

7.3.3. Edinburgh District Asylum (Bangour Village)

Similarly to Kingseat, Bangour Village Asylum was divided into two parts: the medical section, with hospital, admission wards and villas for all patients requiring medical supervision; and the 'industrial' section comprising villas for 'chronic' and convalescent patients. Villas in the medical section comprised an observation (9) and an acute villa (10) for males which were replicated on the female side (observation (7), acute (8)), while the industrial sections comprised four villas for men and five for women. The villas for males were identical structures of 'barrack' style originally built of iron and wood. Those for females were two (19, 20) and three storey (18, 21) stone buildings.

The buildings varied in forms and layouts, thereby to 'destroy all appearance of official residence', and interest was imparted by the 'variety of external treatment in exposed stone, harling, tiled and green slated roofs' ('Bangour Village Lunatic Asylum', 1906: 545). The villas also ranged in size so that more difficult cases were accommodated in smaller dwellings for closer supervision, with acute villas housing 32 patients, whereas villas for chronic patients housed 46–50. The absence of corridors, walls and fences meant that patients leaving the villas and moving between buildings enjoyed the open grounds, exactly as in a domestic house.

Villa 18 for 46 females with chronic mental illness, exhibited a number of domestic features: canted bays on either side of the main elevation: a verandah spanning the middle three bays; wall-head dormers, a characteristic feature of Scottish domestic architecture; grouped windows; and angled chimney stacks (Figure 7-11). The variation in roof line, heights and surface articulation subtly undermined the building's uniformity as an institutional space. The main elevation bears comparison with Edinburgh's stone tenements, often three and four storeys high, but is very large in scale compared with standard bourgeois domestic dwellings. EDLB Minutes state that these villas were built of three storeys, rather than two 'for the sake of economy' (EDLB Minutes, 20th March 1901). Villa 19 for female chronic patients is on a much smaller scale, having only two storeys, and more closely approximates the size of a domestic villa (Figure 7-12). At the rear of the villa is a bartizan, an unnecessary and solely decorative feature, typical of Scots Baronial architecture, which increases the impression of substantial bourgeois dwelling but contrasts uneasily with the stated intention of the EDLB to save costs (Figure 7-13). Although it may have added little to the real cost of the building, it gives the strong impression that economy was not always the overriding priority in the construction of the building.

Villa ten was built as a 'closed' or 'acute' villa for males, intended to accommodate 33 patients and was begun in June 1905 and completed in 1907 (Figure 7-14). The acute block was said to 'supply the minimum accommodation according to the requirements of the Act and is compressed in a simple and economical form' (EDLB Minutes 18th December 1901).

The building material is Scottish sandstone of a cream to pink/orange hue. The stone has a roughly stugged finish and the ashlar blocks are laid in discontinuous, random courses. Dressing stones are of Locharbriggs sandstone which is used for quoins, window surrounds, plinth course, eaves course and other decorative highlights. In scale, the building resembles a large domestic villa and the domestic idiom is emphasised by the two forward-facing gables on the front elevation and the decorative features such as the wallhead dormers on the upper floor which are surmounted with circular-headed gablets finished with cornices and pointed finials. The scale of this villa is much closer to that of a bourgeois domestic villa, as it is only two storeys in height. Again, however, there is much ambiguity surrounding the entrances to the villa. What might be termed the main entrance to the villa is within a single–storey projection at the east of the building

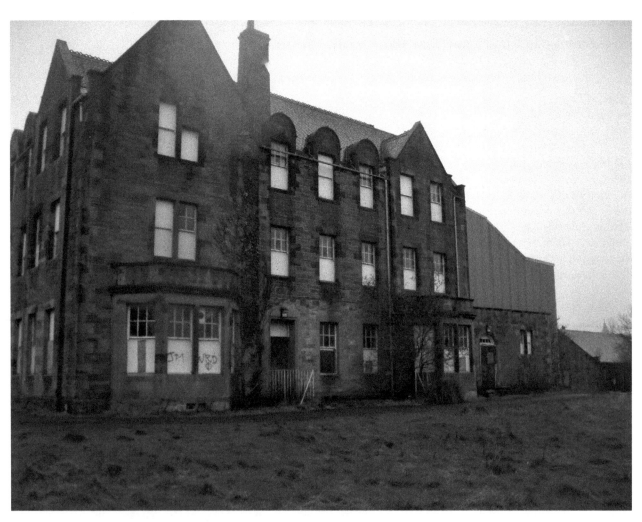

Figure 7-11. Bangour Village Asylum: villa 18. Source: Author's photograph.

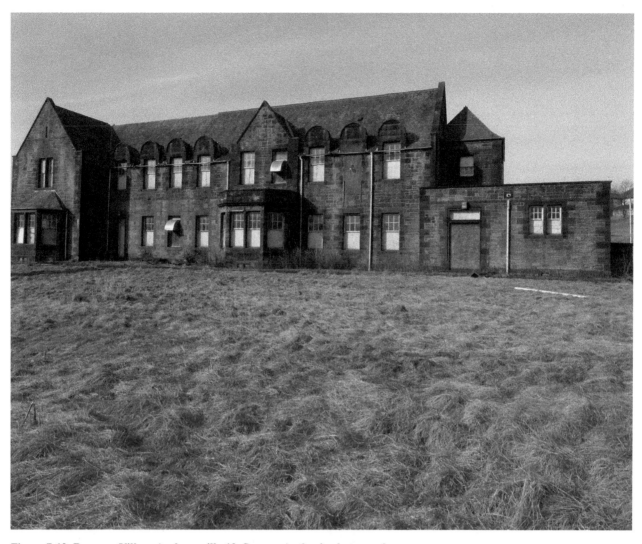

Figure 7-12. Bangour Village Asylum: villa 19. Source: Author's photograph.

forming a porch, and its position within a re-entrant angle means that it is concealed from view when the building is approached from most directions. The main doorway is emphasised with Locharbriggs sandstone dressings which form an elliptical-headed arch and moulded architrave. A second entrance on the south elevation, originally fitted with double-leafed doors, leads to and from a dayroom and can be considered an informal entrance and exit for patients to the verandah. A contemporary photograph of villa eight, the equivalent villa on the female side (Figure 3-22) shows the verandah which appears to be composed of a lean-to glass roof supported by cast-iron pillars. There are two entrances on the north elevation, which is the first elevation to be encountered from the pathway leading round the estate. The north elevation is effectively the back of the house, but is in fact the elevation most visitors, staff and patients would have initially approached from the main path. The soil pipes leading to the sewers are on this elevation, as are the chimneys. Architecturally it is less formal than the main elevation, with a greater variety of forms and greater asymmetricality. One of the entrances on this elevation appears to be an informal rear entrance for patients, while the second is an entrance to the nurses' quarters which is accorded less emphasis than the main entrance in terms of decorative treatment and size. All windows in the acute villa were of normal appearance externally, although some of the windows lit the villa's single rooms which would have been used for the confinement of agitated or disruptive patients, and original plans show that internal shutters were fitted in order to exclude light and prevent breakage/escape. On the first floor, only the single and padded rooms are fitted with air inlets, suggesting that there was a greater concern for ventilation in these smaller spaces, in which the patients may have been unclean or confined for long periods, and the windows may have been closed, preventing 'natural' ventilation. A single air inlet on the north facing elevation ventilates a 'glazed brick duct' of irregular shape that extends along one wall of the padded room. The purpose of this is unclear, but may have provided additional ventilation or a means of removing waste products. The domestic feel of the villa is slightly compromised by a roof ventilator on the eastern side of the building which was fed by flues from lavatories, dayroom, dormitories and stairwell. These small external signs hint at the less than domestic usages of the interior spaces, but the general appearance of the villa as a domestic building is nonetheless retained.

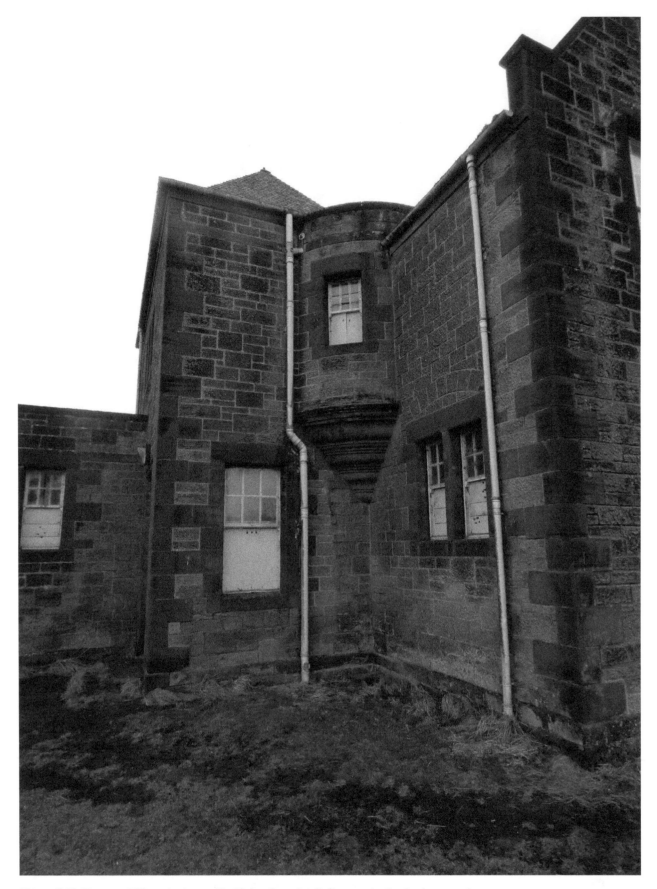

Figure 7-13. Bangour Village Asylum: villa 19, bartizan detail. Source: Author's photograph.

Villas 23, 24, 25, 27 and 28 were five identical homes for men which were built on the higher and more northerly ground at the back of site, each of them with accommodation for 50 patients and the necessary staff (Figure 3-29). Two hundred patients and the requisite staff moved in, in June 1904. The internal arrangements were 'similar to those

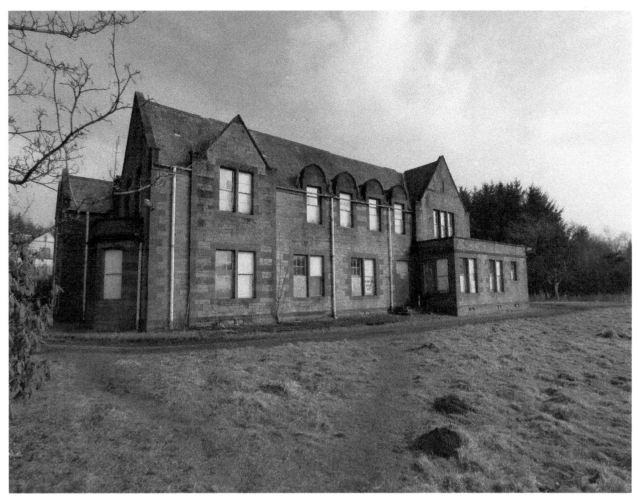

Figure 7-14. Bangour Village Asylum: villa 10. Source: Author's photograph.

in the women's homes' (Keay, 1911). These were the first structures to be built on the site, hurriedly erected while discussions and arguments continued over the main buildings on the site, and were originally of iron and wood with the walls packed with asbestos and the internal surfaces plastered (the structures were later rebuilt in brick and rough cast). However, they were not found to be more economical than stone buildings to construct and maintain, and the experiment was not repeated on the site (Blanc, 1908). These buildings appear to consciously borrow the idiom of barracks, being identical, symmetrical structures of ostensibly temporary materials, using the Edinburgh Council coat of arms within the pediment of the south-facing elevation, in the way that army barracks were wont to do (Figure 7-15). These buildings are very much less domestic in appearance than the women's 'industrial' villas for chronic patients and indeed are of much poorer quality overall. The implication is that the imperative to build 'home-like' accommodation for males was reduced, as they were expected to be working outdoors for much of the time. There is a clear gendered rupture here between the domestic, home-like surroundings that were required for women as guardians and producers of the domestic sphere and the more practical, 'doss-house' style accommodation that was seen as sufficient for working-class men who are not here viewed as central to the production of domesticity.

7.3.4. Renfrew District Asylum (Dykebar)

The four patient villas at Renfrew District Asylum were built between 1905 and 1909 to house 50 patients each, 100 males and 100 females in total, and are similar in design with small variations. The architect of the asylum, Thomas Graham Abercrombie, based in Paisley, was also the designer of domestic houses, churches and schools in the local area. The villas were built for chronic and convalescent patients who were expected to work, while the senile and acute cases and those suffering from bodily illnesses were housed in a separate hospital building, rather than in smaller villas, as was the case at other sites in this study (RDLA Minutes 25th January 1903). RDLA Minutes reveal that the four asylum villas were originally to be built of rough cast brick with tiled roofs. After consulting the Measurer (Quantity Surveyor), the committee was informed that to build the asylum buildings of stone would cost between 8 and 10 per cent more. Nevertheless, the decision was taken, despite the higher cost, to build the asylum, including the villas, of Locharbriggs or other 'good red sandstone' and to use 'good green slates', instead of tiles (RDLA Minutes 24th June, 1903). Although the reason for this decision is not recorded, it can be deduced that strict economy was not always the primary motivation in decisions regarding the construction of the asylum. The

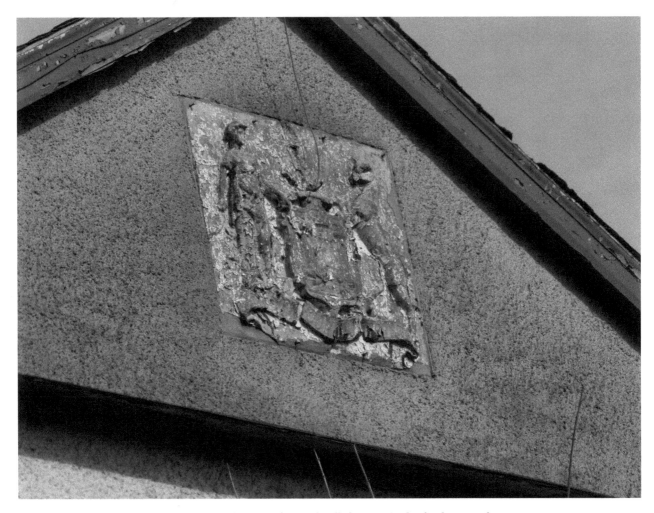

Figure 7-15. Bangour Village Asylum: villa 23, coat of arms detail. Source: Author's photograph.

villas at Renfrew Asylum are of visibly higher quality, relative to the other sites in this study, and are constructed of ashlar sandstone with a variety of subtle decorative details which add to the impression of solid bourgeois villa that the buildings convey (Figures 3-39, 3-41). For instance, there are drip moulds over first-floor windows, several of the windows and doors being architraved in stone, shaped quoins and corniced pediments, tall shaped, corniced chimneys and complex dormer windows with modillioned cornices. The buildings are irregular and asymmetrical in plan with the south front, the most formal façade, consisting of a central section with two cross-wings of different lengths, the asymmetry being increased by the addition of the very domestic canted bay window on the westernmost wing. All the facades of the building are different and most are assymetrical. The quality of the materials and finishes adds to the bourgeois quality of the building, together with features such as dormers, canted bays and the central verandah on the south elevation.

Some factors, however, militate against the villas being seen as domestic. The most prominent of these are the large roof ventilators which were a frequent feature of institutional buildings by means of which vitiated air was removed from the interior, largely through the action of wind through the ventilator (Glaister, 1897: 46-48)

(Figure 7-16). Although roof ventilators were sometimes recommended for domestic houses, they would have been an unusual feature in a domestic setting. It can be seen that at Renfrew, the ventilator is lead-covered and relatively ornate in style, in keeping with the style of the buildings (Figure 7-17). Secondly, although the villas have a number of entrances, none of these qualifies easily as the main entrance to the building. On the south elevation a narrow entrance is almost hidden underneath the verandah, but is not decoratively highlighted. On the north elevation there are three entrances, one, which is porticoed, perhaps has the greatest claim to be considered the main entrance, but is at the rear of the building, and is given none of the grand treatment that one might expect for a substantial building of this size. A further 'rear' entrance is also on the northern elevation, as is a first-floor exit, which was probably intended as a fire escape. Thirdly, as the buildings were intended to house 50 people they are much larger in scale than the average bourgeois villa. The three villas of similar plan, measure 30 x 20 metres, while the laundry villa is of dimensions 25 x 23 metres.[3] The scale of the villas tends to advertise these as institutional rather than domestic buildings.

---

[3] Measurements were obtained for this and other buildings using plans and the measurement tools provided at digimap.com and by google earth.

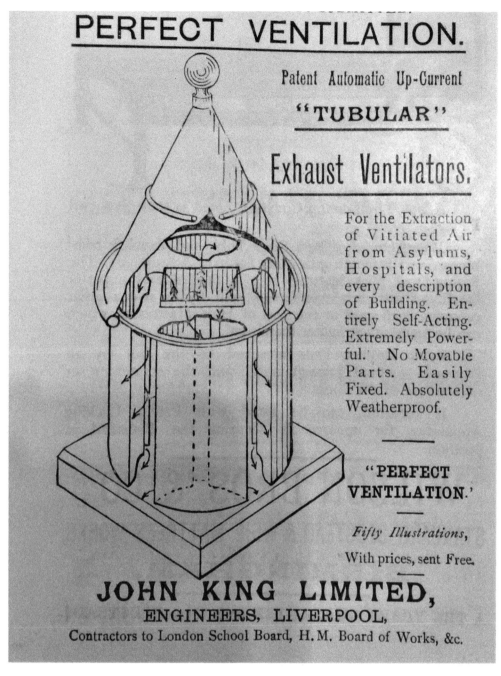

Figure 7-16. Advertisement for roof ventilators. Source: Bibby, G.H. (1896) *The planning of lunatic asylums.* **London: Bradley T Batsford.**

7.3.5. Belfast District Asylum (Purdysburn)

Construction work at Purdysburn Villa Colony began in 1902 and all buildings considered here were completed by 1913. The villas on the site are of four designs. Designs 1A (villas 2, 3 and 6) and 1B (villas 4, 5, 7, 8 and 9, villa 1 being pre-existing on the site) were the work of local architects Graeme Watt & Tulloch. This design was used for all villas which housed chronic and convalescent patients and the original variant, 1A, is considered in Chapter 6. Design 1B was a variation that included a 'sanitary annexe' on the eastern elevation that was introduced against the wishes of the Medical Superintendent William Graham (Figure 7-18). Graham felt that the annexe caused 'asymmetry

and disfiguration of the buildings' and would destroy the buildings' 'homelike character' (BDLA Minutes, 1902:332). Nevertheless, Graham was overruled, most likely because the sanitary annexe, a standard hospital feature, was thought to isolate the harmful gases and germs associated with the sewer system. Design one is of a domestic revival style incorporating elements of 'Queen Anne' and neo-Georgian. The sweeping rooflines, dormers, gables, tall chimneys and white-painted woodwork all derive from popular domestic styles at the period. However, again the sheer size of the villas gives away their institutional character, with design one measuring 23 x 22 metres.

251

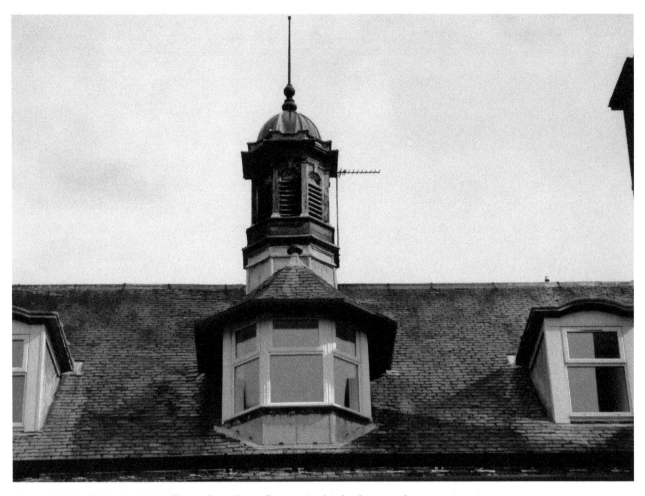

Figure 7-17. Dykebar Asylum: villa roof ventilator. Source: Author's photograph.

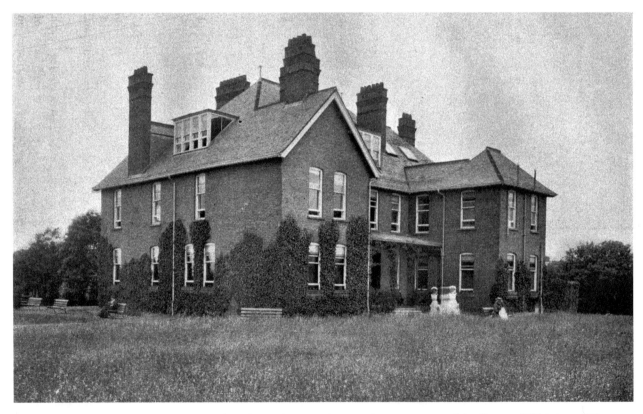

Figure 7-18. Purdysburn Villa Colony: design 1B showing prominent sanitary annexe to right. Source: BDLA Annual Report 1921.

Much more institutional in character were the designs for Villa 10, which was occupied by male 'acute' patients (Design 2) and for Villa 11, which was used for male patients under observation (Design 3) (Figures 7-19, 7-20). These buildings were the work of the foremost asylum architect of his day, G T Hine, with working drawings being prepared by local architects as above. Designs 2 and 3 are rectangular on plan, brick built, two storey buildings. Full height and single storey canted bays give some domestic feel to the villas and each has a verandah on the southern elevation (now replaced in both cases). The observation villa retains a ventilation turret on the roof, not a domestic feature, as discussed above, but one which would have improved the ventilation and therefore the perceived hygiene of the building. The acute villa has a simple frieze marking the boundary between ground and first floors and the observation villa, a plinth which is emphasised with a sandstone course. Otherwise, both buildings are without decorative adornment. This may perhaps be the consequence of having been designed by a professional asylum designer rather than a general architect as was the case for most other villas in this study. G T Hine's villa designs evoke the two-storey pavilions of a traditional asylum in which individual pavilions formed a small part of an integrated whole and are therefore extremely stripped back and simple in form, rather than the free-standing villas designed on domestic lines by the architects on the other sites considered here.

7.3.6. Sixth Lancashire Asylum (Whalley)

The sixth Lancashire asylum at Whalley was built as a 'dual pavilion', composed of two rows of pavilions, men on one side and women on the other, and administration and communal buildings placed down the central spine (Figure 4-20). As a local newspaper report implied, it was a somewhat conservative design in comparison with the compact arrow then more usual in England at this period (*Lancashire Evening Post*, 27th February 1907). The main entrance for patients, staff and visitors was through a formalized gate-screen of railings, piers and arches associated with a substantial lodge, and it is likely that the majority of the estate perimeter was fenced (Cornwell, 2010: 19). The site was almost entirely rectilinear in design, the visitor being led along a largely straight avenue to an open square dominated by the main administration building. Building designs were classical and symmetrical, a repeating theme being the deeply corniced pediment, evoking many generations of institutional building from barrack to hospital (Figure 4-21). Accommodation for men and women was arranged in symmetrical rows, one pavilion behind another, so that the views from dayrooms

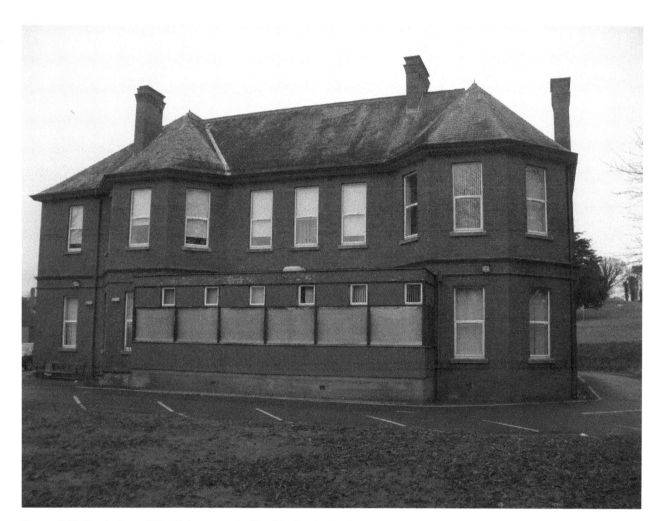

Figure 7-19. Purdysburn Villa Colony: acute villa (10) (Design 2). Source: Author's photograph.

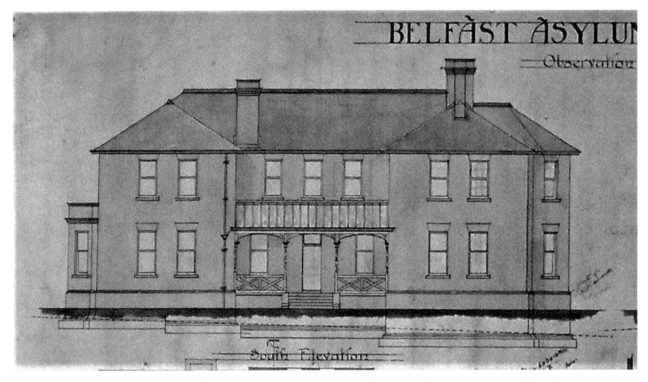

Figure 7-20. Purdysburn Villa Colony: observation villa (11) (Design 3) Source: Architect's drawing held by Estate's Department, Knockbracken Healthcare Park.

were on to other institutional buildings. The pavilions were connected by covered walkways running parallel to the main buildings which were open from above waist level, allowing air to circulate freely, but were roofed to keep out the worst of the weather.

Accommodation pavilions faced south-south-west to obtain the benefits of sunlight, and each was enclosed by a rectangular grassed airing court with a railing over six feet high, hooped at the top for safety reasons, through which the wider grounds were visible but unreachable. There was no apparent intention to practise an open-door system at Whalley, and the main doors to the pavilions may have been intended to be locked. The chronic blocks were without significant features on the main elevation, but a full-height canted bay at the western end of each pavilion provided an architectural flourish, somewhat domestic in nature, that also increased sunlight to the interior at the end of the day. However, full-height sanitary annexes, a distinctive hospital feature, were also prominent on the buildings' exteriors (Figure 4-24). The buildings are much larger than Scottish and Irish villas, 60 x 30 metres and three storeys high and accommodated approximately three times as many patients (148) as the typical villa for chronic patients in a colony asylum. Domestic scale has therefore been altogether abandoned for the chronic accommodation, although pavilions for more acute categories of patients were on a smaller scale.

7.4. Internal layouts, decoration and furnishings

This section will examine the internal layouts of the villas selected above, using extant plans. Contemporary

photographs will also be used to analyse interior decoration and furnishings and this will be supplemented by discussion of layouts, furnishings and decoration from primary sources such as Annual Reports and Lunacy Board Minutes.

7.4.1. Alt Scherbitz, Germany

As above, for the purposes of this section, the analysis will focus on the impressions of visitors from Britain regarding the character of the interiors at Alt-Scherbitz, rather than how they were viewed within the German context. George Beard, visiting in 1880, found the cottages comfortable inside and the patients allowed considerable liberty (Beard, 1880). In 1889, William Letchworth's visit found that furnishing of the observation villas was 'ample and comfortable' and the windows had fine views both 'immediate and distant'. Curtained couches provided a means for female patients to have occasional rest. Bright flowers were on display and there was 'an abundance of health-giving light'. In the sitting rooms were plain chairs and sofas and there were separate sitting and dining rooms. Sleeping apartments were provided with iron bedsteads and the oiled wooden floors were uncarpeted. The villas were divided into three classes, according to the patients' ability to pay and the quality of furnishing therefore varied accordingly, upper class villas containing sofas, bright rugs, mirrors, pianos, writing desks and chests of drawers and having frescoed ceiling and coloured walls. The third-class villa 'had fewer conveniences than others, though it was adequately furnished'. Accommodation was organised as in a domestic dwelling with living accommodation on the ground floor and sleeping apartments above to increase the similarity to home life. Villas were heated by stoves and open fires, which also assisted with ventilation. Although there was no 'costly interior furnishing', the asylum was said to contain 'everything essential to the comfort of the insane'. An ordinary dwelling with homelike furnishings was said to put the patients more at ease and allow them to be 'sooner placed on the road to recovery', while objects of interest 'could agreeably engage the mind'. The succession of villas allowed patients to be removed from the place associated with 'the first period of their disease to entirely new surroundings' (Letchworth, 1889:291-302). It has been pointed out above that Villa G at Alt-Scherbitz was a probable model for villa designs at Purdysburn and Dykebar. Although no original plans exist for villa layouts at Dykebar, it can be seen that the internal layout of Villa G bears a strong resemblance to that at Purdysburn, with rooms opening out of each other rather than from a central corridor, a feature that was almost certainly adopted to improve visibility and therefore assist patient supervision (Figures 4-62, 4-63).

7.4.2. Aberdeen District Asylum (Kingseat)

Villa 4 is the only villa for which plans showing internal layout and interior photographs survive (Figure 7-9). The attendants' cottage at the rear of villa 4 featured a parlour, bedroom, and WC for use by attendants while on duty, and also contained the villa pantry where the slightly isolated location would have made it a little cooler. The right-hand cottage, contained the main entrance way into the building, the WCs, lavatories (wash hand basins) and boot room, which is fitted on three sides with a low bench for boot changing. The sanitary facilities have thus been almost separated from the rest of the building, in an echo of the 'sanitary annexe' that would have been a normal feature of a hospital ward. There appear to have been two further entrances, one into the attendants' accommodation on the left, which also gave access to the 'cottage' and another straight into the stairwell. A corridor leads from the front door straight into the main dayroom, which was lit by a roof light. This corridor also gives access to the sanitary facilities and boot room, for patients, and rooms used by the attendants, such as the brush room, the clothes room and the room used by attendants during the day. None of the other main rooms is accessible from the corridor and, instead, like Alt-Scherbitz, all open out of each other, in an arrangement which departs from the domestic but which would have allowed for better supervision of patients.

The interior plan shows that the front of the building, which faces SSW contains the dayrooms and dining rooms downstairs, the day rooms occupying the left and centre bays, while the dining room is in the right hand bay, nearest the kitchen. The dining room and dayroom appear to be separated by a sliding door, while the two dayrooms were connected by an open archway, hung with curtains that could be drawn together. The interior photograph shows that the room was furnished largely with light, bentwood furniture (minutes show that this was purchased from Thonet brothers in Austria) (ADLB Minutes, 24th November 1903) (Figure 7-21). The ceiling has simple coving and a picture rail runs around the room above head height where it would not cause injury to patients who might fall against the wall. The walls are panelled to dado height and corner fireplaces have allowed more of the external wall to be used for windows, the flues travelling up through the corners of the room. The central dayroom has two fireplaces in each front corner while the dayroom to the left has a single fireplace backing onto the fireplace next door and allowing two rooms to be heated with a single flue. Central heating radiators are also shown. The photograph shows shaded electric lights hanging down from the ceiling. Also shown in the left-hand dayroom is a table (perhaps for bagatelle or billiards) and there is a variety of furniture, upholstered armchairs, bookcase/dresser, plants and plant stands, small tables, a rocking chair, a screen (perhaps to screen patients who were displaying symptoms such as epilepsy or who needed treatment) and a mirror is hung above the fireplace. Pictures are hung on the walls and plants are prominently displayed as table centres and on separate plant stands, and a vase of flowers is on the dresser. The windows are not hung with curtains, but appear to be fitted with blinds. Splayed reveals help the light to be distributed through the very thick walls (1½ feet – fieldwork measurement) and around the room. The floorboards are polished and there are no carpets but a strip of linoleum is laid down the main walkway of the room. The furniture is arranged on two sides of the room to give a free passageway for staff to walk up and down and supervise the room.

Behind the smaller dayroom on the ground floor is a dormitory with eight beds, in a departure from the usual domestic arrangement. All dormitories are lit from the east or the west, and therefore illuminated by rising or setting sun but not well lit during the main part of the day. This would not be a concern since the patients in the colony would generally be out at work during the day. The upper floor consists of four dormitories of eight beds each, each approximately 20x25 feet and a central corridor from which open the bathroom, with two baths and a washhand basin, WC, attendant's room, clothes room, and two single rooms. The corridor appears to have been lit by two roof lights and opens into three of the dormitories. The fourth opens off the third and is the location for an emergency exit leading to the fire escape. The two single rooms (approximately 12ft x 8ft) are lit by a single south-facing window. One has a corner fireplace and the other no fireplace.

The contemporary photograph of the dormitories in the right-hand wing shows that the front dormitory was fitted with a solid door, and in a similar way to the room below, the walls have simple coving at the top and wooden panelling at dado level (Figure 7-22). There are no fireplaces but a radiator is visible in the back dormitory. Again, the windows are not hung with curtains. The polished floorboards are laid with a strip of carpet where patrolling of the ward could take place at night without

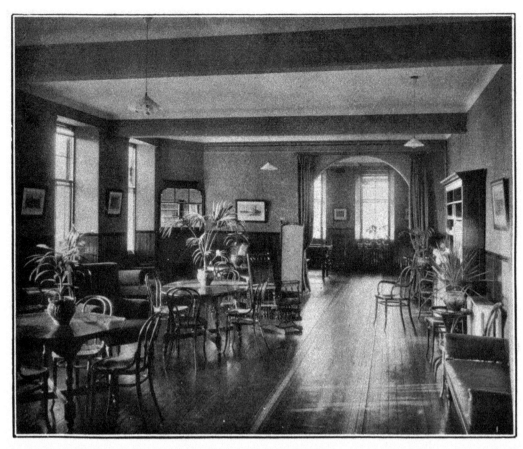

DAY ROOM—MALE COLONY VILLA.

Figure 7-21. Kingseat Asylum: interior villa 4 (male). Source: Kingseat Annual Report, 1904/5 GRHB8/6/1. Courtesy of NHS Grampian Archives.

creating undue noise. The dormitory is divided into two by a wall and connecting archway, forming two rooms of eight beds each. The beds are wooden, with low (possibly to aid observation) solid (so as not to provide ligature points?) head and footboards. The bedding is shown to be generous, two pillows to each bed and a reasonable bulk of blankets and counterpane. Each bed has a chair beside it for the patient's clothes but apart from the chamber p0ts no other furnishing is visible and there are no pictures on the walls. It is possible that this photograph was taken soon after completion and further furnishings may have been added in subsequent weeks and months. The ceiling height upstairs is approximately 3m (or 10 feet), while downstairs it is 3.3 m (10ft, 10 inches) (fieldwork measurements), considerably lower than was usual for a hospital ward, but consistent with a domestic dwelling.

The *BMJ* reported in 1906 that 'the various sections have been furnished in a manner well fitted to secure the efficient care and treatment of the patients. In the day rooms sofas and various kinds of easy chairs have been liberally provided and in many of the day rooms there is a piano. The rooms are abundantly decorated with pictures, plants, and ornaments … the beds are of good design, and are provided with wire and hair mattresses and coverings of good quality' (*British Medical Journal*, 24th November 1906).

7.4.3. Edinburgh District Asylum (Bangour Village)

The interior of Villa 18, the only villa for which an interior photograph has survived, was laid out as a single, unified domestic villa with living accommodation on the ground floor and sleeping and bathroom facilities on the upper floors. The ground floor patient dayrooms were positioned to take advantage of the sunny, south-east-facing main elevation. Unlike a domestic house, however, the main living areas did not open off a central hallway but rather into each other, rendering the control and observation of patients easier, as at the other sites discussed above. The L-shaped day room allowed the room to be cross-ventilated and to receive light from two different directions, although this made patient supervision more difficult because all corners of the room could not be seen from a single point. A contemporary photograph (Figure 7-23) shows that the room was sparsely but comfortably furnished in a restrained domestic style with a relatively elaborate egg-and-dart moulding along the cornice, suggestive of a bourgeois domestic interior despite the expense and potential to trap dust and dirt.[4] The furnishings appear more lavish than those seen in other villa interiors in this study, with

[4] None of the villas at Bangour could be accessed internally during fieldwork due to the dereliction of the site. However, it was possible to see through the windows of villas 18 and 20, both of which still exhibited the egg and dart moulding.

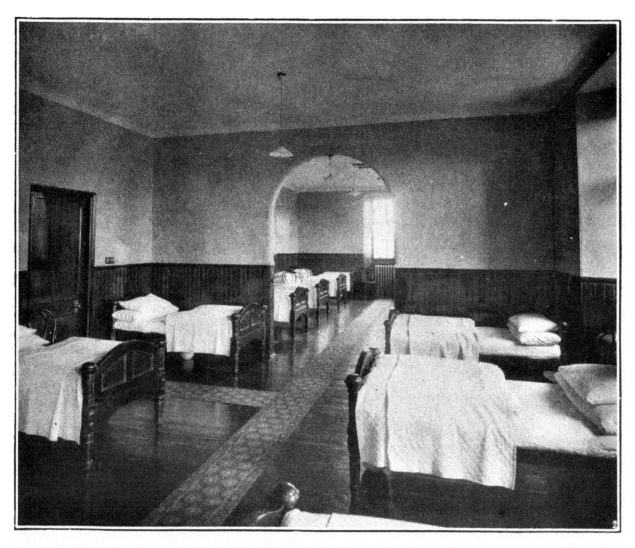

DORMITORY—MALE COLONY VILLA.

Figure 7-22. Kingseat Asylum: interior dormitory villa 4 (male Source: Kingseat Annual Report, 1904/5 GRHB8/6/1. Courtesy of NHS Grampian Archives.

sofas and armchairs upholstered in pale (and difficult to keep clean) colours, bookcases, a large patterned rug and what appears to be a grand piano. There are no pictures on the walls, but this may be because the photograph was taken around the time of opening and pictures had yet to be added to the interior. Although more luxurious than other asylum villas, the Edinburgh villa is still clearly an institutional interior, the rugs being relatively small and the ornamentation sparse. It is notable that the furnishings are distributed unevenly around the room, the carpet in the foreground being positioned at an angle, in an echo of the varied disposition and orientation of buildings around the site.

On the first and second floors, the sleeping accommodation was divided into five dormitories of between six and twelve beds, the small size of which meant that cross-ventilation was not always achieved, as some did not have two external walls. This villa and the other 'industrial' villas all practised the open-door system, with doors kept open during the day and locked at night.

7.4.4. Renfrew District Asylum (Dykebar)

No plans have survived showing the internal layout of villas at Renfrew. A single contemporary photograph survives of the interior of a villa (Figure 3-40). The shape and size of the windows, which differs slightly from the other villas, suggests that this is the laundry villa which was for female working patients. The room is laid out as a sitting or day room (although there is a substantial table and at least one other smaller table in the room, this would not provide enough sitting space for patients to dine at the same time). Chairs are largely individual bentwood seats with and without arms. There are several more comfortable padded armchairs and a padded sofa also visible. A polished wood or linoleum floor is largely free of carpets, two small rugs can be seen. Plants are distributed about the room on tables and plant stands and reading matter is placed on the large central table. The room has a wood panelled dado, possibly to protect the walls from damage by furniture, and there are large wooden panels beside the windows, possibly forming Georgian style internal shutters, or perhaps merely

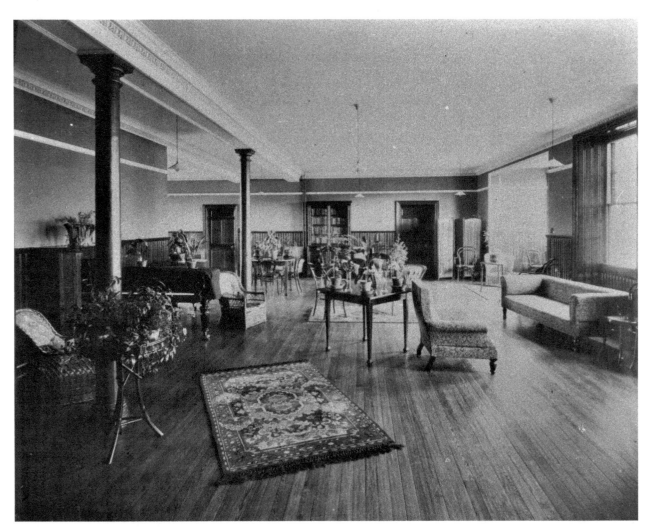

Figure 7-23. Bangour Village: interior of villa 18 c1906. Source: LA LHB44/26/10. Courtesy of Lothian Health Service Archive.

decorative. A picture rail runs around the room above head height, from which at least one picture has been hung and one other framed picture is visible. The very large, small-paned windows are not hung with curtains or valances and, indeed, there are no blinds visible. The overall impression of the room is that considerable attention has been given to producing a genteel, domestic effect, with some of the furniture, especially the large table, appearing to be of high quality. The panelling and picture rail add to the domestic ambience, although the scale of the room and the replication of chairs gives away the space's institutional purpose. Compared with a domestic home of the period, the room lacks the proliferation of pictures, rugs and ornaments that would have been usual, but by the lights of institutional domesticity, a high standard of comfort has been attained.

7.4.5. Belfast District Asylum (Purdysburn)

As has been pointed out above, the interior layout of Design 1 at Purdysburn, particularly Design 1A, bears a strong resemblance to that of Villa G at Alt-Scherbitz, showing the same general arrangement of rooms and the characteristic opening out of one room into another,

rather than off a central hallway or corridor (Figures 7.24, 7.25). The arrangement of rooms in this way puts them increasingly at a distance from exits, reducing the number of points that would need to be supervised by staff. Design 1 also echoes the ambiguity around entrances that is seen in other asylum villas. The 'main' entrance to the villa is on the rear elevation and is also effectively the back door, the only other entrance being a door leading from the yard into the ward scullery. Double glass doors lead out from the dayrooms onto the verandah on each side of the villa, occupying the architectural role of garden entrances, but these are clearly not the principal entrances to the building, since there is one on each side and they are almost concealed beneath the glass verandah. An interior photograph has survived of a dayroom in a villa of design 1 (Figure 6-6) and a further interior photograph of a dayroom in the female hospital wing, which appears to have been used principally as a dining room (Figure 7-26). These photographs show simple furnishings of varied shapes and styles, and a variety of 'objects of interests' including plants, ornaments, books and magazines. Only the absence of pictures on the walls and the large amount of seating detracts from the appearance of domesticity in the villa

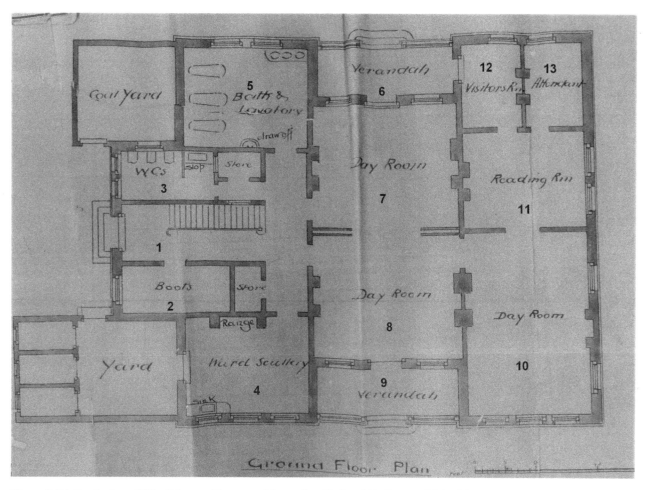

Figure 7-24. Purdysburn Villa Colony: villa ground floor plan (design 1A). Source: PRONI LA/7/29/CB/22 Builder's Specification. Reproduced with permission of the Deputy Keeper of the Records, Public Record Office of Northern Ireland.

dayroom, while the hospital dayroom conveys something of the feel of a café or restaurant.

No interior photographs of the acute and observation villas are extant but plan drawings of interior layouts have survived (Figures 4-11, 4-12, 4-13). The acute villa exhibits some ambiguity around entrances with the 'main' entrance, a rather plain and de-emphasised opening, on the side elevation. Canted bays are used here, to create a domestic feel in the day rooms and dormitories, but, unlike the observation villa, each day room can be accessed from the central hallway. WCs and bathroom are more fully incorporated into the main building, perhaps because patients needed to be more closely attended in these areas, but the WC 'wing' is clearly separated from the service 'wing' by a yard. There is no attendant accommodation on the ground floor, perhaps suggesting that the attendants of acute patients were constantly with their charges. Six single rooms are provided on the first floor, one more than in the observation villa, suggesting that acute patients were expected to be slightly more disruptive. The upstairs is divided into two large dormitories, the lack of separation into smaller spaces, suggesting that these large open spaces allowed patients to be more easily supervised, although the domestic character would have been reduced.

A domestic feel was given to the interior of the observation room by the provision of canted bay windows to two of the dayrooms and accommodation is organised as in a domestic dwelling, with living rooms on the ground floor and dormitories above. However, several measures have been taken to organise the space in order to prioritise patient management rather than domesticity. The ground floor accommodation is organised effectively into two halves with living rooms at the front (south-facing) and service and sanitary rooms at the rear. The WCs and washhand basins have been placed in a block which is isolated on three sides from the rest of the building, for hygienic reasons. Similarly to design 1A, the living accommodation is accessible only through one door from the main corridor, so that the dayrooms can only be accessed through each other. The only other entrance to dayrooms is out through the verandah. Again, entrances are, in general problematic, with no clear main entrance, a side entrance which appears to serve as the main entrance but gives greater access to the accommodation at the rear and one other entrance on the rear elevation, reached through the yard. On the first floor is one very large dormitory of 44 beds, without divisions, and glazed screens are marked in places, all of which would have made observation of the patients easier, but detracts from the domestic feel of the internal spaces. Single rooms have been provided upstairs for patients perceived as more disruptive.

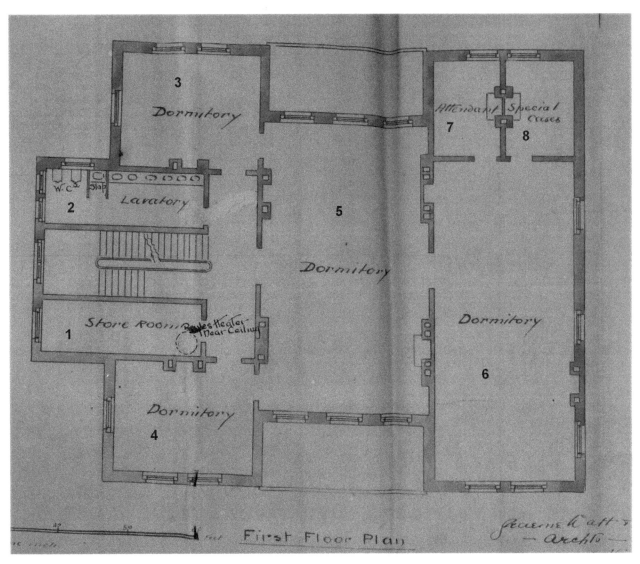

Figure 7-25. Purdysburn Villa Colony: villa first floor plan (design 1A). Source: PRONI LA/7/29/CB/22 Builder's Specification. Reproduced with permission of the Deputy Keeper of the Records, Public Record Office of Northern Ireland.

7.4.6. Sixth Lancashire Asylum (Whalley)

Unlike the colony asylum villas, the interior accommodation of the chronic block at Whalley did not echo the layout of a domestic house, being organised identically on the first two floors, each comprising a large dayroom with western-facing bay, a dormitory of 29 beds, sanitary facilities and a ward scullery. The second floor was laid out as two huge dormitories of 36 and 54 beds, the main rooms organised on the typical plan of a Nightingale ward with tall windows opposite each other, allowing for cross-ventilation and natural light from two directions. WCs and bathrooms were isolated, hospital-style, from the rest of the building in a separate sanitary annexe. The wards were rectangular, allowing easy observation of all parts of the room, with one main entrance into the ward from the covered way and all rooms opening off a central corridor. Although patients moving from room to room would have to pass through the corridor, the small number of rooms made patient supervision relatively easy. Once patients were in the dayroom, for example, there is only a single exit from the room (and the WCs open directly

off it) which would have assisted the control of patient movements. A contemporary image of a chronic ward in use by soldiers shows extremely high ceilings, possibly as much as the 15 feet recommended by Nightingale to give patients healthful amounts of air, and the effect of sunlight pouring into the ward from all sides (Figure 7-27). The walls had rounded arrises, thought to assist air circulation and aid cleaning, but—despite plain dado and picture rails—no panelling or cornicing of the domestic kind seen at Bangour was evident, suggesting that such finishes were seen as unnecessary, or dirt traps and were dispensed with, despite the more domestic feel that these features might have given.

7.5. Discussion and conclusion

It can be seen from the foregoing that the colony asylum, in some ways, represented a return to the domestic values that had informed asylum reform during the late eighteenth and early nineteenth centuries, when the Tukes proposed small-scale home-like environments as the appropriate locale for the 'moral treatment' of the

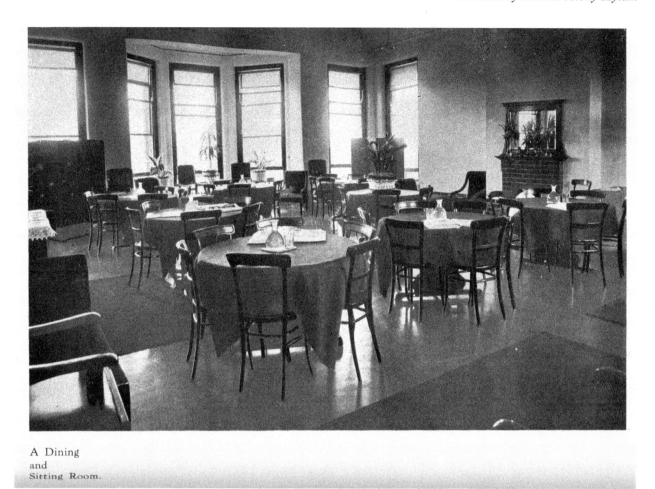

A Dining
and
Sitting Room.

Figure 7-26. Purdysburn Villa Colony: hospital dayroom, female wing. Source: BDLA Annual Report, 1921.

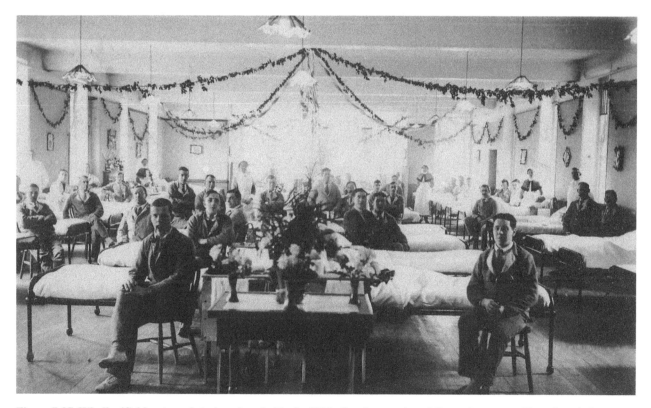

Figure 7-27. Whalley/Calderstones interior, chronic block c1915 after the opening of the asylum as a military hospital. Source: Cornwell, R.B. (2010) The history of the Calderstones hospital railway 1907-1953. Accrington: Nayler Group Ltd. With permission of Val Valovin.

insane. The colony asylum, however, turned away from the outward-looking, public style of asylum architecture, often accused of being 'palatial', which provided the concrete symbolism of municipal benevolence at the end of the nineteenth century, towards a more inward-looking, private architecture whose focus was on the patients. The colony asylum represented an attempt to replicate domestic spaces: in architectural style, in scale, in layouts, and in decoration and furnishing. However, colony villas represented a particular version of domesticity, more closely related to the bourgeois environments of the rising middle classes than the stigmatised homes of the poor. Often closely resembling middle-class suburban villas in architectural style, the spacious, sunlit interiors of asylum villas, filled with comfortable furnishings and 'objects of interest', were intended to have a refining effect on patients and to render them more tranquil and contented and more willing to engage in productive work (SLC 1896:80; 1882:66).

However, there were many tensions produced by the attempt to render asylum villas more home-like which are revealed by a close analysis of buildings and spaces. Although economy must be considered a factor in any building project, asylum builders were under considerable pressure to deliver buildings that both appeared and were in fact, economical and represented good value for the ratepayers' expenditure. The many delays in the construction of Bangour Village, caused to a large extent by redrawing the plans several times to make them more economical, is but one example of this drive to save costs. However, the villas as actually built do not always demonstrate strict parsimony in styles and finishes. Styles range from the very simple and unornamented villas 1-4 at Kingseat, to the ashlar stone and drip moulds of the substantial villas at Dykebar (the ashlar stone entailing a considerable premium in cost over brick), and the bartizans of Bangour. Simplicity of style was, in any case, seen as a domestic virtue at this period, with cleaner lines and more subdued decoration part of the 'domestic revival' and many asylum villas would not have been out of a place in a suburban setting (Girouard, 1977: 5-37; Stamp, 1980: 2-4). There is a clear distinction between asylum villas and the pavilions of the traditional asylum, represented here by Whalley. Architecturally Whalley's pavilions for chronic patients are considerably plainer and more institutional in style than most of the asylum villas, and are largely lacking in detail or articulation. It is also noticeable that the only asylum villas in this study designed by an asylum specialist, Purdysburn designs 2 and 3, are less domestic in external aspect than most other villas we have seen, as might be expected from a professional asylum architect who was not accustomed to designing domestic houses. Although the asylum villas are very large in scale when compared to a domestic villa, as they housed up to 50 patients, the scale is dwarfed in comparison to Whalley's chronic blocks for 148 patients. Internal room sizes, while these are often much larger at the asylum villas than would be usual for a domestic house, are again much smaller, (with the exception of the Purdysburn observation villa),

than the pavilion dayrooms and dorms at Whalley which housed up to 54 patients in one room.

Although we have seen that Scottish Lunacy Commissioners explicitly connected freedom and domesticity in their annual reports, asylum villas do show evidence of attempts to control the movements of patients through the disposition of rooms. The layout of internal spaces in asylum villas shows a distinct preference for the type of layout seen at Alt-Scherbitz, which most likely provided the inspiration. Many asylum villas chose a layout consisting of rooms which open out of each other, rather than off a central corridor as in a domestic house, reducing the number of exit points which needed to be controlled. However, this may also have made it easier to pursue the 'open-door' policy which was the colony asylums stated objective. Under this layout, control of patients' movements could more easily be provided by staff rather than by locking doors, despite the relatively large number of rooms. The central corridor arrangement seen at Whalley, ostensibly making control of patient movements more difficult, is not likely to have been an issue for supervision because of the small number of rooms, and the single exit from each room.

With few exceptions, the rooms of asylum villas are divided and arranged along domestic lines, with dayrooms on the ground floor and dormitories and other sleeping rooms on first and second floors. Furthermore, living areas are often divided into distinct areas, with most villas providing more than one downstairs dayroom and a separate dining room, while Purdysburn Design 1 provided a reading room and visitors' room in addition. Most villa rooms are simple rectangles but the dayrooms in villas 18 and 21 at Bangour were L-shaped. The division of space into small rooms would have increased the need for staff in order to supervise them, as would the unusually-shaped rooms at Bangour, but provided a less institutional feel and a closer approximation to domestic living spaces. By contrast, at Whalley, the accommodation was arranged with dorms and undifferentiated dayrooms on ground and first floors (the second floor is all dorms) and the large, open spaces would have made it easier for small numbers of staff to supervise large numbers of patients, although home-like feeling is sacrificed.

Attention has been drawn at each site to the ambiguity surrounding entrances to asylum villas. The positioning, decorative emphasis and hierarchy of entrances is one of the most noticeable departures of asylum villas from what would be expected at a domestic house. It is often hard to identify a 'main' entrance as these are usually not placed prominently on the 'main' elevation but at the rear or side of the building and are not given the decorative emphasis one might expect. At some villas there are two or three entrances, none of which appears to have primacy. This apparent reluctance to designate one of the clearest signifiers of a domestic house, the front door, suggests that the implications of providing a threshold over which ownership could be symbolically assumed, either by staff or patients, were problematic for the asylum regime, although it is unclear whether this was intentional. Although the patients were provided with a space that was 'home-like' and granted a certain amount of freedom, this appears to have been one of the points where freedom became subordinated to the hierarchy of the asylum, as both patients and staff were discouraged architecturally from viewing this home as 'theirs'.

Another visible tension between the domestic and the institutional arises out of hygiene considerations. For the most part, effective ventilation and 'sunning' was achieved in asylum villas through positioning of the villa building, window placing and size and through the provision of ventilation grilles and flues, much as might have been the case in a domestic house (although asylum authorities with large acreages of land at their disposal can be presumed to have had more choice about the siting and orientation of individual buildings than private developers). However, some villas (all villas at Renfrew, design 3 at Purdysburn and medical villas at Bangour) have roof ventilators, a feature associated with public and institutional buildings rather than domestic houses, and which demonstrates the buildings' hygienic properties while detracting from their domesticity. Similar in this respect, is the provision of sanitary annexes on some villas at Purdysburn (Designs 1B and 3) which, as we have seen, was done against the wishes of the Medical Superintendent. Although a sanitary annexe was a hygiene measure, standard in hospitals and provided at all the pavilions in Whalley asylum, Dr Graham felt that it destroyed the homelike character of the villas at Purdysburn. Villas at Kingseat and Bangour achieved some of the effect of a sanitary annexe by housing these facilities in a single storey extension but without the corridor separating the annexe from the main building, thus retaining a domestic appearance to the villa.

Hamlett has suggested that the late nineteenth century saw an increasing concern with hygiene in internal asylum decoration (Hamlett, 2015: 25), and some of the simplicity and lack of clutter that we see in villa interiors may be accounted for by this. However, some internal features seem to have been included for their domestic feel, in defiance of the fact that they would have rendered interiors more difficult to keep clean and dust free. Dado panelling is a feature at all the Scottish and Irish villas, and additional moulding, above picture rail height is also common. Bangour villas have particularly elaborate ceiling moulding of the egg and dart style. This contrasts with the simple, painted wall divisions, rounded arrises and minimal moulding at Whalley which is more in keeping with hospital styles.

We have also seen a distinct difference between the types of accommodation offered to male and female patients at Bangour Village and this echoes the tendency to situate male accommodation on higher (and better ventilated) ground which we saw at Purdysburn and Bangour. Male patients are accommodated at Bangour in 'barrack-like' quarters of relatively low quality, while the female patients

lived in high-quality, stone villas of domestic aspect. The reasons for this division are not recorded but this was a period when Scotland differed from England and Wales in the active employment of female nurses on male wards in asylum hospitals (Arton, 1998: 64). The reasons for doing so, betray some of the cultural attitudes surrounding women at the time and the ways in which women's traditional association with the domestic was being constructed and professionalised. Female nurses were said to be more sympathetic and kindly and more efficient (ADLB Minutes 28th July 1903). But critically, they were also said to have a 'refining influence on male society' and it was thought that association with female nurses would have a beneficial effect on male patients (Halliday, 2003: 265). Female nurses, and by implication female patients, were associated with the gentleness, comfort and refinement of the domestic sphere, a sphere that usually excluded working-class men. The difference in accommodation also highlights the difference in occupation between men and women in the asylum. While women at Bangour were employed in laundry, in the kitchens and at sewing and knitting, largely domestic, indoor activities, 40 per cent of the male patients were employed on the land (EDLB Annual Report 1908), effectively acting as labourers for the asylum estate, and spending far less time indoors than the women. Nonetheless, at most of the other sites in this study, the accommodation for men and women was broadly similar in character.

The material practices of the Scottish colony asylums and Whalley may be seen as illustrative of regionally specific attitudes to the insane poor and their care. The colony asylums speak of a Scottish medical culture which arguably placed a high value on patient freedom and individuality, while imposing a paternalistic standard of bourgeois domestic living intended to elevate patient conduct and to induce calm and order. The spatial organisation of the village asylum promoted individuality and mental health by maintaining small patient groups, as well as by replicating the character of individualising domestic spaces. A concern with individuality extended even to the choice of furniture: armchairs were chosen which would render each patient 'comfortable and isolated,' in contrast to benches which would seat five or six together 'increasing their irritability and excitement' (ADLB Minutes, 28 July 1903). Individuality was to be encouraged both by the preservation of domestic scale and by environmental variety. The diversity of the village asylum, with variation in siting and surroundings, architectural styles and materials, alongside the lack of regularity of the buildings' disposition on a site, were frequently identified as implicitly individualising and antithetical to the usual homogenising asylum architecture and layout.

The asylum at Whalley opened initially as a military hospital and no photographs of the interior in use as a general asylum exist, since the buildings were never used for their intended purpose during the period covered by this study. Somewhat instructive, however, are surviving images of the interior of Claybury Asylum, taken in around 1893, the year of the institution's opening (Figures 7-28, 7-29).[5] When compared with the photograph of a villa interior at Bangour Village, at first sight the two institutions would appear to have made comparable efforts to create home-like interiors. The Claybury images were captured about a decade earlier than the Bangour image, and the wallpaper and valanced curtains betrays this. Bangour's painted finishes and window blinds are more consistent with hygienic practices at the end of the century. Claybury appears to have more 'domestic' clutter in terms of pictures, ornaments, birdcages etc, but the rooms shown are nevertheless unmistakeably institutional due to the arrangement of chairs and tables in a linear fashion, replicating the linear design of the compact arrow asylum. The dayroom for chronic patients is vast, housing 70 patients and was their living room when they were not outside. The dayroom at Bangour may be viewed as a much more successful approximation to a bourgeois interior, despite being rather more sparsely furnished and decorated. The furnishings are comfortable, even luxurious, and with the dining function separated into a different room, this is

clearly a sitting room, if an over-sized one. However, in addition the arrangement of furniture and floor coverings appears to have been rendered deliberately informal, with tables, chairs and carpets placed at angles, in an echo of the varied, individual style of the colony asylum layout itself. There appears to be a deliberate continuity here between the architecture of the colony asylum, in terms of variety of aspect and 'random' distribution, and the internal furnishing.

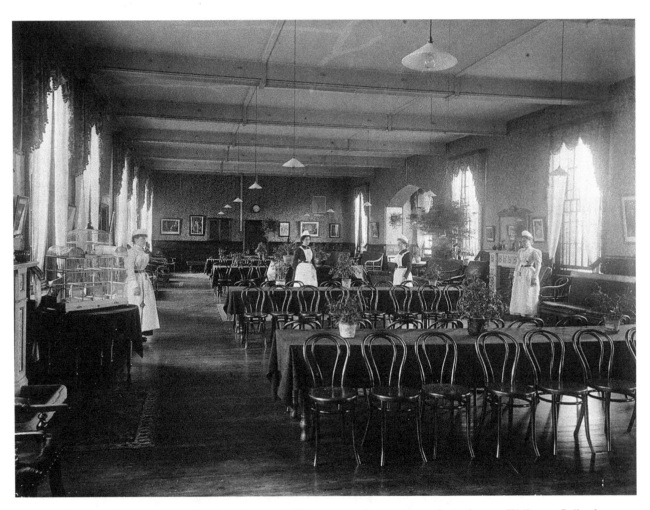

Figure 7-28. Essex County Asylum, Claybury (opened 1893): dayroom for chronic patients. Source: Wellcome Collection, Attribution 4.0 International (CC BY 4.0). Tentatively labelled 'dining room' by Wellcome.

[5]Although tentatively labelled by Wellcome, the location of the Claybury images may be securely identified using window and door openings as a guide and cross referencing with historic plans.

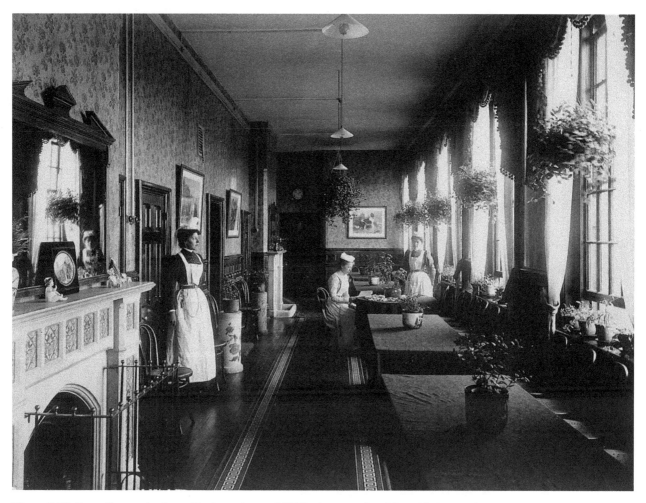

Figure 7-29. Essex County Asylum, Claybury (opened 1893): dayroom for sick and infirm patients. Source: Wellcome Collection, Attribution 4.0 International (CC BY 4.0). Tentatively labelled 'a nurses' day-room' by Wellcome.

8

Discussion

'Home life, with its domestic surroundings and interests, has numerous attractions, for the loss of which nothing can fully compensate .... The enjoyment by the insane of a liberty, the same in kind as that enjoyed by their sane neighbours, increases their physical and mental well-being; and another marked advantage in this mode of care lies in the fact that it gives patients a full opportunity of realising and developing their individuality.' (SLC 1895: xl)

The above extract from the 1895 report of the Scottish Lunacy Commissioners, referring to the benefits of 'boarding out' of patients within village communities, alludes to the paradox at the heart of asylum care in the late nineteenth century. As asylums became filled with ever greater numbers of insane patients, the buildings became ever larger and more 'institutional', detracting from the atmosphere of 'home' which was characteristic (or intended to be so) of the reformed asylums of the early nineteenth century. Of particular concern to Scottish asylum authorities was the loss of liberty and individuality that this entailed, which they felt to be detrimental to physical and mental health. The adoption of the colony asylum, with accommodation separated into villas, can be seen as a response to these concerns, and this chapter will explore the connections between the physical layout, buildings, interior furnishings and spaces and the wider aims of asylum authorities to provide hygienic, home-like spaces in which the freedom and individuality of patients was maximised.

The gradual abandonment of the asylum project in the second half of the twentieth century has been accompanied by a historiography which paints a thoroughly dystopian picture of the accumulation of 'chronic' cases in ever larger institutions. Andrew Scull appropriated the terms 'warehouses' and 'museums of madness' to describe the vast buildings which were used to segregate society's unwanted by the end of the nineteenth century (Scull, 1979). Although the asylum project had begun with high hopes, it is Scull's contention, followed by the majority of scholars of madness, that by the turn of the century therapeutic pessimism prevailed, based on the Morelian theory of degeneration and a resurgence of interest in Larmarckian evolution (Scull 2015: 243). According to this reading of medical discourses, hereditary weakness was caused by the poor habits and lax morals of the degenerate; mental illness was the ultimate penalty for breaking moral and hygienic laws. Society's duty was, therefore, simply to sequester the insane to prevent reproduction of the 'unfit' in asylums built as quickly and as cheaply as decorum would allow (Scull 1979: 277-279).

This study challenges the prevailing historiographical orthodoxy which suggests that, by the end of the nineteenth century, an initial therapeutic optimism had evaporated and asylums were being constructed as 'warehouses' to sequester the unwanted (Waddington, 2011: 326; Freeman, 2010; Gold and Gold, 2015: 25; Pietikäinen, 2015: 134-136; Scull, 2015: 223, 2017: 105-106; Shorter, 1997: 65). This implies a detachment from the asylum project not supported by the close analysis of the buildings and primary sources in this study, which reveals both deliberate attention to the therapeutic effect of buildings and spaces, and a less conscious embedding of material practices within their local cultural contexts. Previous scholarship has used the word 'warehouses' as an evocative term to describe various aspects of the late nineteenth-century asylum system. 'Warehouse' has been used to imply the accommodation of unwanted, chronically ill patients who were removed from public view and kept for long periods in ever larger, cheaply-constructed institutions that were architecturally dull and repetitive (Dale & Melling, 2006: 39; Waddington, 2011: 326; Wallace & Gach, 2008: xxx). However, the systematic assessment of the asylum buildings in this study suggests that most do not conform to the epithet 'warehouses', and indeed a variety of motivations were embodied in the construction of the colony asylum. It is possible to read from the designs and layouts, together with contemporary published and unpublished materials, a range of complex attributes, both practical and symbolic, that reflect contemporary attitudes to the insane and their therapeutic treatment, but also to the poor more generally and to the role of environment in generating health or illness at this particular juncture.

The following chapter is divided into six sections. Firstly, I will consider two factors that can be considered to be significant in the construction and siting of colony asylums, namely hygiene and rural location, before turning to some less obvious considerations that arise from the links that can be drawn between asylum materiality, contemporary cultural trends and ideas about how to treat the mentally ill. The ways in which the colony asylum was made to appear less 'asylum-like' and more 'home-like' will be considered followed by an exploration of the bourgeois values that were appealed to in the construction of a home-like environment. This will then lead to a discussion of the spatial segregation of buildings and patients within the colony asylum and what were seen to be the natural corollaries of this, the promotion of individuality and the consequent release of vitality that was essential for good mental and physical health.

8.1. The colony asylum and hygiene

The growing concern with hygiene as an important attribute of buildings and spaces can be traced to the mid-nineteenth century and before, but the early 1900s saw an increase in the number of publications on the subject. Hygiene, which, at this period, broadly signified disease prevention, had been gradually linked to concerns about the environmental causes of racial degeneration, arising from a belief in the interconnection of mind and body. One of the standard medical works on the topic, Parkes' *Manual of Practical Hygiene*, makes it clear that hygiene was not understood in merely physical terms, 'Taking the word hygiene in the largest sense, it signifies rules for perfect culture of mind and body. It is impossible to dissociate the two. The body is affected by every mental and moral action, the mind is profoundly affected by bodily conditions. For a perfect system of hygiene we must train the body, the intellect and the moral faculties in a perfect and balanced order'(Parkes, 1887:xvi-xvii). Hygiene in this period applied to a much wider range of environmental issues than it does today, with Parkes advising on soil conditions, water supply, sewage systems, ventilation, the heating of homes, the choice and cooking of food, exercise etc, as well as the admission of light into buildings. Contrary to the assertion that asylums of this period were 'warehouses', an analysis of the sites in this study soon revealed that they had been built with considerable attention to questions of hygiene, and that this entailed careful planning and often expense. The siting and orientation of the buildings in the colony asylums under study, the size, spacing and arrangement of windows, the interior glazing and the simplicity of interior spaces suggest that the management of light was a highly significant consideration in the design of the asylum. Light-filled rooms could bring vitality, both moral and mental, to weakened patients, light purified the spaces in which they lived ensuring that disease-causing organisms were kept at bay, and light promoted cheerfulness and raised spirits, providing an environment where the inherent weakness of the mentally ill patient could be strengthened. The provision of light-filled rooms within the asylum can also be seen as a symbolic display. The provision of large windows and light-filled rooms manifested the humanity and modernity of the asylum authorities, demonstrating to potential patients, their families and the general public not only that the asylum was a place of health but that it was a place that was open to observation, and the gaze of the proper authorities, deterring potential abuses. The asylum is characterised through light-filled spaces as a place of humane treatment where no patients are hidden away in darkened rooms. Not part of this public image, however, is a powered understanding of light as facilitating observation and surveillance of patients by staff together with policing of socio-sexual categories. Light allowed observation to extend into the most intimate parts of patients' lives and allowed large groups of patients to be monitored visually at all times by relatively small numbers of staff. An analysis of light provision demonstrates how care for the wellbeing of patients elides seamlessly into control and reinforces hierarchical relationships within the asylum and the wider society within which the asylum is situated.

However, as an enlightenment project, asylum buildings were not only places of light, but also had to be seen to be so, and thus hygienic, healthy and able to promote mental healing. Central to this was the need to position discursively the asylum in opposition to the prison. Where the prison had bars, locks and single cells, the asylum had open doors, and unbarred windows, correlating it with the forms and practices of a domestic environment. But most crucially of all, where the prison was dark, or perceived to be so, the asylum was filled with light. Through the provision of light-filled spaces the asylum authorities attempted to demonstrate the provision of an environment that was not only sane and healthy but also humane and compassionate.

Discourses of light and darkness at this period constituted patients as degenerate in eugenic terms, by dint of their madness, part of the indiscriminate mass of the underclass who were to be removed from contaminating association with the healthy. Analysis of light as a material and discursive practice, nuances our understanding of the network of power relations in which staff, patients and asylum doctors were embedded. These power relations demonstrate a range of attitudes to the insane poor, which go far beyond overt physical and mental control. Asylums were not only sites of power because doors were locked, because patients were confined, or because they thought they were being watched, but also because patients were discursively positioned as morally, mentally and physically lacking. Patients were constituted in sometimes contradictory ways, both as a social threat to be controlled, and as objects of pity who were to be treated with enlightened care and brought back to sanity through exposure to a healthy environment.

It is clear from much of the contemporary literature about asylums and from a study of buildings themselves that hygiene of various kinds was a significant concern for asylum authorities in all locations in Britain and Ireland. We have seen that at Whalley in Lancashire, which was built as a 'barracks' design with large numbers of patients accumulated together in vast wards, that hygiene was nevertheless an important consideration and the built evidence suggests that hygiene was, in fact, prioritised over the desire to provide a 'home-like' setting for patients (although, as we have seen the hygiene of the site chosen was severely compromised by the need for a large expanse of flat land). In particular, internal spaces were laid out similarly to a 'Nightingale' hospital ward giving access to light and cross-ventilation and ceilings were high allowing for large volumes of air to circulate. However, there were unique features to the hygienic surroundings provided in the colony asylum, which meant that the colony could lay claim to some hygienic advantages. The ability to site individual buildings in relation to the topography, and the fact that asylum buildings could be sited at some distance from each other, rather than in a predetermined pattern, allowed asylum builders to take advantage of high points in the ground, allowing for better ventilation of spaces and for better access to light and air. Given that respiration was seen as one of the main sources of 'vitiated' air, the limiting of patient numbers within internal building spaces was likely to mean a lower volume of vitiated air and therefore easier ventilation of the rooms and wards. The smaller size of internal rooms, while ceiling heights were often maintained at 12 feet and above, allowed for better natural lighting of internal spaces, with all the advantages that entailed.

The construction of asylum buildings as hygienic spaces can be said to have been motivated by the sanitary revolution that had been ongoing since the mid-nineteenth century, inflected by an understanding of the environment of the poor as noxious and disease-producing and thereby detrimental to mental as well as physical health. Hygiene was therefore a characteristic of the *institutional* as opposed to the *domestic* space (as this applied to the poor) and had been a prime concern of asylum builders for decades, justifying the removal of the poor from their disease-ridden environments. Although there were some changes in the application of hygienic principles at this period, including increased provision of natural light through windows of a larger size (Figure 7-2), hygiene was not in itself a distinctive feature of the colony asylum, but was applied in some form to all asylums and institutional buildings.

The colony asylum appears to have arisen out of a different environmental concern, produced by the asylum movement itself. By this late stage of the asylum project, the aggregation of patients within asylums, was seen to cause significant problems that were detrimental to the mental and physical health of the poor. As the numbers of insane grew ever higher, existing asylum buildings which had been constructed as models of healthy and hygienic environments were extended and new asylums proliferated, causing overcrowding and consequent outbreaks of disease such as colitis, dysentery, typhoid, tuberculosis and pneumonia (ELC Report 1896:20). The colony asylum can therefore be seen partially as a response to disease produced by the asylum system itself by dispersing asylum buildings and dividing patients into smaller groups.

However, the hygienic advantages to the colony asylum system are rarely mentioned as the most significant ones by asylum authorities. William Graham, the medical superintendent of Purdysburn, praised the 'hygienic efficiency' of the newly-completed asylum, and the Lancashire deputation to Germany pointed out that 'nothing … is more insanitary than the massing of human beings together in a limited area. The more they are spread out, as a question of sanitation, the better', when they praised the dispersed layout of Alt Scherbitz (BDLA Annual Report 1911; Report of a Lancashire deputation, 1900: 67). Few others, however, were minded to emphasise

these issues, which may have appeared standard concerns for responsible institutional authorities by this period. An alternative motivation for favouring the colony asylum has been raised by several scholars, namely that colony asylums were a means of removing the poor insane to distant rural sites where they could not affect the healthy population through inter-breeding. The next section will therefore consider the positioning of the colony sites in the study and the possible reasons for choosing rural areas, often far outside the nearest centres of population.

8.2. The colony asylum and rural location

Generative spatial rationalities, which expressly endow environments with the ability to generate health and/or virtue have a lengthy provenance. Chris Philo identifies a 'moral geography' associated with the influential Quaker asylum 'The Retreat' (opened 1796), which prioritised healthy situation, the availability of land for exercise and employment and 'retirement' from the nearest urban centre (seen as a source of 'mental disturbance') in contrast to earlier asylums whose urban sites were, like those of infirmaries, equated with better access to medical care (Philo 2004: 430-525). Philo suggests that the during the course of the nineteenth century a medical takeover of the asylum resulted in a blurring of boundaries between medical and moral which justified the location of asylums in rural sites on a number of grounds. These included the health of patients and the asylum as source of infection, but also a deeper cultural sense of 'moralised natural spaces' symbolising and enacting the harmonious juncture of nature and humanity (Philo 2004: 526-650). In Scotland and Ireland the trend over time was to locate asylums ever further outside urban centres. Before the 1880s no asylum building in Scotland, the striking exception being Perth District Asylum, was located more than five kilometres from the nearest urban settlement from which it drew patients. Irish asylums were all built less than 3 km from the nearest urban centre until the building of Portrane, 18 km outside Dublin in 1902 and Purdysburn, 7 km outside Belfast. Previous scholarship has suggested that the reasons for such trends elsewhere lie in ideas of hereditarianism and the nascent pseudoscience of eugenics. It has been suggested that, in England and Wales, degenerationist thinking during the later decades of the nineteenth century led to a downgrading of the importance attributed to the environment in the treatment of mental illness. As greater importance began to be given to the inheritance of mental abnormality, previous therapeutic optimism was shaken by the belief that many patients were not susceptible to improvement and would remain in the asylum for life. This strand of pessimism can clearly be discerned in medical writing of the period and has been noted by numerous scholars of Victorian approaches to mental illness and disability (Fennell, 1996: 46; Forsythe, 2001; Wright, 2001: 191-192; Freeman, 2010). For example, Matthew Jackson's study of the Sandlebridge colony for the feeble-minded, founded in Cheshire in 1902, finds that in the period up to the introduction of the Mental Deficiency Act of 1913 insanity and feeble-mindedness were increasingly attributed to hereditary rather than environmental causes. While acknowledging the tension between hereditarian and environmentalist explanations of racial decline, Jackson emphasises that rural colonies effectively segregated 'socially dangerous defectives' in places where they could not reproduce (Jackson 2000: 63). John Radford and Deborah Park have also suggested that custodial institutions for the mentally deficient in the U.S., Britain and Canada in this period were primarily 'manifestations of eugenically-driven social policy', the implication being that cost saving was also a prime driver in the rural, colony form of institution (Radford, 1991; Radford & Park, 1995). However, the present research suggests that continuing in the early nineteenth-century tradition, rural locations continued to be seen as healthy and desirable asylum locations in and of themselves. For example, Kingseat was praised for the quiet, country life it offered and its 'pure, bracing air', attributed to its high elevation (ACDLB Annual Report 1905). The 'extensive view of mountain scenery' that the site offered, followed in a long therapeutic tradition of concern with the vistas available to hospital and asylum patients, views that were endowed with stimulating, soothing or healing properties (Hickman, 2013: 22-39). Because of the relative seclusion of these sites, patients had considerable freedom to walk in the grounds without fear that they might escape, despite the lack of walls and gates, and therefore greater opportunities to enjoy views and fresh air than might have been possible elsewhere. At Purdysburn, several additional plots were purchased, over a period of years after the estate was initially acquired for the BDLA, (and to the consternation of some councillors) in order to provide for the patients, 'open-air exercise and labour' which were the 'best curative powers in connection with insanity' (*Belfast Newsletter*, 14th January 1902).

It is also clear that in Scotland, and elsewhere, the impulses to sequester and economise were wedded to a desire to provide as much agricultural land as possible for asylum patients—ideally one and a half acres per male patient by 1904, whereas in 1857 a quarter of an acre per patient had been seen as sufficient, and that this was an important factor in the sudden rise in asylum estate size after 1890, somewhat before eugenic approaches to racial decline were being discussed with any great seriousness.[1] The extra land afforded 'the means of healthy occupation' and of making the patients' lives more like those 'of sane persons' (Ross 2014:189-217). Farm work was seen to be 'a natural, healthy and sane interest which tends to promote recovery or at all events contentment and easy management' and was stated to be more mentally stimulating than other types of outdoor work because it was more varied, than, for example, work on the grounds (ACDLB Annual Report 1909). It must be borne in mind that asylum patients provided free labour for the farm, where otherwise labour would have had to be bought in, raising the cost to ratepayers of asylum care. There can be

little doubt, however, that there was a genuine belief, no doubt rooted in a romanticised attitude towards rural life, that farm work provided a therapeutic means of occupying mental patients, the Medical Superintendent of Kingseat commenting in 1908,

> 'The chronic patient working on the farm, who is, comparatively speaking more or less sociable with his fellows … I cannot imagine a happier existence for this man, whose powers of earning a living wage have been ruined by mental disease, than the life in one of the parole villas of the Asylum' (ACDLB Annual Report, 1908)

It must also be stressed that, despite the rise in numbers of chronic inmates, large numbers of patients left each asylum every year, the majority deemed cured, but even if not so, assessed as being sufficiently well to live again in their communities. For example, during the first five years that Renfrew asylum was open, between 1909 and 1914, 515 patients were directly admitted,[2] and 243, roughly half, were discharged (Dykebar Annual Reports 1910-1914). Although this leaves a large number of patients who were long-term residents, an almost equally large number were temporary residents of the asylum and were clearly not treated as a genetic threat to society, with high discharge rates being seen as desirable rather than otherwise. The 'hard hereditarian' approach to curbing degeneracy, by discouraging the reproduction of the 'unfit' through sterilisation or segregation and promoting the marriage of the 'fit' through legislation appears to have been little pursued by medical officials and those concerned with public health. More prevalent was a 'soft hereditarian' approach, Lamarckian/Morelian in its basis, which emphasised the importance of environmental factors in harming the offspring of the morally weak and held that in order to improve working class 'stock' reformers should address the environment and/or the personal failings of those tending to degeneracy (Snelders, Meijman, & Pieters, 2007:219-236; Woiak, 1998:30-71). Nicholas Rose has pointed to a 'strategy of social hygiene' taken up by the medical profession at this period which used the findings of social investigators as evidence for the interaction between environment and health. Physical deterioration of the population was blamed on over-work and lack of sunshine, outdoor exercise and fresh air and could be addressed by environmental reform and education. The 'neo-hygienist' approach became public policy and although, after 1900, this was increasingly influenced by eugenicist proposals to sequester the degenerate, this motivation never became a prime driver. Internal colonies were proposed, not only to limit the reproduction of the unfit, but also as a solution to urban poverty and overcrowding and a means of bringing under-used agricultural areas back into production (Rose, 1985: 82-88). Eugenic motivations for removing asylums into rural areas should not be over-emphasised, therefore. It is more likely, in the case of the colony asylum, where

---

[1] It is usually agreed that eugenics 'took off' as a political doctrine in the first decade of the twentieth century (Rose, 1985: 75)

[2] This figure excludes a number of chronic patients who were transferred from other asylums when Renfrew opened.

the sites were largely purchased in the period before eugenic thought became more influential, [3] that the prime motivations were twofold: firstly the attraction of high elevations, fresh air and hygienic environments and secondly the opportunity to render patients productive as outdoor labourers. William Booth's 'Farm Colony', for the unemployed proposed:

'a settlement of the Colonists on an estate in the provinces, in the culture of which they would find employment and obtain support. As the race from the Country to the City has been the cause of much of the distress we have to battle with, we propose to find a substantial part of our remedy by transferring these same people back to the country, that is back again to "the Garden!"' (Booth, 1890: 92).

This was based on an understanding of urban environments as detrimental to health, as much as it was on a belief that the unemployed should be encouraged to be productive. Booth's labour colonies were themselves part of a European tradition, as we have seen, of returning the poor to the land, but his ideas were hugely influential in the period after 1890 and were productive of several experiments in the colonisation of the unemployed (Brown, 1968: 357). However, it is possible that the fact that colony asylums were driven much further into rural areas in search of larger expanses of agricultural land and male patients were encouraged to become farm workers, may also have been a point of sensitivity. The equation of institution for the insane, with the more familiar 'labour colony' for the unemployed, may have seemed unduly harsh and indeed this is a possible reason why the terms 'village' and 'villa colony', were used in preference to 'labour colony' to describe the new layouts. Although, as we have seen, the asylum layout was often divided into two parts, one described as 'medical' and the other as 'industrial' or 'colony', denoting that patients in the latter area of the asylum were working.

8.3. The colony asylum as 'home-like'

The main factors cited by contemporaries, both asylum authorities and architects, in favour of the colony can be divided into the following categories:[4]

The colony was thought to be more 'home-like': the buildings were similar to ordinary private dwellings in size, architectural style, internal arrangements and grouping. Continual reference is made to the 'scattered'

and 'irregular' layout of buildings, particularly at Bangour, and the 'variety' both in the materials, treatments and styles of the buildings and the environment of each building due to their distribution about the sites. Also frequently commented upon is the 'simple', 'natural' nature of the villas and their freedom from architectural pretension.

The colony gave greater freedom to patients, both in appearance and actuality: no walls surrounded the sites, nor were individual buildings fenced off. The open door system was practised, which meant that the majority of patients were free to go in and out of rooms and buildings during the day. Although this system was not entailed by the architecture, and standard asylum layouts could also practice the open door system, the stand-alone nature of the villa buildings and the absence of corridors meant that patients passing from building to building were not constrained by walls or locked doors, and therefore were either self-regulating or were subject to additional supervision. It was felt that the appearance of restraint was, in itself, antithetical to patient contentment and, therefore, the absence of visible walls and fences was symbolically, as well as practically significant.

The colony allowed patients to be more easily classified, because of the provision of smaller spaces: although the nature of the classification varied between commentators. Some thought that patients should be divided according to their diagnosis with noisy or dirty patients separated from the quiet and clean, others that patients should be grouped according to their 'tastes, habits, interests and occupations', with farm labourers or laundry workers living in the same villa. In practice, the classification of patients tended to be driven by a combination of these factors, with acutely manic patients separated from the seriously depressed in the medical section villas, while chronic or recuperating patients were housed in 'industrial' villas according to their occupation, laundry workers occupying a separate villa from dressmakers, for example.

The colony avoided the aggregation of large numbers of patients: both the buildings and their internal spaces broke down patient numbers into small groups, which was considered important in defeating a herd mentality and promoting patient individuality. Individuality was associated with vigour and vitality (and good mental health), where aggregation of large numbers of patients was seen to render them listless and apathetic (Palmer, 1887: 169; Burdett, Vol 1, 1891: 159). Aggregation of patient numbers was also considered physically unhealthy, due largely to the vitiated air produced in confined spaces.

The colony was predicted by some to be more economical to construct than other asylum types, due to the lack of connecting corridors and surrounding walls and because centralised heating systems were unnecessary. In practice the cost of colony asylums was highly variable, Kingseat being comparatively cheap (£253 per bed) but Bangour much more expensive (£387 per bed, putting Bangour in the highest third when compared with English asylums)

---

[3] The estates were purchased in the following order: Purdysburn (1895), Bangour Village (1897), Kingseat (1899) and Renfrew (1902).

[4] The advantages of the colony asylum layout have been summarised from the following sources: *Aberdeen Daily Journal*, 13th September 1901:4; Hine, 1901, *British Medical Journal*, 24th November 1906; *Journal of Mental Science*, 1900 (46): 87-109; 1905 (51): 681-710; *British Architect*, 12th September, 1902:182; 26th May, 1905:376-377; 5th October, 1906: 247-248, 13th October 1906:972-974; Report of Edinburgh Deputation, 1897; *The Builder*, 10th November 1906:545-547; Blanc, 1908; Rhodes, 1897; Report of Lancashire deputation, 1900; Sibbald, 1897.

('The First British Village Asylum', 1906; Keay, 1911; ELC 1910: 258-265).[5] The colony also allowed for additional accommodation to be more easily added after the initial construction phase.

However, overarching these considerations was another important motivation for adopting the colony as a layout, the fact that the colony was as little like an asylum as possible. As we saw above, the colony asylum can be considered to have been a response to some of the hygienic issues affecting the asylum system itself which was beset by problems with overcrowding and disease. But it was not only overcrowding and disease that made the old-style asylums appear increasingly unattractive. There was a strong antipathy within Scottish asylum culture to the aggregation of large numbers of patients, and large, 'barrack' style English asylums were pointed to as examples of the kind of monotonous architecture that was to be avoided. From the mid-nineteenth century onwards it was suggested that an ideal asylum might resemble 'a large English homestead, or some large industrial community', 'a farming or industrial colony', or might be composed of 'separate houses, in which the patients are distributed according to their dispositions and the features and stages of their disease' (Browne, 1837: 185; Lindsay, 1857: 115). Scottish authorities praised Alt Scherbitz for avoiding the 'monotonous uniformity' of asylum buildings, implying that 'barracks' architecture rendered the inhabitants dull and passive (*Report of an Edinburgh deputation*, 1897: 28).

The goal of the colony asylum was 'the assimilation of the life of a community of lunatics to ordinary life in a country village' and Sibbald and his Edinburgh colleagues agreed that it rendered 'the conditions of life the same as sane people in an ordinary rural community' (*Report of an Edinburgh deputation*, 1897: 17; Sibbald, 1897: 20). The equating of asylum conditions with those of ordinary life hinged on several factors. Firstly, the colony was constructed to architecturally resemble an ordinary asylum as little as possible. The colony had 'an absence of the appearance of an institution' and the architect of Bangour also praised its 'absence of institutional character'. Among the characteristics which allowed this to be achieved, were the absence of the traditional visual 'markers' of the asylum. Usually mentioned are the lack of surrounding walls but the field survey of Bangour and Purdysburn shows that gate lodges and screens were also eschewed at some sites. Additionally, the architecture of the asylum buildings itself was 'simple' and 'picturesque' rather than 'grand or imposing' (Sibbald, 1897). In this respect, the colony distinguishes itself sharply from the tradition of institutional building, in which the building itself is of a scale and decorative splendour sometimes described as

'palatial', and hence constitutes a visual expression of the charity and benevolence of the relevant authority. That this was clearly understood by contemporaries is exemplified by a comment in the *British Medical Journal* which praised Kingseat for prioritising the patients rather than the buildings:

'It is recognized by the Aberdeen municipal authorities that insanity cannot be cured by bricks and mortar, even in the most massive doses. We earnestly commend their method to the notice and imitation of certain public bodies in England, which appear to think that the solution of the lunacy problem is to be found in covering as much ground as possible with palatial buildings. In this, as in other things, their motto would seem to be *Ad majorem Concilii gloriam*[6]. In the Kingseat Asylum the foremost consideration has been the greatest good of the sufferers for whose relief it is intended.'('The First British Village Asylum', 1906)

In fact, the lack of pretension of colony asylum buildings defeated the expectations of some commentators to the extent that it was seen as a sign of the lack of generosity of asylum authorities. A visitor to Bangour commented that, 'On entering the grounds, the visitor ... soon finds himself at the administration block, generally the most commanding portion structurally of public institutions, but in this case constructed by the board in one of its fits of parsimony, and looking pretty much as if it were trying to sink out of sight in offended dignity' ('The Bangour Asylum', 1906) (Figure 3-16). An imposing architecture was popularly seen as synonymous with appropriate public spending on the poor and the colony asylum, therefore, ran counter to expected norms. Colony buildings were on a small scale, decoratively simple and informal in aspect, corresponding more closely to the desired aspects of middle-class houses, being without pretension but evoking 'home'. In addition, the villas of the colony exemplified 'variety' rather than the 'monotony' or 'uniformity' that was held to be characteristic of the monolithic asylum building. For example, the villas of Bangour used 'a variety of external treatment in exposed stone, harling, tiled and green slated roofs. A fair architectural effect is obtained by simple variations in form, without superimposed decorative details' ('Bangour Village Lunatic Asylum', 1906).

Variety was obtained by means of materials, finishes, orientations and positioning of buildings, variations in internal layouts and external forms and the exploitation of variations in terrain and aspect. Additionally, however, the buildings were not decoratively elaborate, frequently being described as 'plain', 'unpretentious' or 'natural', and the lack of decoration being commented on (e.g. 'The New Asylum at Kingseat', 1901, 'Bangour Village Lunatic Asylum', 1906). This can be seen both as a desire to emphasise due economy being brought to bear, but also is very likely intended to show the contrast with the

---

[5] The per bed costs here include land, buildings and furnishings, but patient numbers for Kingseat were 472 in 1906 and for Bangour were 873 in 1911. Since the administration, kitchens and other communal buildings were in each case constructed for larger numbers, it was felt that the eventual cost in each case would be lower when further villas were added to the sites.

[6] 'To the greater glory of the Council'

traditional asylum building, which were often, by contrast, elaborate and detailed decoratively.

Although the term 'village' was habitually used to identify the colony layout in Scotland, descriptions often equate the colony asylum to a city suburb (by implication middle class) and this is the architectural style and register that the villas most consistently evoke. Although the dispersed style may have aimed to be more 'home-like', the substantial villas of the colony asylum resemble the comfortable homes of the better off, more than they do the rows of byelaw housing, the poorer Scottish city tenements or even worse, the dank and dark courts and alleys, that were more typical of the housing of the poor. Archive and field analysis of the buildings shows that materials and features were used in asylum villas, such as bartizans at Bangour, dressed stone at Renfrew and 'Old English' timbering at Kingseat that could not have been justified on the grounds of economy, and rather belie the claims to simplicity and plainness that were often made. Furthermore, interiors were sometimes furnished in a way which appeared lavish, even to contemporaries, a case in point, being the dayroom in Bangour Villa 18 with its grand piano and egg and dart moulding around the upper walls. The provision of such high-quality environments for the insane poor was not always met with approval or even equanimity. No doubt to the surprise of the assembled company, the former Prime Minister Lord Rosebery, who was invited to open Bangour in 1906, complained that the villas were 'sumptuous homes for the insane ... laid out as daintily as they could be for the blood royal' and asked rhetorically 'why do all this for the intellectually dead?' ('Lord Rosebery on the insane and their cost', 1906). A visitor to Kingseat from the *BMJ* commented that the villas gave the impression of 'a private dwelling inhabited by persons of cultivated taste', but cautioned that the homes were 'perhaps a trifle luxurious. The patients with the stigmata of degeneracy writ large upon them and their cheap 'slops'[7] hanging in ungainly folds about their awkward limbs, produced a curious effect of incongruity with the suburban aestheticism of their environment' ('The First British Village Asylum', 1906). The attempt to avoid the resemblance to an asylum and to instead use the domestic bourgeois home as a model requires some explanation, given the low esteem in which the 'degenerate' insane were often held at this period, exemplified by the comments quoted above. Working class housing was not the model used here, and the strict requirements of economy were not adhered to in the way that the historiographical orthodoxy claims for the so-called 'warehouses' of the late nineteenth and early twentieth centuries. At first sight, the traditional asylum also would appear to meet many of the cultural and social needs associated with asylum provision, making a clear statement about the charity of the asylum builders and allowing for the provision of hygienic spaces. In the next section, therefore, we will make a deeper analysis of the cultural and social context for the choice of the colony as an asylum layout and argue that the environmental effects aimed at in asylum planning are more complex than is usually argued.

8.4. The colony asylum and bourgeois values

The architecture of asylum villas may be seen (and indeed was seen) as representing a type of accommodation that was most often to be found in the middle-class suburban housing estate. Some villas approximate more closely to this ideal than others, the plainer Kingseat and Bangour villas, for example, evoking Scottish styles which would certainly have required some embellishment to fulfil bourgeois requirements. However, all the sites offer good examples of the villa style that would not have been out of place in a suburban setting. The interiors are often even more evocative of a higher standard of living than would have been enjoyed by patients returning to everyday life outside the asylum. These standards were enacted, as we have seen, in the face of some opposition, both within the asylum system and outside it, relating both to expense and the perceived appropriateness of providing in this way for patients of low social class and even lower social standing due to their perceived degeneracy or hereditary weakness. Interiors, in particular, sometimes prioritised a bourgeois living standard above the demands of hygiene. The egg and dart moulding in the dayroom of Villa 18 at Bangour would have been a trap for dust and dirt and much plainer wall treatments are used at Whalley where interior hygiene seems to have been a greater priority and indeed even at other colony sites, particularly Purdysburn and Kingseat. The use of such a moulding despite the threat to hygiene and the additional expense it represented, suggests that there were compelling reasons for its inclusion in the decorative scheme at Bangour. As we have seen, Scottish Lunacy Commissioners explicitly connected 'homelike' environments of a high quality with the tranquillity and contentment of patients and their willingness to work (SLC 1882: 66).

The resemblance to home was said to lead to happier and more productive patients and this was expressly contrasted with 'the institutional asylum life, which is always irksome and leads to irritability and the need of an increased staff of attendants' (SLC Report, 1884:111). The smallest improvement in domestic environment was claimed to have an effect on the disposition of patients. For example, an increase in the 'number of plants and other articles of decoration' at Fife and Kinross asylum 'would have a beneficial effect on the patients by giving a more homelike appearance to the wards' (SLC Report, 1896:70). The introduction of easy-chairs in the lunatic wards at Aberdeen Poorhouse and 'of a better class of furniture generally, would give the rooms a more home-like and comfortable appearance which would have a good influence on the patients' (SLC Report, 1897:103). At a time when mental illness could only be defined as a departure from social norms (and many would argue, can still only be defined thus - e.g. Szasz, 1961), environment was seen to play a key part in acting on patients to produce behaviour that conformed to expectations, not only of

---

[7] Cheap, mass-produced clothing

correct behaviour in broad social terms, but to expectations that were heavily inflected by the values of the dominant authorities within the asylum system, the middle classes. The asylum environment, therefore, while nominally 'appropriate' to the social class of the insane poor, in fact expressed a discursive construction of bourgeois values as aspirational for patients and inherently both health-producing and health-signifying.

Middle-class practices (or those associated with 'working people of the better class', whose practices were seen as emulating the middle classes) such as the correct use of dining implements and the serving of tea by older women in asylums were also advocated on the grounds that they were 'refining'. Indeed, the introduction of female nurses to male wards was also intended to produce a 'refining' effect on male patients by modelling and policing such practices, thereby producing the tranquillity and adherence to social norms which was desired (SLC Report, 1896:80).

In addition, the freedom from discipline which was associated with home-like rather than institutional surroundings was thought to lead to an increase in individuality and productivity. Commissioners noted, in relation to boarding-out, that, 'home influences, the acquirements of domestic habits long in abeyance ... have the effect of drawing out sociable instincts, and of revealing and developing a latent capacity for work and usefulness ... patients begin to think and act for themselves' (SLC Report, 1897:120). Although specific comments on the interior environments at the sites in this study are few, it is noteworthy that material objects were viewed as significant in promoting individuality as well as behaviour that conformed to social norms. The pattern of the tea-cups at Alt Scherbitz was praised for its variety, while armchairs at Kingseat were for individual patients rather than bench seats for five or six (*EDLB Report* 1897:27; ADLB Minutes, 28 July 1903).

Insofar as contemporary photographs have survived of the interiors in this study, these impress by the relative comfort of the furnishings used, particularly Bangour with its upholstered fabric sofas, glass bookcases and strategically disposed carpets. All the interiors show a concern for varied disposition and types of furniture and ornaments, with plants, mirrors and pianos usual elements in the design. Although the interiors must often be viewed as more sparse than a genuine domestic interior of the period, they are at a far remove from the workhouse or the prison of the period, in which the regularity of identical human units seated at long benches appears to have been common. As we have seen, there was a tendency for traditional asylum interiors to replicate the linear, repetitive mode of spatial organisation often seen in institutions, despite their relatively high level of comfort. Seating in the colony asylum, by contrast, is usually individual, sometimes for two or three, and the size, furnishing and decoration of the rooms gives the impression of a comfortable middle-class home in which individual choice and taste has

been expressed, without the excess clutter (and hygiene problems) this might have entailed. In addition, the domestic scale and architectural design of the buildings and the interior spaces of the colony asylum was seen to give it a distinct advantage relative to the traditional asylum building in fostering a home-like setting. Although domestic furnishings could be used in any type of asylum structure, the scale and layouts of the colony asylum would readily have lent themselves to the kind of facsimile of home living that was being attempted. Because of the smaller size of villas and interiors, and smaller numbers of patients accommodated, the colony would have provided closer approximations to the *ersatz* family in its carefully constructed spaces and greater opportunities for patient liberty and individuality to be expressed.

The materiality of the colony asylum thus reflected the bourgeois values of appropriate sociability, liberty, individuality and vitality as those likely to render the inhabitants of the asylum 'useful', if not necessarily cured. Asylum authorities were reflecting a contemporary concern with ideals of middle-class domesticity, that was expressed through the kind of domestic revival architecture to which the asylum villas often allude. This period (1860-1914) saw a flowering of domestic architecture and the development of 'the first truly middle-class architecture in Britain' (Creese, 1966; Bolsterli, 1977; Girouard, 1977, Stamp, 1980: 3). The new domestic designs rejected aristocratic styles and pastiche and catered for a middle class which was growing in numbers, assurance and influence. The new architecture had its roots in the Romanticism of the early nineteenth century but also drew its influences from simple vernacular buildings that owed their forms to materials and craft practices. The domestic revival looked towards rural styles and expressed the wish to live in close contact with 'Nature', shunning contemporary industrialisation. In the forefront were thinkers such as Ruskin and Morris who sought to revive craft traditions in a rejection of the mass-production of the machine age, Morris's Society for the Protection of Ancient Buildings actively preserving a vanishing world of rural dwellings (Stamp, 1980: 2). Domestic architects prioritised the 'Picturesque', in other words the antithesis of the 'formal, symmetrical, grand house of the Palladian tradition', but instead houses that were sympathetic to their surroundings, asymmetrical, eccentric and charming (Stamp, 1980:2-3). The middle-class domestic dwelling at this period, therefore, can be seen as a material expression of a certain conjunction of emotions, desires and aspirations for bourgeois living. The domestic home expressed a romanticised rural-leaning way of life and a freedom from formality and constraint, and the architecture itself was seen as capable of evoking these emotions. Voysey commented in 1911,

'Do we not all desire peace, repose, protection, warmth, cheerfulness and sincerity, open, frank expression and freedom from chafing convention in our homes? There are certain...qualities, like grandeur, pomp, majesty and exuberance which are suitable only to comparatively few. In the category of qualities of general need we should put repose, cheerfulness, simplicity, breadth, warmth, quietness in storm, economy of up-keep, evidence of protection, harmony with surroundings, absence of dark passages or places, evenness of temperature, making the home a frame to its inmates, for rich and poor alike will appreciate these qualities.' (Voysey, 1911; quoted in Stamp, 1980:36)

The contemporary and influential German commentator on the domestic revival, Hermann Muthesius, talks of the home becoming a 'retreat from the ever-increasing turmoil of life' where the inhabitants are 'restricted by no social trammels' (Muthesius, Volume I, 2007[1904-5]:xxvi). Muthesius praises English domestic designs (similar architectural developments took place in Scotland)[8] for their individuality and variety which he clearly feels reflect an aspect of 'English' character, allied to the desire to escape the restrictions of formality (Figure 8-1). He emphasises that England 'stands apart from the countries of the continent of Europe, [and] it is a world

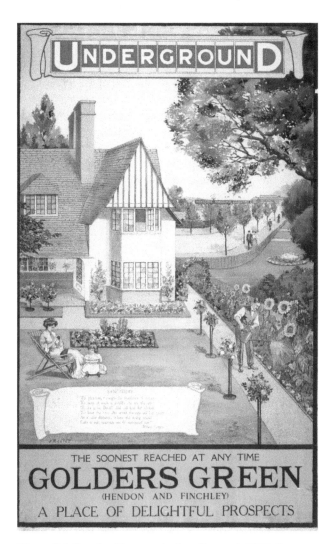

Figure 8-1. London Transport advertisement, 1908. Source: © TfL from the London Transport Museum collection.

---

[8] The most celebrated architect of the domestic revival in Scotland was Charles Rennie Mackintosh.

of its own displaying an individuality of a quite special character in every aspect of culture' (Muthesius, Volume I, 2007[1904-5]:1).

In summary, then, the rejection of the 'palatial' style of asylum architecture that would have been more common in England and elsewhere at this period can be seen as a desire to avoid some of the problems of overcrowding and consequent disease that were affecting the asylum project by splitting up the patient cohort into smaller numbers. It can also be seen, however, as a desire to elevate the behaviour of patients by exposing them to the forms and practices of the middle-class home. Higher quality decorations and more individualised furnishings were seen as liable to produce more acceptable behaviour in patients and render them more amenable and better able to be productive. Although the asylum villas by no means constitute perfect examples of the domestic revival form, the adoption of bourgeois suburban styles for asylum accommodation, rather than the formal pavilion that was more common in England, suggests that asylum authorities were discursively accessing, whether consciously or not, values that were being newly expressed in a developing domestic architectural idiom. The asylum villa evokes a domestic world of peace, seclusion and retreat, surrounded by nature, but also harks after a simplicity and freedom that was seen as less possible within the restrictive formality and 'irksome' routine of the conventional asylum building, just as the suburban middle-class home provided freedom from the contraints of formality in the public social sphere. The adoption of bourgeois styles and environments as therapeutic for the insane poor suggests that these were seen as normative and inherently health-producing, whereas working class practices and environments were continually cast as unhealthy and, indeed, morally suspect.

8.5. The colony asylum and spatial segregation

In this section we will examine the layouts used in the colony asylum in further detail, with particular focus on the 'garden city' layout that was used at Kingseat. We have seen in the preceding section that on the scale of villas themselves, domestic architecture, spaces and furnishings were used as an 'antidote' to an asylum system which was characterised by the construction of large pavilion buildings connected by corridors and which borrowed much from the hospital as architectural and spatial idiom. As we have seen, the asylum system was beginning to raise a number of problems, particularly disease and overcrowding, that echoed the perceived problems raised by aggregating large numbers of poor in urban areas. The asylums, like the urban slums, were potential centres of disease and could act in a detrimental way on the mental, moral and physical health of individuals by crowding together the poor insane into herds. One contemporary response to the urban slums, the garden city, achieved a level of conjuncture with a response to the problem of traditional asylums, the colony asylum, with the building of a garden city for the insane at Kingseat. Both the garden city and the colony asylum can be seen as proposing environmental solutions to the problems of disease and overcrowding, by dispersing patients/inhabitants around a rural site and thereby allowing greater hygienic access for light and air, but also implicitly fostering the development of individuality and vitality.

Ebenezer Howard's garden city, which sought to address the dangers of degeneration, overcrowding and disease represented by the urban slums, is a likely source for the layout of the asylum at Kingseat, outside Aberdeen, which, as we have seen, strongly resembles Howard's garden city template. The essential structure echoes his southwest facing circle sector situated close to a railway line, with paths radiating from a central point and concentric rows along which villas are placed. Villas are situated within broad bands of green space, with extensive tree planting following the lines of pathways and different sections of the site are separated by large open recreation grounds that are positioned similarly to those in Howard's diagram. A walled garden, workshops, conservatory and administration buildings all find their parallels to Howard's scheme in the way they are sited and oriented in the Kingseat layout. However, within the parameters of Howard's scheme there has been some room for individual expression, the villas are all orientated slightly differently and vary in layout and style, rather than the regular crescent rows that Howard envisaged in his Grand Avenue (Figure 5-16). Although no other colony asylum in this study bears such a close resemblance to Howard's scheme, there are reasons to believe that Howard's garden city ideals were considered in the planning of other sites. For instance, the *Illustrated London News* claimed in 1906 that the Lunacy Board for Edinburgh had erected 'A Garden City for Lunatics' (*Illustrated London News*, 13th October 1906). The original design for Bangour was completed by 30th June 1898, a few months before the publication of *To-morrow*, and although Alt Scherbitz was ostensibly the inspiration for the design, the early design does not follow that of Alt Scherbitz to any recognisable extent. Apparently more influential was the 'cottage home' model of dispersed villas for orphans in which villas are arranged in a rough circle around a central open space (Figure 5-11). However, the layout was substantially altered by the time the main buildings on the site came to be built, from 1904 to 1906, taking more account of the topography, spreading the villas more widely across the site and creating a less regular and more scattered layout with larger expanses of open space (*Glasgow Herald*, 11th May 1898) (Figures 3-12, 3-15). It is possible, therefore, that the developing designs took some account of garden city ideals, which were themselves beginning to draw away from Howard's prescriptive designs, and that this is reflected in some of the journalistic coverage of the asylum's opening. As the garden city project progressed, there was an increasing awareness by Howard and others, that strict diagrammatic forms needed to give way to a much greater freedom in terms of forms and layouts. For example, the second edition of *To-morrow*, renamed *Garden Cities of To-morrow* reduced the number and

centrality of Howard's schematics, captioning them as 'diagrams only' and asserting that the 'plan must depend on site selected' (Howard, 1902:22). This instruction appears to be a rather terse summary of Howard's proof amendments, which muse that what he is providing is 'A diagram, not a map. A sketch, not a filled-in picture. A suggestion of possibilities, not a mould into which Society is to be run' (HALS DE/Ho/F4/1 Revised volume of *To-morrow* annotated by Howard, c1899). The remaining asylums, Renfrew, which was constructed between 1905 and 1909 and Purdysburn (main phase 1909-1913), were designed within a cultural context in which garden city ideals had made great progress and Letchworth Garden City had taken shape. The diagrammatic forms suggested by Howard, had by this time been more or less abandoned in practice, while the ideals of open space, high quality dwellings and aesthetic and rational planning remained. Renfrew consists of a central hospital and administration building with villas distributed around it in an irregular fashion taking advantage of the topography. Purdysburn, by contrast, was originally envisaged as a layout which shows some similarities to Howard's original garden city scheme, with a north-east to south-west oriented site, and administration and hospital buildings at the north-east corner with villas positioned along circular and radiating paths. This design differs considerably from the asylum as actually built, which makes greater use of the topography to situate villas on high ground, and also separates male and female accommodation more distinctly (Figures 4-3, 4-5). The impression is more random and scattered than the regular pattern of the original plan and although most of the villas are of almost identical design and materials, their irregular distribution across the landscape gives each an individual character.

Just as Letchworth Garden City came to be built with a 'loose and informal aspect' rather than the strict linear plan originally envisaged, the colony asylums in this study were ultimately built with greater freedom in the design than was originally proposed, both to take advantage of topography but also in situating buildings with greater irregularity across the landscape. In this, they constitute the antithesis of what was considered the monotony and ugliness of contemporary working class housing. This monotony was undesirable, not only in aesthetic terms, but also because aesthetically impoverished and repetitive environments, had a deleterious effect on morals and behaviour, and because they suppressed individuality:

> 'how hard it is to make a home of a dwelling exactly like a hundred other dwellings, how often it is the dullness of the street which encourages carelessness of dirt and resort to excitement … it is the mean house and the mean street which prepare the way for poverty and vice' (Barnett and Barnett, 1915, quoted in Creese, 1966: 252).

The colony asylum also expresses the antithesis of the overcrowded asylum with its corridor-linked pavilions, symmetrical in design and repetitive in architectural character, restricted by its size to uniform, level ground, as at Whalley, and arranged in such a way that pavilions were close together and orientated identically with relatively limited open spaces between them. The contemporary pavilion asylum can be seen, therefore, as the institutional equivalent of byelaw housing, and subject to the same kind of objections, that it was repetitive, dull and monotonous and liable to affect patient health and behaviour in a negative way. The descriptive term often used for such an asylum was 'barracks'. Medical discourses were often critical of the 'barracks' asylums, built on a huge scale with large rooms and long corridors; indeed, 'barrack-like' became a kind of shorthand for the very antithesis of the domestic in asylum planning. The Scottish Lunacy Commissioners declared in their 56th report that Bangour Village was 'an advance on the old 'barrack' type of institution[9] and an approximation towards the normal mode of life of human beings' (SLC, 1914: xxviii), permitting better classification, greater freedom and greater facilities for work and exercise in the open air. The barrack asylum system was also criticised by Lindsay, the Murray Royal Superintendent, who held that 'the practical tendency of the age [is] to *diffuse*, not to mass, the sick and dependent' (Lindsay, 1871 (original italics), quoted in Sturdy, 1996: 11). The barracks reference was intended to convey regularity, monotony, symmetry and the crowding together of large numbers of patients, who were positioned by the architecture and layouts as passive, mentally dull, identical units to be brought under a unifying discipline. Burdett (1891: 103) describes one such barrack asylum, Leavesden near London, as 'well arranged for the storage (we use the word advisedly) of imbeciles'. An antipathy to aggregating large numbers of patients within such barrack-style institutions appears to have originated at an early stage in Scotland, partly fuelled by the comparison with English asylums. In 1857, W. Lauder Lindsay, Medical Superintendent of Murray Royal Asylum at Perth, advised that '[w]e must have no Colney Hatches[10] in Scotland, huge, overgrown, unmanageable establishments, whose interior rivals the gloom and monotony of a prison' (Lindsay, 1857: 114). He objected to 'isolated, single, symmetrical masses of building', preferring:

'... a series of buildings studded over the grounds, resembling in general character and appearance a large English homestead, or some large industrial community; we look forward to the time when a pauper asylum will partake of the character of a farming or industrial colony; when we shall have a large proportion of its inmates living in cottages under the charge of intelligent and kind attendants ...'(Lindsay, 1857: 115; also McCandless, 1979)

---

[9] This is despite the fact that the male accommodation on the site was of a distinctly 'barrack-like' architectural quality. However, the Bangour male villas were built for relatively small numbers, 50 patients each, and apparently escape censure for this reason.
[10] Colney Hatch, the asylum for Middlesex, opened in 1851 for 1,255 patients as one of the largest asylums in its day, but was dwarfed by later English asylums.

The fact that more than 40 years elapsed before the 'village' type of asylum layout took shape in Scotland, can be attributed to the lack of models in Britain, and perhaps an unwillingness to experiment with asylum design among conservative district asylum authorities. It was not until a German colony for the insane at Alt Scherbitz emerged and appeared to be a practical and successful model that Scottish district asylum builders broke away from English styles in asylum design. However, it is clear that at Kingseat and possibly elsewhere, the garden city was another important influence and that the distribution of dispersed villas around a rural site allowing greater access to air, light and by implication, freedom and individuality, tapped into the same vein of antipathy to overcrowding and monotony that drove the garden city movement. The development of colony asylum designs, from Kingseat, with its fairly rigid adherence to Howard's model, to Bangour and possibly Purdysburn, which can be seen as much looser interpretations of the general ideals, echoes a development within the garden city movement itself. In the terms of Margot Huxley, a 'dispositional' spatial rationality which produced docile subjects through ordered arrangements that would 'foster correct comportments' was ultimately rejected by the garden city movement as productive of the very moral problems that it was intended to combat. The kind of disciplinary structure that was entailed by Howard's strict diagrammatic forms thereby gave way to a 'generative' spatial rationality in which the quality of the environment in a broad sense, rather than the hierarchical, grid-like arrangements of buildings and streets, was intended to bring about moral and physical health (Huxley, 2006). It was in this sense that the garden city, ultimately had much in common with the late nineteenth and early twentieth-century asylum project in Scotland.

8.6. The colony asylum, liberty and individuality

In this section, it will be argued that distinct conceptions of liberty and individuality prevailed within Scottish asylum culture which had an influence on the adoption and implementation of the colony asylum in Scotland (and to a limited extent in Ireland), in contrast to its much more limited acceptance by asylum authorities in England and Wales. Despite the lead set by English alienists in the early-nineteenth century, a quantitative comparison of the *Reports of the Commissioners in Lunacy* (England and Wales) (ELC) and the *Reports of the General Board of Commissioners in Lunacy for Scotland* (SLC) carried out for this study, suggests that discourses of liberty and freedom relating to asylum patients were more fully developed in Scotland by the end of the century. On average, the SLC reports refer to 'liberty' or 'freedom' eight times as often as the ELC reports in the period 1880–1910 (Figure 8-2). A qualitative assessment suggests that Scottish Commissioners pushed forward an agenda where patient freedom was prioritised, with almost all references to freedom/liberty occurring when offering praise for asylums giving greater freedom to patients. The English Commissioners, although making a handful of approving

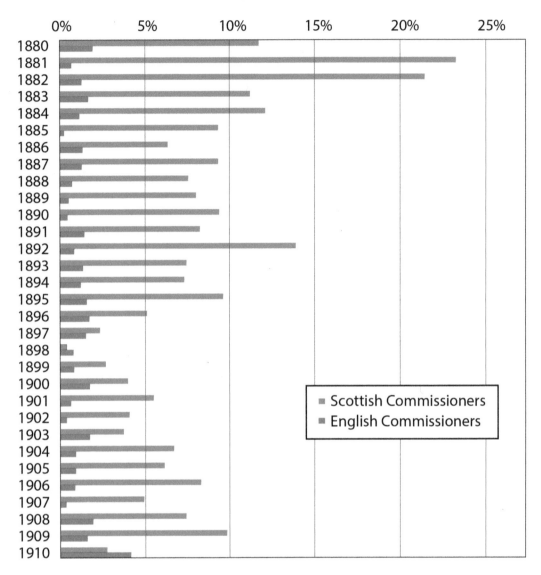

Figure 8-2. References to 'liberty' or 'freedom' in annual reports of Scottish and English Lunacy Commissioners. References have been adjusted to be proportional to report length (Scottish reports are generally roughly half the length of English reports) by expressing the number of references as a percentage of the number of pages. Source: data obtained by using terms 'liberty' and 'freedom' to search digital versions of Lunacy Commissioners' reports at https://parlipapers.proquest.com.

references, more commonly referenced patient freedom in relation to suicide (where a patient had taken advantage of an implicitly excessive freedom to harm themselves), lunacy legislation (the protection for individuals against wrongful incarceration) and, most commonly, the characteristics of a well-run asylum (freedom from odours, disease, excitement and complaints). This emphasis may have reflected the legalistic concerns of the ELC visiting panel, three of six being practising barristers, in contrast to the SLC, whose legal members did not take part in visiting asylums (*Report of Royal Commission, Volume VIII*, 1908: 210). Andrews (1998: 63) suggests that the SLC enjoyed a better relationship with medical superintendents and among themselves than did the ELC, and were not criticised, as were the ELC, for their resistance to 'new treatments'.

The SLC firmly positioned itself as an advocate of non-restraint in its 23rd annual report: 'it is now held wrong, not only to use any form of mechanical restraint of the person, but even to put restriction of any other kind on the liberty of a patient, which cannot be shown to be necessary either for his own welfare or the safety of the public' (SLC, 1881: xxxi; also Ross, 2014). Modifications to asylums at this stage were intended to remove their prison character and to 'assimilate them to the arrangements of private houses'. It was stated that fenced or walled 'airing courts' had disappeared at most public asylums, and that the practice of locking ward doors had given way to an 'open door' system reliant on the supervision of attendants to exercise control over patients (SLC, 1881: xxxi–xxxv). The open-door system was thought to diminish the patient's desire to escape, in the same way that removing shackles and chains had been thought by early advocates of non-restraint to induce calm. Another strand in allowing liberty for patients was a more extensive use of parole, by which some patients were permitted to walk or work in or beyond the grounds of the asylum. Previous scholarship has questioned the real extent of these changes (Halliday, 2003: 130), pointing to how an apparent liberty served other, more subtle forms of control (Ross, 2014: 238–9), but it is argued here that the ideological support for the liberty of patients did have real effects in the ways that the site and buildings were laid out and administered. The absence of corridors, walls and fences meant that patients leaving the villas and moving between buildings enjoyed the open grounds, in contrast to sites such as Whalley, where the airing court system had been retained and where the entire estate was surrounded by a barrier.[11] Difficulties in managing patients outdoors (and in the 'open' villas, the claim was that patients were free to move outdoors at will), therefore had to be addressed either by vesting more trust in the patients or by increasing attendant supervision, rather than relying on the built environment. The interior layouts of villas at Bangour, Purdysburn and Kingseat, where rooms open into each other, rather than off a central corridor, as at Whalley, suggest that control over patients was exercised through the layout of the rooms rather than by locking doors. The Lancashire Asylums Board commented that dormitories in Alt Scherbitz were arranged so that smaller rooms opened off larger ones to facilitate supervision (LAB 1900: 27), and this is the system practised, both on ground and upper floors, in most of the villas for which plans are available, apparently in imitation of Alt Scherbitz. Glass panels in the doors not only increased the amount of light within the building, but allowed for staff to supervise one room from another. By contrast, when rooms opened off a central corridor, as at Whalley, a staff member would have to be present in each room, or rooms would have to be locked to prevent patients entering unsupervised spaces, although the arrangement of interior space into a small number of very large rooms may have been a method of enabling supervision with a smaller number of staff. It can be readily appreciated, therefore, that increased supervision did not necessarily mean less freedom for patients, since the visibility of spaces had the potential to increase staff confidence in the open door system. Being able to observe patients as they moved from room to room may have been an important spatial support for the policy of keeping doors unlocked. On the whole, however, the colony asylum had relatively high staff to patient ratios in practice: on average one to 11 by day and one to 46 by night at Bangour, for example, which was considered a high ratio for the period, and indeed the colony system was sometimes criticised for its high staffing requirements (Steen, 1900).

The physical freedom of patients can be linked symbolically, as well as physically, to the 'variety' exhibited by the asylum buildings, their styles and materials and their

disposition about the site. Although the open-door system and the colony system were not dependent on each other, and indeed the internal layout described above could have been applied in a pavilion, the villa form did offer some advantages in terms of supervision without the need for locking doors, due to the smaller size of internal spaces. There were also perhaps some drawbacks, in that patients exiting a villa were not contained within the corridors and wards of the larger asylum. However, in a larger sense the villa colony exemplified freedom from constraint, patterning and uniformity with buildings that could be tailored to the topography, to the surroundings and to different categories of patient. In a similar way, patients themselves were to be freed from the rigidity and formality of routine, the restraint of locked doors and boundary walls and the tyranny of other patients in which the needs and wishes of the herd would dominate.

It is suggested here that a concern with freedom and liberty in the colony asylum was bound up with a concern for the expression of individuality and that the form of the colony asylum was considered to give greater latitude for patient individuality. Dr Charles Angus in his first annual report for Kingseat asylum stated: 'Experience has shown that individuality is prone to be lost in a crowd, and with the loss of individuality goes loss of initiative and mental energy. Appeals to the personal initiative are more successfully made to patients living in small communities …' (Kingseat Annual Report 1904-5).[12] Scottish asylum culture arguably placed a high value on patient freedom and individuality, while imposing a paternalistic standard of bourgeois domestic living intended to elevate patient conduct and to induce calm and order. The spatial organisation of the village asylum promoted individuality and mental health by maintaining small patient groups, as well as by replicating the character of individualising domestic spaces. Individuality was to be encouraged both by the preservation of domestic scale and by environmental variety. The diversity of the village asylum, with variation in siting and surroundings, architectural styles and materials, alongside the lack of regularity of the buildings' disposition on a site, were frequently identified as implicitly individualising and antithetical to the usual homogenising asylum architecture and layout. Conversely, the architecture and layout of the Whalley pavilion suggests that patient individuality was minimised here, and that the needs of the hierarchy to manage 'unitised' patient bodies, or to keep the hospital environment free from disease, were prioritised over the provision of idealised 'home-like' surroundings.

It is also clear that the garden city pioneers were concerned with the quality of individuality and how this

---

[11] It should be noted that Renfrew was unusual among the colony asylums in this study in that the estate was enclosed by a barrier, an 'iron fence'.

[12] This is a very similar statement to that made by the Lancashire Asylums Board on visiting Alt Scherbitz. The LAB asserted that the smaller numbers in each villa led to the preservation of the individuality noted as a key requirement for sanity: 'Individuality is lost in a crowd, and the increasing loss of the sense of individuality in a lunatic goes *pari passu* with a loss of initiative and of mental energy, in short of mind' (Report of a Lancashire deputation, 1900: 64).

could be encouraged by the reduction of overcrowding and segregation of buildings within a settlement. Ebenezer Howard understood the city as a source of ill health for specific physical reasons, particularly poor ventilation, smoke, dirt and overcrowding. In this he replicated the 'city as unhealthy' trope put forward by the social explorers, but he also stated that society was 'most healthy and vigorous' where there were free and full opportunities for both individual and combined effort, making perhaps an unconscious elision between physical health and the metaphorical health of society conceived as a growing organism. Howard's conception of health is thus continually associated with his ideas relating to freedom of the individual. Here the assertion of individual freedom allows for a release of 'pent-up energy' which helps society to flourish and releases 'vitality' which is the life force that is suppressed under unequal economic conditions. For Howard, one of the major consequences of social reform along garden city lines was that:

'A new sense of freedom and joy is pervading the hearts of the people as their individual faculties are awakened, and they discover in a social life, which permits alike of the completest concerted action and of the fullest individual liberty, the long-sought-for means of reconciliation between order and freedom, — between the well-being of the individual and of society'(Howard 1898:143).

Howard and the asylum builders both saw a healthy and flourishing society as one which promoted individuality, releasing the energy and vitality that was deadened by the monotony and uniformity of asylum materiality and urban slum living alike. The preservation of individuality was noted as a key requirement for sanity by contemporary medical thinkers, because the aggregation of patients and slum-dwellers alike reduced vitality and resistance to vice. Key to preserving vitality, individuality and mental health were high quality environments. For example, Thomas Clouston, envisaged the individual as a vitalist system possessing a finite amount of 'energy' where one organ or function could not be 'overpressed' without 'the risk of stealing energy from other organs and functions' (Clouston, 1906: 157). Surplus energy gave the brain a quality of 'resistiveness' which allowed it to combat unhealthy surroundings. On the other hand, healthy surroundings were capable of generating the vitality which was essential to mental health. Clouston saw 'Mind' as 'the highest form of energy known to us' and equated individuality with the resourcefulness that arises from vitality (Clouston 1911:94). Poor environments were a danger to the high-level functioning of the brain and could potentially be transmissible through the generations, and this was an argument for treating environment as being of the highest importance:

'On [the] brain cells act the highest and subtlest of all forms of environment, viz., those of emotion, of passion and of beauty. No one can deny that the worst effects on the individual of certain unfavourable environments,

such as bad social conditions and alcohol, are on the brain. If the securing of good environment will not only benefit the individual, which no one can deny, but will also improve posterity through the transmission of their beneficial effects, then indeed we have an argument for improved human environments which is irresistible' (Clouston, 1906: 64).

Environment, to Clouston, signified a wide range of external influences, extending from alcohol to bad air, and it had a strong moral component. Insofar as asylum treatment was concerned, Clouston was clear that healthy and pleasant environments could be 'healing' to the insane and asylum surroundings should be clean, cheerful, bright, elegant and tasteful in order to counteract the 'tendency to degeneration in habits and ways'(Letchworth 1889:313-330). Clouston's recurring prescription—in addition to pharmaceuticals and dietary changes—for all forms of mental illness was fresh air. Children at hereditary risk of developing insanity 'should have lots of fresh air, and … well-ventilated class-rooms … Make them colonists, sending them back to nature'(Clouston 1898: 688-689).

8.7. Conclusions

When seen in conjunction with contemporary primary documents and published materials relating to the care of the insane, the evidence of buildings, interiors and layouts contradicts the assertion that late nineteenth and early twentieth-century asylums were merely 'warehouses' for the unwanted. Colony asylums do not appear to represent solely a means of control, by containment and surveillance, of some of the most weak and vulnerable in society. However, it is important to note that there is often considerable tension between contrasting goals set out for/by the asylum builders. Considerations of hygiene/ domesticity, liberty/security, comfort/economy often conflicted and the physical remains of the asylums provide evidence of this. There is often a difference between the discursive construction of patients and the spaces they inhabit and the reality. For example, patient freedom is often emphasised whereas patients were not in fact free to leave the asylum and would be recovered if they 'escaped', attendants even having to pay the cost of recovery out of their wages (NRS MC14/4 *General Rules and Instructions for Nurses and Attendants*, Dykebar, 1912). This particular tension around the discursive construction of asylum life as bourgeois domesticity, contrasting with the need to position patients within an institutional hierarchy, is exemplified by the recurring ambiguity surrounding villa entrances. Many, if not most, of the asylum villas do not have a clear main entrance. Entrances are often partially hidden, architecturally minimised, moved to the 'back' of the building, and/or multiplied, making it unclear where the building is to be entered, or who is to enter where. In many of the buildings, all entrances appear to be architecturally positioned as 'service' entrances. This suggests that despite the expressed ambition of asylum authorities to render the villas 'home-like' in bourgeois terms, and to elevate the social practices of patients and staff, they remain in some important ways, constructed as lower class. The threshold of the asylum villa appears to be an emblem of control that cannot be entrusted to the working classes, either staff or patients. A strongly architecturally signalled main entrance would be a sign of authority for those inside the villa, both staff and patients, a signal that the inhabitants were able to say who should enter and who should leave. The fact that such a sign is avoided and blurred by masking, multiplying and diminishing entrances suggests that there was a point where the asylum builders baulked at the simulation of suburban domestic life they were creating. The villa entrances signal that all who entered the villas were in fact entering as discursively constructed servants or children, subordinated to the villa design and subject to its elevating qualities, but not in charge of it.

Nonetheless, it is clear that the architecture and spaces of the colony asylum reflected a desire to build institutions that were as little like institutions as possible and that this stemmed from a particular understanding of insanity as a product of poor environments, such as the dark and dirty slum with its unsegregated spaces. Within the asylum, the insane poor could be exposed to the 'special advantages to be found in modern hospitals; which include. . .the light, pure air, warmth, bathing, and other conveniences that form essential features of the building' (*JMS* 1871 (16): 527). Discourses of hygiene constituted the insane poor as pitiable, weakly, lacking in vitality and strength and prone to degeneracy. Discursively positioned alongside thin, spindly and blanched plants, the patients were to be stimulated into healthy development by the light and air-filled asylum, given strength and energy and their healthy moral and mental processes revived. Asylum builders of the late Victorian and Edwardian periods were facing, as we have seen, similar problems to those who sought to combat urban overcrowding and disease through planning and housing reform, such as the garden city. A recurrent theme is the low mood and lack of energy of slum inhabitants, entailing a symbiotic relationship with their environment that was detrimental to mental as well as physical health. The tendency of the poor to mental ill health was, it was argued, triggered or exacerbated by poor environment and these poor environments were, in turn, caused by their inhabitants' degenerate practices. Mental, physical and moral health were irrevocably connected within these discourses, which were informed by a medical understanding of mental illness as broadly somatic in origin. While poor environments were responsible for causing disease, environmental improvements could lift up the poor from their degraded physical and mental condition.

The advantages offered by the colony asylum were, in many cases, practical. For example, the segregation of villas and their distribution about a rural site gave greater perceived access to health-giving light and air. Large windows and glazed doors allowed light to illuminate interiors, kill germs and raise spirits. But in other ways the physical attributes of the colony asylum can be seen as part of a less conscious effort to discursively position the asylum

as a place of health and liberty. The locating of colony asylums deep in the countryside has often been seen as a sign of the desire to sequester the unwanted. However, it can equally be viewed as resulting from a persistent belief in the therapeutic nature of rural areas, and in particular healthful rural air, and a desire to provide more acreage to employ patients in the outdoors. Both these aims arise out of a romanticised view of a countryside which was threatened by industrialisation. The wedding of asylum villa to bourgeois domestic house at this period is a telling one, because it speaks of the rising middle classes' desire for rural peace, freedom and escape from formality and routine, expressed through the new architecture of the middle-class home. The bourgeois family, through the architecture and spaces of the colony asylum, becomes symbolic of sanity and social order. The reviled traditional asylum, by contrast, symbolises the overcrowding and disease that ensue from the aggregation of bodies. .

It is clear, therefore, that the provision of high-quality environments was of great importance in the construction of the colony asylum. The 'hard hereditarian' approach to mental illness in which environmental considerations are no longer important and the function of asylum buildings is merely to contain 'patients' as cheaply as possible, does not appear to have prevailed here.

However, the question of why the colony asylum was more readily adopted in Scotland than in England remains to be addressed.[13] There were clear differences between the accommodation offered to chronic patients at Bangour (Edinburgh) and at Whalley (Lancashire). At Bangour, an environment was created that resembled, if imperfectly, a bourgeois domestic house in its furnishing and layout, while the division into relatively small rooms emulated the individualised spaces of a domestic interior. The Bangour villa dispensed with visible emblems of patient control such as corridors and airing courts, and the interior was arranged to facilitate patient supervision without the need for locking rooms. The Whalley pavilion was three times as large and the interior layout grouped patients together in huge dormitories and dayrooms, exceeding the scale of hospital wards and perhaps suggestive of army barracks. The aspiration to be 'home-like' was here subordinated to the hygienic requirements of the hospital, with wards designed to maximise cross-ventilation and natural lighting, and sanitary facilities withdrawn into separate annexes. The Whalley pavilion was designed to enable patients to be controlled with the minimum of attendant supervision, with corridor connections between buildings,

---

[13] Of the three asylums that were built in Ireland in the period 1899-1914, Antrim (1899), Portrane (1904) and Purdysburn (1902-1912), only Purdysburn was built on the colony model (Antrim and Portrane were built to the echelon design that was more common in England). It is likely that the medical superintendent William Graham, who received some of his medical training in Edinburgh, was influenced by Scottish ideas on the treatment of mental illness, indeed it is highly likely that he would have attended classes by the eminent psychiatrist Thomas Clouston, whose views on the importance of environment to the treatment of mental illness have already been alluded to. The Irish example of a colony asylum should therefore be seen in the context of Scottish influences on the medical profession in Ulster.

fenced airing courts and huge rectangular rooms all making for easy surveillance.

It may be argued that Enlightenment concepts such as liberty and individuality have been subject to local inflection, which may help to explain variations in material evidence between Scotland and England/Wales. Dalglish (2001) analyses changes in nineteenth-century rural Scotland shaped by an ideology of agricultural 'Improvement', noting that a fundamental element of Improvement was the emphasis on both the individual and private property, a structuring disposition which replaced an earlier emphasis on community. Pre-Improvement domestic space was characterized by unpartitioned dwellings focused on a shared central hearth, while Improved dwellings were increasingly divided. Everyday activities became segregated and associated with different spaces, making the 'ideology of the individual knowable' (Dalglish, 2001: 23). Key to the success of Improvement ideology was a conception, with its roots in the Scottish Enlightenment, specifying stages of development through which society is carried by the initiative of the individual: 'There is … in man a disposition and capacity for improving his condition, by the exercise of which, he is carried from one degree of advancement to another' (Millar, 1771, quoted in Dalglish, 2001: 19). The success of Scottish capitalism has been attributed to refashioning the 'habits, attributes and attitudes' of a backward workforce through Improvement, while the European-wide advance of capitalism was inflected in Scotland by features of Calvinism lending individual conscience an elevated position and resulting in 'constant self-criticism and a need to do better' (Whatley, 2000: 98–9). Calvinism 'envisaged a social order that radiated outward from the self-disciplined individual' and which, regardless of individual adherences, produced a cultural climate north of the border that placed high value on individual identity and striving (Gibson, 2006: 35). The increasing division of domestic space within the rural dwellings of the poor, as identified by Dalglish (2001), suggests that material practices were seen as directly formative of desired attributes, leading to increased wealth production and capitalist accumulation.

An analysis of the architecture, spaces and discourses of Scottish asylums of the early-twentieth century suggests that the emphasis on the individual was not only a feature of the historical development of Scottish capitalism, but had thoroughly permeated discourses of poverty and insanity. The ethic of Improvement was discernible in the attitude to the poor insane in Scotland, seen less as a problem of contagion, to be contained, and more as one of inefficiency: of unproductive persons whose latent initiative was to be promoted through addressing their individuality. Individuality, in the sense of personal initiative, had become a quality—associated with productive work—to cultivate in the poor as a means of lifting them out of the related problems of poverty and mental disease. Even in chronic patients who were not expected to recover, a strong cultural imperative existed to raise them up from the drab homogeneity thought to be the corollary of insanity. This attitude led to material changes in how the poor were accommodated and treated in asylums. The planned variety of environments and spaces afforded by the village asylum system, together with the spatial separation of patients into small groups, reflected the seeming will of Scottish asylum culture to engage the individuality of patients. This will can be seen as deriving from a long tradition of Calvinist-inspired Improvement directed towards the majority, arguably a distinctive driver in the development of Scottish modernity, and it found ideal material expression in Continental European-inspired village schemes for the colonisation of the poor, which provided inspiration for both the colony asylum and the garden city.

Howard's garden city design may have been attractive to a Scottish professional sector whose faith in the power of environment to be therapeutic was intensifying, underpinned by a resurgence of interest in Lamarckian approaches to evolution based on the inheritance of acquired characteristics. At Kingseat asylum builders appear to have been drawn by the utopian resonances of his ideas, seeking, through his forms, to attain a higher level of social functioning for the groups and individuals under their care. Huxley's 'vitalist' spatial rationality in which environments are shaped in order to 'foster the progressive development of humanity' speaks to asylum space at Kingseat and to garden city spaces, both of which sought to constitute a better humanity through the harnessing of 'vitalistic life forces' that, in both cases, could be released through the spatial disaggregation of bodies. Despite the spatial exclusion and bodily discipline associated with asylum siting, there is a sense in which the drive to constitute subjects through asylum spaces was focussed as much on inclusion as it was on exclusion. While actually bound, patients were discursively constituted as individualised subjects situated within bourgeois, suburban spaces in which 'freedom' released the vitality which was seen as cohesive to social order. In this, the asylum and the garden city reach an identity of purpose which could account for the choice of garden city as asylum model.

The apparent rigidity and prescriptiveness of Howard's diagrams led him to draw back from his own schematics over time in favour of an understanding of the garden city that was looser and emphasised the flexibility of his geometrical sketches. If the form of the garden city was replicated at Aberdeen it suggests that the asylum builders were seeking to access, through the planning out of lines and curves, a series of elusive qualities that were not fully entailed by this particular arrangement of constructed buildings, spaces and connecting pathways, but formed part of its symbolic resonance, evoking the idealised society conveyed by Howard in his writings. The division of the traditionally unitary asylum building into a number of separate villas of differing designs, finishes and orientations is emblematic of Howard's marriage of opposites, combining heterogeneity with cohesion. Although the garden city had been proposed by Howard as a solution to the problems of urban overcrowding, disease and unconstrained growth, and not a solution to the problems of a growing asylum population, there were profound similarities in the problems faced by asylum builders and urban reformers and a congruence in the cultural context that gave rise both to the garden city ideal and to idealised asylum spaces.

Howard's work combines a practical economic analysis with some highly evocative writing on the benefits of wedding town with country that include romanticised assessments of the benefits of country living, the beauty of nature and easy access to fields and parks, pure air and water and bright homes and gardens. Howard's understanding of the city as unhealthy was based on well-rehearsed contemporary discourses to which he added ideas of an emotional and spiritual dependency on nature which may have resonated among asylum builders seeking meaningful approaches to designing asylum buildings, spaces and layouts. Howard offered the promise of harnessing the power of the natural environment in favour of good health through the deliberate and planned activity of human beings. His garden city ideal encapsulated the power of environment to influence how people live, think and feel and is unambiguous about the possibility that high quality environments can have powerful effects on both individuals and society. Howard's cultural understanding of health penetrates through the viscerality of bodily illness to deeper perceptions of the nature of mind and spirit, appropriating these as the comforting metaphors of successful societal functioning. If asylum builders in Scotland did choose Howard's prescription for a better society they would have been allying themselves with a utopian vision of society in which the hope of improvement had not subsided and where therapeutic optimism survived.

9

Conclusion

This study has been an analysis of the four colony asylums in Scotland and Ireland that were all directly or indirectly inspired by the asylum of Alt- Scherbitz in Germany. A contemporary traditional-style asylum in Lancashire has also been studied as a point of comparison. The sites, except Whalley where little of the original site survives, were visited in person, and a wealth of primary sources consulted, both published and unpublished. This produced an extremely rich and varied range of sources to draw from in analysis and interpretation of the material culture of each site. As we have seen in the preceding chapter, a number of conclusions have been drawn about the colony asylum and asylum cultures in England, Scotland and Ireland, which will be summarised below, before moving to a consideration of the particular contribution made by this study to asylum scholarship.

An analysis of the colony asylum suggests that the historiographical contention that late nineteenth-century asylums were built as 'warehouses' to sequester the insane as cheaply as possible, is an over-simplification and is not applicable to the asylums that were part of the present study. Although asylum authorities were expected to exercise economic restraint, there are surprising examples of ostentation in both buildings and interiors, and it appears to be untrue to assume that asylum authorities were always guided by such epithets as that of Henry Tuke 'It is wise to avoid anything in the way of costly embellishment calculated to prejudice the mind of the ratepayer on entering the building' (Tuke, 1889:12).

The colony asylum buildings were built as hygienic spaces, being orientated in order to make full use of light and air for this purpose, and are fitted with windows, glazed partitions, flues and ventilation devices, as well as sanitary annexes in some cases. This was thought to produce practical benefits for patients in terms of the elimination of disease-causing organisms and the removal of vitiated air but it has also been suggested that there were important symbolic benefits, particularly to the provision of light-filled spaces, which discursively constructed asylum authorities as humane and caring. Light was also thought to be an important source of vitality and it has been shown that the vitality of patients was a prime concern, lowered as it was thought to have been, by poor environments outside the asylum.

It has also been shown that, although the environments inhabited by the poor were a concern, the asylum project itself was, at this period, understood as a threat to health, because of the aggregation of large numbers of patients in overcrowded conditions. The splitting up of patients into smaller groups within buildings that could be positioned on a site in ways that optimised their exposure to light and air, can be seen as a response to this problem.

This study has also challenged the understanding that asylums were built in rural areas in order to sequester the insane and prevent them proliferating through reproduction. It has been shown that, at least as important as the desire to sequester, were the therapeutic benefits thought to derive from rural situation, clean country air and, for male patients, the opportunity to work in the outdoors. The need to provide larger and larger acreages for this purpose constituted a strong 'push' into the countryside for early twentieth-century colony asylums.

The colony asylum was seen as more home-like and less institutional than the traditional asylum style, which was criticised for its architectural monotony, aggregating large numbers of patients together in a way which increased their tendency to be dull, passive and herd-like. However, we have seen that it was not the ordinary working class street which was the model to be aimed at, but the bourgeois home, which the asylum villas resemble, both architecturally and in their internal spaces. The attempt to resemble such dwellings is, at times, prioritised over economy, and we have seen from the Lunacy Commissioners reports that the artefacts of bourgeois living were seen as positively affecting and refining the behaviour of patients, making them calmer and more productive. Aspects of the architecture, placement and furnishing of the villas emphasise variety and individuality, seen as the antithesis of the drab homogeneity of the typical asylum. The disaggregation of patients into smaller, more domestic spaces, appropriately furnished was seen to encourage individuality and initiative, which in turn released the vitality that not only made patients easier to manage but also signified conformity with social norms and a return to good mental health. The particular architecture and furnishings that are favoured suggest an equation of therapeutic environments with the bourgeois home which has here become the model for sane and healthy living in contrast to working-class homes and environments which are continually vilified as productive of disease and mental ill-health.

Spatial segregation of patients and of buildings within the colony asylum has been seen here to be a response both to overcrowding and disease within poor urban environments and to similar problems within the asylum system itself. Ebenezer Howard's garden city was a utopian solution to the problems of urbanisation that was readily adopted by asylum builders at Kingseat, who were seeking environmental solutions to the problems raised by aggregations of the unhealthy. The garden city, and the garden city asylum, both provided answers to the problems of monotonous and impoverished environments both in the asylum system and without, which suppressed individuality and were detrimental to health, both mental and physical.

This study has concluded by postulating that a distinct asylum culture existed in Scotland at the turn into the twentieth century, for which the main evidence is the wholesale adoption of the colony or village asylum for new asylum building in the period 1900-1914. In England, trends that led to segregation of asylum accommodation never resulted in the adoption of the colony as the prevalent style of asylum, with only one colony being built by an asylum authority (for epileptic patients) before World War One. It has been suggested here that there was a greater concern within Scottish asylum culture with the liberty and individuality of patients and a greater antipathy towards the monolithic style of asylum, which led to the adoption of the Alt Scherbitz model once this had been proven workable. These findings undermine the prevailing understanding that the material response to insanity was similar across Europe and suggests that local variations may have much to tell us, not only about insanity and its treatment but also about regional attitudes to the working classes and the poor.

This study has been the first full length study of the material culture of the colony asylum in Scotland and Ireland, including architecture, internal layouts, spatial location of buildings, spatial distribution of buildings, topography and interior decoration and furnishings. For most of the asylums included here, this study is the most detailed account available of their construction, buildings and furnishings. This study also includes a short account of the colony asylum which has situated it, for the first time, fully within a European tradition of colonisation of the poor. This study has taken an inter-disciplinary approach, incorporating scholarship from historical archaeology, historical geography, architectural history and social history in order to set out the historiography of asylum environments in the early twentieth century in Scotland and Ireland. The research has also looked at all aspects of asylum environments, including those that have not previously been the subject of study within the discipline of archaeology, such as spatial location.

In terms of methodology, this study has been unusual in integrating archaeological, historical and geographical methods to analyse asylum buildings and sites. Site visits have been made in all cases, allowing appraisals to be made of architecture and spaces that have added additional depth to the study. It is only by studying the buildings themselves that some issues become apparent that are unclear or obscured in documentary evidence. For instance, management committee minutes for the asylums are replete with the rhetoric of economy, and if these were the only source for understanding asylum sites, one would have to assume that they were built as cheaply as possible. It is only by visiting the sites themselves and examining other types of evidence with care, that the picture becomes clearer, that economy was one consideration among many, and was sometimes dropped in favour of other, apparently more pressing requirements.

An analytical and empirical approach was taken to building appraisal, including locating buildings in relation to topography, determining building heights and using map evidence to assess the layout and distribution of buildings on each site. A similar approach was used with building plans to assess the layout and usage of rooms and other spaces on each floor of a villa building. In particular, a methodology was developed for assessing how well a building was lit, using the percentage of window space relative to floor space. This is a simple method which could be used for any building and correlates with building regulations of the period, allowing asylum buildings and individual rooms within them, to be compared against a domestic standard. At a period when the admission of light into buildings was becoming increasingly important, this has been a useful means of assessing how windows and light were managed within buildings of this type. Site visits also proved useful for assessing styles and ornamentation of buildings in order to determine how they met or departed from contemporary expectations in relation to middle-class domestic dwellings, an assessment which is difficult to make from documents alone, or even photographs which do not easily convey finishes and details. Site visits also enabled more phenomenological assessments of the 'village-like' feel of the sites to be made. Although these subjective responses have not been included in the study, they have been influential to an assessment of the asylum builders aims as credible and sincere. The attempt to create a certain kind of atmosphere is still palpable at the sites, even those that are now derelict or highly altered.

This study has also been unusual in treating both material and textual evidence as part of wider social discourses relating to attitudes to the poor, as well as to medical discourses. The evidence analysed conveys information about cultural beliefs and attitudes that may be intended or is more often unintended. For example, the provision of light within asylum buildings can be understood as symbolic of humane approaches to mental illness as well as having a practical function in eliminating disease-causing organisms. The segregation and distribution of asylum buildings and furnishings can be understood as reflecting attitudes to individuality that are closely to connected to ideas of health and vitality. Buildings and material evidence, often in preference to documentary evidence, have been central to the interpretations of asylum environments throughout this study, in the belief that numerous and sometimes conflicting discourses are distilled in the choices that are made about what buildings to construct and what furniture to purchase and that additional significance accrues to these material manifestations.

There are several substantive findings of this study that can be considered as contributions to the literature on asylum materiality. The overarching theme of this study has been the contention that early twentieth-century asylums, at least as far as the colony asylum is concerned, were not built as 'warehouses' as has frequently been claimed. The frequent corollary of this, that environmental approaches to the treatment of insanity had fallen out of favour by this stage, has also shown to be much exaggerated in the case of the asylums in this study. Indeed the material and textual evidence suggests that environment continued to be an important concern and that various types of environmental approach to the treatment and management of insanity were pursued with vigour and imagination, including such current ideas as the 'garden city'. Changes in the understanding of light and its contribution to physical and mental health were implemented in asylum buildings. Light and air have previously been understood by scholars as important factors in the construction of therapeutic environments because of their effect on physical health. This study has shown some of the ways that light and air were specifically of concern to builders of institutions for the mentally ill, whether it be the use of open air treatment for active insanity, or the provision of 'cheerful' light-filled spaces that elevated mood and increased the vitality of the insane poor. This study has suggested that there were perceived to be strong links in this period between physical, mental and moral health and that 'vitality' was a key component in all these aspects being associated with the strength to be productive, the emotional and psychological energy to conform to social norms and the initiative to resist the temptations of drink and vice. The colony asylum has been shown to be a distinctive institutional solution to the problem of aggregating patients in large numbers, not only because this was a risk in terms of disease and overcrowding, but also because bringing patients together in large numbers reduced individuality and vitality, and led to a herd-like mentality, detrimental to mental health. This research has also built on the work of Hamlett, Guyatt and others, which has shown that the furnishings and decorations of asylum interiors were intended to be calming and therapeutic for patients, rendering them more productive, but has also shown that asylum builders worked with several, sometimes competing, aims that, on occasion, compromised the home-like feel of asylum buildings . It has been demonstrated here how committed asylum authorities were to replicating at the colony asylum a bourgeois version of domesticity which was considered to be refining and to improve behaviour. This has been connected to the wider social construction of domesticity and a burgeoning bourgeois domestic architecture, resulting from the rise of the middle classes whose distinctive ideas of home as, for example, a place of freedom from irksome formality, are repeated in asylum environments. It has also been connected to a fundamental change over the centuries in the social orientation of asylum buildings in Scotland and Ireland. Scottish and Irish asylums originated as outward-looking 'palaces' reflecting to onlookers the wealth, prestige and charity of benefactors. By the period of this study, the emergence of colony asylums as inward-looking domestic spaces in which the focus of the architecture and furnishings was now on the patient experience, demonstrated an ideological shift which ultimately paved the way to the de-institutionalisation of the late twentieth century.

Bibliography

Primary Sources (unpublished)

Aberdeen, Central Library (ACL)
ACL Lo 363.2 Aberdeen City District Lunacy Board Minutes (November 1901 – October 1907)

Aberdeen, Sir Duncan Rice Library, NHS Grampian Archives (GA)
GA GRHB8/6/1 Kingseat Annual Reports (1904-11, 1913-1916)

GA GRHB8/6/8 Kingseat Hospital Commemorative booklet (1979)

GA GRHB8/1/1 Kingseat case notes male admissions (1904)

GA GRHB8/1/2 Kingseat case notes female admissions (1904)

GA GRHB8/6/2 Scrapbook of newspaper cuttings (1904-1975)

Belfast, Public Record Office of Northern Ireland (PRONI)
PRONI HOS/28/1/1/6-11 Belfast District Lunatic Asylum Management Committee Minutes, 1895-1913

PRONI HOS/32/1/9 Printed prospectus of Belfast Mental Hospital, June 1924

PRONI LA/7/29/CB/22 Builder's Specification for Villas 2 and 3 including floor plans, 1902

Belfast, Knockbracken Healthcare Park, Estates Department
Plans and elevations of Purdysburn, signed by architects, unarchived and largely undated (most of these were photographed at the beginning of my research and a large number are no longer held at Knockbracken, leaving my own photographs as the only available record)

Belfast, Queen's University Medical Library (ML)
ML RC450.N8.B5 Belfast District Lunatic Asylum Annual Reports (1829-1947)

Edinburgh, National Records of Scotland (NRS)
NRS RHP49135 Plan of villa 20 for chronic patients Bangour Village (Aug 1904)

NRS RHP49136 Plan of villa 20 for chronic patients Bangour Village (Aug 1904)

NRS RHP49140 Plan of villa 19 for chronic patients Bangour Village (Aug 1904)

NRS RHP49143 Plan of villa 21 for chronic patients Bangour Village (Aug 1904)

NRS RHP49146 Plan of villa 18 for chronic patients Bangour Village (Aug 1904)

NRS RHP49147 Plan of villa 18 for chronic patients Bangour Village (Aug 1904)

NRS RHP49149 Plan of villa 10 for acute patients Bangour Village (Nov 1904)

NRS RHP49150 Plan of villa 10 for acute patients Bangour Village (Nov 1904)

NRS MC14/4 General Rules and Instructions for Nurses and Attendants, Dykebar (1912)

Edinburgh, Edinburgh University Library, NHS Lothian Archive (LA)
LA LHB44/1/1-16 Edinburgh District Lunacy Board Minutes (11th December 1899-10th December 1915 (1903, 1906, 1907 missing))

LA LHB44/3/3-10 Bangour Village Annual Reports (1907-1923) (1910, 1913 missing)

LA LHB44/6/3 Edinburgh War Hospital pamphlet (1915-1920)

LA LHB44/26/5 Proposed plans of Bangour Village (n.d.)

LA LHB44/26/10 Interior photographs of Bangour Village (n.d.)

LA P/PL44/B/E/2 Postcard of Bangour Village, general view looking east (n.d.)

LA P/PL44/B/E/6 Postcard of acute villa (n.d.)

LA P/PL44/B/E/7 Postcard of administration block (n.d.)

LA P/PL44/B/E/25 Image of hospital block under construction (n.d.)

Edinburgh, Library of Historic Environment Scotland (LHES)
LHES 08582 Perth District Asylum Villa (2001)

LHES B19820 Bangour Village Hospital (c1906)

LHES C14149 Bangour Village Villa 7 (1993)

LHES C14153 Bangour Village Villa 9 (1993)

LHES C14155 Bangour Village Villa 10 (1993)

LHES C14172 Bangour Village Villa 18 (1993)

LHES C14174 Bangour Village Villa 19 (1993)

LHES C14176 Bangour Village Villa 20 (1993)

LHES C14177 Bangour Village Villa 21 (1993)

LHES C14185 Bangour Village Villa 28 (1993)

LHES C14189 Bangour Village Coat of Arms Villa 23 (1993)

LHES D76961 Kingseat Aerial View (2001)

LHES E52764 Dykebar, Doorway of Admin block (2004)

LHES E52770 Dykebar, Villa (2004)

LHES E52794 Banff District Asylum Villa (2004)

Glasgow, Mitchell Library, NHS Greater Glasgow and Clyde Archives (GGCA)

GGCA AC18/8/1-3 Renfrew District Lunacy Board Minutes (Oct 1901-July 1914)

GGCA AC18/1/1 Dykebar Annual Reports (1909-1924)

GGCA AC18/3/1 Dykebar Letter Book (1909-1910)

Hertford, Herts Archives and Local Studies (HALS)

HALS DE/Ho/F1/5 Notes of speech by Ebenezer Howard 'City of Health and how to build it' (c1890-1891)

HALS DE/Ho/F4/1 Revised volume of *To-morrow, A peaceful path to real reform*, annotated by Ebenezer Howard (c1899)

Preston, Lancashire County Archives (LCA)

LCA CC/HBM/2-3 Lancashire Asylums Board Minutes (29th November 1900-29th May 1913)

LCA DDX 1254/1/1/8 Whalley Asylum plans (1912)

Schkeuditz, Sächsisches Krankenhaus Altscherbitz

Images stored in Altscherbitz Traditionskabinett (Museum)

Primary Sources (published)

'Bangour Village Lunatic Asylum' (1906), *The Builder*, (November 6th), pp. 545–547.

'In the Belfast slums' (1907) *British Medical Journal*, (February 2nd) pp. 283–284.

'Lord Rosebery on the insane and their cost' (1906), *The Lancet*, (October 27th), pp. 1160–1163.

'The Bangour Asylum' (1906), *The British Architect*, (October 5th), pp. 247–248.

'The First British Village Asylum' (1906), *British Medical Journal*, (November 24th), pp. 1498–1502.

'The International Home Relief Congress.' (1904), *Journal of Mental Science*, 50(210), pp. 521–523.

'The New Asylum at Kingseat' (1901), *The Aberdeen Daily Journal*, (September 13th), p. 4.

Bateman, S. F., & Rye, W. (1906). *The history of the Bethel asylum at Norwich built by Mrs Mary Chapman in the year 1713*. Norwich: Gibbs & Waller.

Beard, G. M. (1880) 'The Asylums of Europe', *Boston Medical and Surgical Journal*, 103(26), pp. 605–608.

Belfast Corporation (1929) *The Belfast Corporation 1929, Local Government in the City and County Borough of Belfast*. Belfast: R Carswell & Son.

Besser, D. L. (1881). 'Die Irren-Heil- und Pflege-Anstalt Alt-Scherbitz , den literarischen Veröffentlichungen des weiland Professor Dr Köppe.' *Archiv Für Psychiatrie Und Nervenkrankheiten*, *11*(3), pp. 804–809.

Bibby, G. H. (1895) *The Housing of Pauper Lunatics*. London: Bradley T Batsford.

Bibby, G. H. (1896). *The Planning of Lunatic Asylums*. London: Bradley T Batsford.

Blanc, H. J. (1908) 'Bangour Village Asylum', *RIBA Journal*, XV(10), pp. 309–26.

Booth, W. (1890) *In Darkest England and the Way Out*. London: Salvation Army

Brodie, D. (1881) 'The conditions necessary for the successful training of the imbecile', *Journal of Mental Science*, 27(117), pp. 18–31.

Browne, W. A. F. (1837) *What Asylums were, are and ought to be*. Edinburgh: Adam and Charles Black.

Bucknill, J. C. and Tuke, D. H. (1879) *A Manual of Psychological Medicine*. London: J & A Churchill.

Burdett, S. H. C. (1891) *Hospitals and Asylums of the World, Volume 1*. London: J & A Churchill.

Clouston, T. S. (1879) 'An asylum or hospital-home for two hundred patients: constructed on the principle of adaptation of various parts of the house to varied needs and mental states of inhabitants; with plans &c', *Journal of Mental Science*, 25, pp. 368–388.

Clouston, T. S. (1906) *The Hygiene of Mind*. London: Methuen.

Clouston, T. S. (1911) *Unsoundness of Mind*. London: Methuen.

Clouston, T. S. (2005) 'Phthisical insanity.', *History of psychiatry*, 16 (Pt 4 (no 64)), pp. 479–95.

Commissioners in Lunacy (1870) *Suggestions and instructions in reference to (1) Sites (2) Construction and arrangement of buildings (3) Plans of lunatic asylums*. London: HMSO

Conolly, J. (1847) *The construction and government of lunatic asylums and hospitals for the insane*. London: John Churchill.

Conolly, J. (1856) *The treatment of the insane without mechanical restraints*. London: Smith, Elder & Co.

Easterbrook, C. C. (1907) 'The sanatorium treatment of active insanity by rest in bed in the open air', *Journal of Mental Science*, 53 (October), pp. 723–750.

Ewart, C. T. (1892) 'Epileptic colonies', *Journal of Mental Science*, 38(161), pp. 212–222.

Galton, F. (1904) 'Eugenics: Its definition, scope and aims', *The American Journal of Sociology*, 10(1), pp. 1–25.

Galton, S. D. (1893) *Healthy Hospitals*. Oxford: Clarendon Press.

Glaister, J. (1897) *A Manual of Hygiene for Students and Nurses*. London: The Scientific Press Ltd.

Graham, W. (1901) 'Recent Lunacy Legislation: retrogression or progress?', *Journal of Mental Science*, 47, pp. 687–702.

Graham, W. (1911). Psychotherapy in mental disorders. *Journal of Mental Science*, *57*, pp. 617–628.

Hammond, W. A. (1863) *A treatise on hygiene, w ith special reference to the military service*. Philadelphia: J B Lippincott & Co.

Hine, G. T. (1901) 'Asylums and Asylum Planning', *RIBA Journal*, (8), pp. 161–180.

Howard, E. (1898) *To-morrow: a Peaceful Path to Real Reform*. London: Swan Sonnenschein & Co Ltd.

Howard, J. (1791) *An account of the principal lazarettos of Europe; with various papers relative to the plague: together with further observations on some foreign prisons and hospitals; and additional remarks on the present state of those in Great Britain and Ireland*. London: J Johnson, C Dilly and T Cadell.

Keay, J. (1911) 'Bangour Village', *Journal of Mental Science*, 57(April), pp. 408–411.

Kirkbride, T. S. (1854) 'Remarks on the construction, organization and general arrangements of hospitals for the insane', *American Journal of Psychiatry*, 11(2), pp. 122–163.

Labitte, G. (1861). *La Colonie de Fitz James, succursale de l'asile privé d'aliénés de Clermont (Oise), considérée au point de vue de son organisation administrative et medicale*. Paris: J. B. Baillière et Fils.

Letchworth, W. P. (1889) *The Insane in Foreign Countries*. New York and London: G P Putnam's Sons.

Lindsay, W. L. (1857) 'The Scottish Lunacy Commission', *North British Review*, 27(53), pp. 106–126.

Locke, J. (1824[1725]) *An essay concerning human understanding*. London: Thomas Davison, Whitefriars.

Lockwood, F. W. (1898) 'The Sanitary Administration of Belfast', *Proceedings of the Institute of Sanitary Engineers*, pp. 36–58.

Loudon, J. (1845) *The Suburban Horticulturist, or, an Attempt to Teach the Science and Practice of the Culture and Management of the Kitchen, Fruit, & Forcing Garden to those who have had no previous knowledge or practice in these departments of gardening*. London: William Smith.

Macgibbon, D. and Ross, T. (1887a) *The castellated and domestic architecture of Scotland from the twelfth to the eighteenth century. Volume One*. Edinburgh: David Douglas.

Macgibbon, D. and Ross, T. (1887b) *The castellated and domestic architecture of Scotland from the twelfth to the eighteenth century. Volume Two*. Edinburgh: David Douglas.

Macpherson, J. (1905) 'Morison Lectures, Lecture VI: The causes and treatment of insanity', *Journal of Mental Science*, 51, pp. 471–490.

Mearns, A. and Union, L. C. (1883) *The Bitter Cry of Outcast London: An Inquiry into the Conditions of the Abject Poor*. James Clarke & Company.

Mort, F. (1912). *Renfrewshire*. Cambridge: Cambridge University Press.

Muthesius, H. (1979) *The English House*. Edited by D. Sharp. Crosby Lockwood Staples.

Muthesius, H. (2007[1904]) *The English House, Volume I [Das englische Haus]*. London: Frances Lincoln Ltd.

Nightingale, F. (1860) *Notes on Nursing*. London: Harrison.

Nightingale, F. (1863) *Notes on hospitals*. Third. London: Longman, Green, Longman, Roberts and Green.

Norman, C. (1904) 'Gossip about Gheel', *Journal of Mental Science*, 50(208), pp. 53–64.

O'Hanlon, R. W. M. (1853) *Walks among the poor of Belfast*. Belfast: McComb, Phillips, Mayne

Owen, R. (1858). *A Supplementary Appendix to the first volume of the life of Robert Owen containing a series of reports, addresses, memorials and other documents referred to in that volume. 1803-1820. Volume 1A*. London: Effingham Wilson.

Paetz, A. (1893). *Die Kolonisirung der Geisteskranken in Verbindung mit dem Offen-Thür-System: ihre historische Entwickelung und die Art ihrer Ausführung auf Rittergut Alt-Scherbitz*. Berlin: Verlag von Julius Springer.

Palmer, G. E. (1887) 'Colony System of caring for the insane', *The American Journal of Insanity*, XLIV, pp. 157–169.

Parkes, E. A. (1887) *A Manual of Practical Hygiene*. London: J & A Churchill.

Powell, E. (1961) *Opening speech at annual conference*. London: National Association for Mental Health.

Purdom, C.B. (1913) *The Garden City: A study in the development of a modern town*, Letchworth: J.M.Dent & Sons Ltd.

Report of a deputation appointed to visit asylums on the continent with recommendations regarding the building of a new (sixth) Lancashire asylum (1900). Preston: Lancashire Asylums Board.

Report of a deputation from the Edinburgh District Lunacy Board appointed to visit certain asylums in France,

Germany and England, recommended by the General Board of Lunacy (1897). Edinburgh: James Turner & Co

Rhodes, D. J. M. and McDougall, A. A. (1897) *Treatment of Imbeciles and Epileptics: Report to the Chorlton and Manchester Joint Asylum Committee on the best methods for the care and treatment of imbeciles and epileptics.* Manchester: Poor Law Officers' Journal.

Rhodes, J. M. (1905) 'The Provision of Suitable Accommodation for the Various Forms of Insanity', *Journal of Mental Science,* 51, pp. 681–710.

Richardson, B.W. (1876) 'Hygeia, a city of health', London: Macmillan & Co.

Robbins, E.Y. (1886) 'How to warm our houses' *Popular Science Monthly,* Iss 30, p.239

Royal Institute of Public Health (1901) *Transactions of the Congress held in Aberdeen, 2nd to 7th August, 1900.* London: Baillière & Co.

Sibbald, J. (1897) *On the Plans of Modern Asylums for the Insane Poor.* Edinburgh: James Turner & Co.

Steen, R. H. (1900) 'The Evolution of Asylum Architecture , and the Principles which ought to control Modern Construction', *Journal of Mental Science,* 46(192), pp. 87–109.

Tuke, H. (1889) *The past and present provision for the insane poor in Yorkshire.* London: Churchill.

Tuke, S. (1813) *Description of the Retreat, an institution near York, for insane persons of the Society of Friends containing an account of its origin and progress, the modes of treatment and a statement of cases.* Philadelphia: Isaac Pierce.

Tuke, S. (1815) *Practical hints on the construction and economy of Pauper Lunatic Asylums.* York: William Alexander.

Wallis, J. A. (1894) 'On the Separate Treatment of Recent and Curable Cases of Insanity in Special Detached Hospitals, with Plan and Description of Buildings about to be Erected for this Purpose at the Lancaster County Asylum, Whittingham', *Journal of Mental Science,* 40(170), pp. 335–344.

Winslow, F. (1867) *Light: its influence on life and health.* London: Longman, Green, Reader & Dyer.

Newspapers, journals and parliamentary papers

Academy Architecture (Library of Historic Environment Scotland)

BBC News (closure of Calderstones hospital) (http://www. bbc.co.uk/news/uk-england-lancashire-39421399) [28th March 2017]

Belfast Health Journal (Linenhall Library, Belfast)

British Architect (RIBA Library)

British Newspaper Archive (www.britishnewspaperarchive. co.uk)

Aberdeen Free Press

Aberdeen People's Journal

Aberdeen Weekly Journal

Aberdeen Journal

Belfast Newsletter

Belfast Telegraph

Burnley Express

Cambridge Daily News

Daily Record

Edinburgh Evening News

Glasgow Herald

Lancashire Daily Post

Lancashire Evening Post

Manchester Courier

Manchester Evening News

Manchester Guardian

Morning Post

Reading Mercury

Scotsman

Sketch

St Andrews Citizen

Weekly Irish Times

Yorkshire Post

British Medical Journal (http://journals.bmj.com)

British Journal of Psychiatry/Journal of Mental Science (1855-1914)

Building News (RIBA Library)

Illustrated London News (British Library)

Irish Builder (QUB Library)

Irish Times (http://www.irishtimes.com)

Parliamentary Papers (https://parlipapers.proquest.com)

Correspondence and communication on public lunatic asylums in Ireland (1827) London: House of Commons

Report from the Select Committee on provisions for better regulation of madhouses in England (1815-1817). London: House of Commons

Report from the Select Committee on the lunatic poor in Ireland (1817) London: House of Commons

Report of the Inter-departmental Committee on physical deterioration (1904). London: HMSO.

Report of the Royal Commission on Physical Training (Scotland) (Volume 1) (1903). Edinburgh: HMSO.

Report of the Royal Commission on Physical Training (Scotland) (Volume 2) (1903). Edinburgh: HMSO.

Report of the Royal Commission on the care and control of the feeble-minded, Volumes I-VIII (1908) London: HMSO

Reports of General Board of Commissioners in Lunacy for Scotland (1859-1914). Edinburgh: HMSO

Reports of the commissioners in lunacy to the Lord Chancellor (1846-1914) London: House of Commons

Reports of the inspectors of lunatics (Ireland) (1901-1916). Dublin: HMSO

Reports on District, Local and Private Lunatic Asylums in Ireland (1843-1900) *Dublin: HMSO*

Returns of the total amount of accommodation now existing in each district lunatic asylum in Ireland ... of the amount of accommodation which will be provided by the four district lunatic asylums now in course of construction (1867) London: House of Commons

Sixteenth report from the Board of Public Works, Ireland (1848) London: HMSO

RIBA Journal (RIBA Library)

The Builder (RIBA Library)

The Lancet (QUB Medical Library)

Secondary Sources (unpublished)

Arton, M. (1998) *The professionalisation of mental nursing in Great Britain, 1850-1950*. Unpublished PhD thesis, University College, London.

Darragh, A. (2011) *Prison or palace? Haven or hell?* Unpublished PhD thesis, University of St Andrews.

Delargy, R. (2002) *The history of the Belfast District Lunatic Asylum 1829-1921*. Unpublished PhD thesis, University of Ulster.

Halliday, E. C. (2003) *The Hospitalisation of the Scottish Asylum 1880-1914*. Unpublished PhD thesis, University of Stirling.

Hurn, J. D. (1998). *The history of general paralysis of the insane in Britain, 1830 to 1950*. Unpublished PhD thesis, University of London

Longhurst, P. (2011) *The Foundations of Madness*. Unpublished Bachelor's dissertation, University of Sydney.

Jenkins & Marr (1997) *Kingseat Village Proposals*. Unpublished report for Grampian Healthcare NHS Trust.

McLaughlan, R. (2014). One dose of Architecture, taken daily: Building for Mental Health in New Zealand. Unpublished PhD thesis, Victoria University, Wellington.

Newman, C. J. (2010) *The Place of the Pauper: A Historical Archaeology of West Yorkshire Workhouses*. Unpublished PhD thesis, University of York.

Reuber, M. (1994) *State and Private Lunatic Asylums in Ireland: Medics, fools and maniacs (1600-1900)*. Unpublished thesis submitted for the degree of Doctor of Medicine, University of Cologne.

Richardson, H. (1988) *Scottish Hospitals Survey*. Unpublished survey held by Historic Environment Scotland.

Ross, K. A. (2014) *The Locational History of Scotland's District Lunatic Asylums, 1857-1913*. Unpublished PhD thesis, University of Glasgow.

Rutherford, S. (2003) *The Landscapes of Public Lunatic Asylums in England, 1808-1914*. Unpublished PhD thesis, De Montfort University, Leicester

Sonntag, M. (1993) *Zur sozialen Lage und ärztlichen Betreuung pscyhiatrischer Patienten im höheren und hohen Lebensalter in der Zeit von der Reichsgründung 1871 bis 1933 - unter besonderer Berücksichtigung der Erfahrungen in der Provinzial-Irren-Anstalt Rittergut Alt-Scherbitz*. Unpublished thesis submitted for the degree of Doctor of Medicine, University of Leipzig.

Sturdy, H. C. G. (1996). *Boarding-out the insane, 1857-1913: a study of the Scottish system*. Unpublished PhD thesis, University of Glasgow.

Woiak, J. (1998). *Drunkenness, Degeneration and Eugenics in Britain, 1900- 1914*. Unpublished PhD thesis, University of Toronto.

Secondary Sources (published)

200 Years of the census in Lancashire (2001), Report for the Office of National Statistics.

Aalen, F. H. A. (1987) 'Public housing in Ireland, 1880–1921', *Planning Perspectives*, 2:2, pp. 175–193.

Adams, A. (1996) *Architecture in the Family Way: Doctors, Houses, and Women, 1870-1900*. Montreal & Kingston: McGill-Queen's University Press.

Allmond, G. (2016) '"The outer darkness of madness": an Edwardian Winter Garden at Purdysburn asylum for the insane poor.' In: M. Dowd and R. Hensey, eds. *The Archaeology of Darkness*. Oxford: Oxbow Books.

Allmond, G. (2016) 'Light and darkness in an Edwardian institution for the insane poor - illuminating the material practices of the asylum age.' *International Journal of Historical Archaeology, 20 (1), pp.1-22.*

Allmond, G. (2017) 'The First Garden City? Environment and utopianism in an Edwardian institution for the insane poor' *Journal of Historical Geography, 56 (Jan), pp.101-112*

Allmond, G. (2017) 'Liberty and the Individual: the colony asylum in Scotland and England' *History of Psychiatry*, 28 (1), pp.29-43

Allmond, G. (2018) '"Levelling up the lower deeps": the hygiene of light and air in an Edwardian asylum'. In: G. Laragy, O. Purdue and J. Wright, eds. *Urban Spaces in Nineteenth Century Ireland*. Liverpool: Liverpool University Press.

Andrews, J. (1998). *"They 're in the Trade ... of Lunacy They 'cannot interfere'- they say ": The Scottish Lunacy Commissioners and Lunacy Reform in Nineteenth-century Scotland*. London: Wellcome Insitute for the History of Medicine.

Arnold, D., Ergut, E. A. and Ozkaya, B. T. (2006) *Rethinking Architectural Historiography*. London and New York: Routledge.

Bailey, R. M., McKean, C., Walker, D. M., Gow, I., Gray, I. M., & Thomas, J. (1996). *Scottish Architects' Papers: a source book*. Edinburgh: The Rutland Press.

Ballantyne, A. (2006) 'Architecture as evidence', in Arnold, D., Ergut, E. A., and Ozkaya, B. T. (eds) *Rethinking Architectural Historiography*. London and New York: Routledge, pp. 36–49.

Banham, R. (1984) *The architecture of the well-tempered environment*. London: Architectural Press.

Barnett, C. S. A. and Barnett, S. A. (1915) 'The Church and Town Planning', in *Practicable Socialism*. London: Longmans Green.

Bartlett, P. and Wright, D. (1999) *Outside the walls of the asylum: The history of care in the community 1750-2000*. London and New Brunswick: Athlone Press.

Bashford, A. (2004) *Imperial hygiene: a critical history of colonialism, nationalism and public health*. Basingstoke: Palgrave Macmillan.

Baugher, S. (2001) 'Visible charity: The archaeology, material culture, and landscape design of New York city's municipal almshouse complex, 1736–1797', *International Journal of Historical Archaeology*. Springer, 5(2), pp. 175–202.

Baugher, S. (2009) 'Historical overview of the archaeology of institutional life', in Beisaw, A. M. and Gibb, J. G. (eds) *The archaeology of institutional life*. Tuscaloosa: University of Alabama Press, pp. 5–16.

Beevers, R. (1988) *The Garden City Utopia, A Critical Biography of Ebenezer Howard*. Houndmills and London: Macmillan Press Ltd.

Beisaw, A. M. and Gibb, J. G. (2009) *The archaeology of institutional life*. Tuscaloosa: University of Alabama Press.

Berrios, G. E. and Freeman, H. L. (1991) *150 Years of British psychiatry, 1841-1991: Volume I*. London: Gaskell.

Beveridge, A. W. (1991) 'Thomas Clouston and the Edinburgh school of psychiatry', in GE Berrios and H. Freeman (eds*)*, *150 Years of British psychiatry 1841-1991: Volume I*, London: Gaskell, pp.359-388.

Blau, E. (1982) *Ruskinian Gothic: The Architecture of Deane and Woodward*. Princeton, Guilford: Princeton University Press.

Bolsterli, M. J. (1977) *The early community at Bedford Park: 'Corporate happiness' in the first garden suburb*. London and Henley: Routledge & Kegan Paul.

Boschma, G. (2003) *The Rise of Mental Health Nursing. A History of Psychiatric Care in Dutch Asylums, 1890-1920*. Amsterdam: Amsterdam University Press.

Bourdieu, P. (1970). The Berber house or the world reversed. *Social Science Information*, 9(2), 151–170.

Brown, J. (1968) 'Charles Booth and Labour Colonies, 1889-1905', *Economic History Review*, 21(2), pp. 349–360.

Brown, T. (1980) 'Architecture as therapy', *Archivaria*, 10(4), pp. 99–124.

Bryder, L. (1988) *Below the magic mountain: A social history of tuberculosis in twentieth-century Britain*. Oxford: Clarendon Press.

Burke, P. (2008) *What is cultural history?* Cambridge: Polity.

Bynum, W. F. and Porter, R. (1993) *Companion encyclopedia of the history of medicine, volume I*. London and New York: Routledge.

Carr, G., Jasinski, M. E. and Theune, C. (2017) 'The Material Culture of Nazi Camps: An Editorial', *International Journal of Historical Archaeology*. https://doi.org/10.1007/s10761-017-0444-z

Carpenter, A., Loeber, R., Campbell, H., Hurley, L., Montague, J., & Rowley, E. (2015). *Civic, institutional and military architecture. Art and architecture of Ireland, Volume IV*. Dublin: Royal Irish Academy.

Carter, S. (2003) *Rise and shine: Sunlight, technology and health*. Oxford and New York: Berg.

Casella, E. C. (2001) 'Landscapes of punishment and resistance: a female convict settlement in Tasmania, Australia', in Bender, B. and Winer, M. (eds) *Contested Landscapes: Movement, Exile and Place*. Oxford, New York: Berg, pp. 103–120.

Casella, E. C. (2007) *The archaeology of institutional confinement, The American experience in archaeological perspective*. Gainesville: University Press of Florida.

Clarke, L. (1993) 'The opening of doors in British mental hospitals in the 1950s', *History of Psychiatry*, 4, pp. 527–551.

Cook, L. J. (1991) 'The Uxbridge Poor Farm in the Documentary Record', in Elia, R. J. and Wesolowsky, A. B. (eds) *Archaeological Excavations at the Uxbridge*

Almshouse Burial Ground in Uxbridge, Massachusetts. Oxford: British Archaeological Reports International Series No 564, BAR Publishing, pp. 40–81.

Cornwell, R. B. (2010) *The History of the Calderstones Hospital Railway 1907-1953.* Accrington: Nayler Group Ltd.

Cotter, J. L., Moss, R.W., Gill, B.C. and Kim, J. (1988) *The Walnut Street prison workshop.* Philadelphia: Athenaeum of Philadelphia.

Cotter, J. L., Roberts, D. and Parrington, M. (1993) *The buried past: An archaeological history of Philadelphia.* Philadelphia: University of Pennsylvania Press.

Creese, W. L. (1966) *The Search for Environment: The Garden City before and after.* New Haven and London: Yale University Press.

Dale, P. and Melling, J. (2006) *Mental Illness and Learning Disability Since 1850: Finding a Place for Mental Disorder in the United Kingdom.* Abingdon, New York: Routledge.

Dalglish, C. (2001). Rural Settlement in the Age of Reason. *Archaeological Dialogues*, 8(1), 2–48.

Deacon, H. (2000) 'Landscapes of Exile and Healing: Climate and Gardens on Robben Island', *The South African Archaeological Bulletin*, 55(172), pp. 147–154.

De Cunzo, L. A. (1995). Reform, respite, ritual: An archaeology of institutions; The Magdalen Society of Philadelphia, 1800-1850. *Historical Archaeology*, 29(3), i-168.

Donnelly, M. (1983) *Managing the mind: A study of medical psychology in early nineteenth-century Britain.* London and New York: Tavistock Publications.

Dörries, A. and Beddies, T. (2003) 'The Wittenauer Heilstatten in Berlin: a case record study of psychiatric patients in Germany, 1919–1960', in *The confinement of the insane: international perspectives.* Cambridge and New York: Cambridge University Press, pp.149-172.

Driver, F. (1990). Discipline without frontiers? Representations of the Mettray reformatory colony in Britain, 1840–1880. *Journal of Historical Sociology*, 3(3), 272–293.

Driver, F. (2004). *Power and pauperism: the workhouse system, 1834-1884* (Vol. 19). Cambridge: Cambridge University Press.

Durie, A. J. (2006) *Water is Best: The Hydros and health tourism in Scotland 1840-1940.* Edinburgh: John Donald.

Edginton, B. (1994) 'The well-ordered body: the quest for sanity through nineteenth-century asylum architecture.', *Canadian bulletin of medical history = Bulletin canadien d'histoire de la medecine*, 11(2), pp. 375–386.

Edginton, B. (1995). 'Architecture's Quest for Sanity'. *Journal on Developmental Disabilities*, 4(1), 12–22.

Edginton, B. (1997) 'Moral architecture: the influence of the York Retreat on asylum design', *Health & Place*, 3(2), pp. 91–99.

Edginton, B. (2003) 'The Design of Moral Architecture at The York Retreat', *J Design Hist*, 16(2), pp. 103–117.

Engstrom, E. J. (1997) *The Birth of Clinical Psychiatry: Power, Knowledge and Professionalization in Germany, 1867-1914.* University of North Carolina.

Engstrom, E. J. (2003) *Clinical psychiatry in imperial Germany: A history of psychiatric practice.* Ithaca: Cornell University Press.

Eraso, Y. (2010). "A Burden to the State": The reception of the German "Active Therapy" in an Argentinean "Colony-Asylum" in the 1920s and 1930s. In W. Ernst & T. Mueller (Eds.), *Transnational Psychiatries: Social and Cultural Histories of Psychiatry in Comparative Perspective, c1800-2000*, pp. 51–79.

Evans, R. (1982) *The Fabrication of Virtue: English prison architecture, 1750-1840.* Cambridge: Cambridge University Press.

Farnsworth, P. and Williams, J. S. (1992) 'The archaeology of the Spanish colonial and Mexican Republican periods: Introduction', *Historical Archaeology*, 26(1), pp. 1–6.

Farquharson, L. (2016). A 'Scottish Poor Law of Lunacy? Poor Law, Lunacy Law and Scotlands parochial asylums. *History of Psychiatry*, 28 (1), pp.15-28.

Feister, L. M. (2009) 'The orphanage at Schuyler mansion', in *The archaeology of institutional life.* Tuscaloosa: University of Alabama Press, pp. 105–116.

Fennell, P. (1996) *Treatment Without Consent: law, psychiatry and the treatment of mentally disordered people since 1845.* London and New York: Routledge.

Fennelly, K. (2014) 'Out of sound, out of mind: noise control in early nineteenth-century lunatic asylums in England and Ireland', *World Archaeology*, 46(3), pp. 416–430.

Fennelly, K. (2019) An Archaeology of Lunacy: Managing madness in early nineteenth-century asylums. Manchester: Manchester University Press.

Fennelly, K. and Newman, C. (2016) 'Poverty and Illness in the "Old Countries": archaeological approaches to historical medical institutions in the British Isles', *International Journal of Historical Archaeology*, 21(1), pp. 178–197.

Forsythe, B. (2001) 'Hope and suffering at the Devon county pauper lunatic asylum at Exminster, 1845-1914.', *Southern history*, 23, pp. 116–147.

Foster, J. L. H. (2013). What can Social Psychologists Learn from Architecture? The Asylum as Example.

Journal for the Theory of Social Behaviour, 14(2), pp. 131-147.

Foucault, M. (1961) *Folie et déraison: histoire de la folie à l'âge classique*. Paris, Plon.

Foucault, M. (1965) 'Madness and Civilization, trans. Richard Howard', *New York, Pantheon*.

Foucault, M. (1977) *Discipline and punish: The birth of the prison*. London and New York: Allen Lane.

Freeman, H. L. (2010) 'Psychiatry in Britain, c.1900', *History of Psychiatry*, 21(3), pp. 312–324.

Freund, D. (2012) *American Sunshine: Diseases of Darkness and the Quest for Natural Light*. Chicago: University of Chicago Press.

Gach, J. (2008) 'Thoughts toward a critique of biological psychiatry', in Wallace, E.R. and Gach, J. (eds) *History of psychiatry and medical psychology*. New York: Springer, pp. 685–693.

Garman, J. C. (2005). *Detention castles of stone and steel: Landscape, labour and the urban penitentiary*. Knoxville: University of Tennessee Press.

Gibson, S. K. (2006). Self-reflection in the consolidation of Scottish Identity: A case study in family correspondence, 1805-50. In P. Buckner & R. D. Francis (Eds.), *Canada and the British World: Culture, Migration and Identity* (pp. 29–44). Vancouver and Toronto: University of British Columbia Press.

Gieryn, T. T. F. (2002) 'What buildings do', *Theory and Society*. Springer, 31(1), pp. 35–74.

Giles, K. (2014) 'Buildings Archaeology', in Smith, C. (ed.) *Encyclopedia of Global Archaeology*. New York: Springer, pp. 1033–1041.

Girouard, M. (1977) *Sweetness and Light: The Queen Anne Movement, 1860-1900*, Oxford: Clarendon Press.

Gittins, D. (1998) *Madness in Its Place: Narratives of Severalls Hospital 1913-1997*. London and New York: Routledge.

Godbey, E. (2000) 'Picture me sane: photography and the magic lantern in a nineteenth-century asylum', *American Studies*, 1(Spring 2000), pp. 31–69.

Goffman, E. (1961) *Asylums: essays on the social situation of mental patients and other inmates*. New York: Anchor Books.

Gold, J. and Gold, I. (2015) *Suspicious Minds: How culture shapes madness*. New York and London: Free Press.

Grant, F. (2013) *Glasshouses*. Oxford: Shire Publications.

Grauer, A. L., McNamara, E. M. and Houdek, D. V (1998) 'A history of their own: patterns of death in a nineteenth-century poorhouse', in A.L , Grauer and P. Stuart-Macadam (eds), *Sex and gender in paleopathological perspective.Cambridge: Cambridge University Press*. pp. 149–164.

Guyatt, M. (2004) 'A semblance of home: mental asylum interiors 1880-1914', in McKellar, S. and Sparke, P. (eds) *Interior design and identity*. Manchester University Press, pp. 48–71.

Hall, P. and Ward, C. (2014) *Sociable Cities: the 21st-century reinvention of the Garden City*. Abingdon, New York: Routledge.

Hamilton, S. and Martin, D. (2013) *The burn, the fever and beyond ...* Belfast: Stephen Hamilton.

Hamilton, S. and O'Donnell, H. (2013) *Purdysburn Hospital*. Belfast: Stephen Hamilton.

Hamlett, J. (2010) *Material Relations: Domestic interiors and middle class families in England*. Manchester: Manchester University Press.

Hamlett, J. (2015) *At Home in the Institution: Material life in asylums, lodging houses and schools in Victorian and Edwardian England*. Basingstoke, New York: Palgrave Macmillan.

Hamlett, J., Hoskins, L. and Preston, R. (2013) *Residential Institutions in Britain, 1725-1970: inmates and environments*. London and Vermont: Pickering & Chatto Limited.

Harrison, J. F. (1969). *Robert Owen and the Owenites in Britain and America: The quest for the new moral world*. London: Routledge and Kegan Paul Ltd.

Hashimoto, A. (2013). A "German world" shared among doctors: a history of the relationship between Japanese and German psychiatry before World War II. *History of Psychiatry*, 24(2), 180–195.

Hendrie, W. F., & Macleod, D. A. D. (1991). *The Bangour Story. A History of Bangour Village and General Hospitals*. Edinburgh: Mercat Press.

Hickman, C. (2005) 'The Picturesque at Brislington House, Bristol: The Role of Landscape in Relation to the Treatment of Mental Illness in the Early Nineteenth-Century Asylum', *Garden History*, 33(1), pp. 47–60.

Hickman, C. (2009) 'Cheerful prospects and tranquil restoration: the visual experience of landscape as part of the therapeutic regime of the British asylum, 1800-60.', *History of Psychiatry*, 20(80 Pt 4), pp. 425–441.

Hickman, C. (2013) *Therapeutic Landscapes: A History of English Hospital Gardens Since 1800*. Manchester: Manchester University Press.

Hide, L. (2014) *Gender and Class in English Asylums 1890-1914*. Basingstoke, New York: Palgrave Macmillan.

Hopkinson, R. G., Petherbridge, P., & Longmore, J. (1966). *Daylighting*. London: Heinemann.

Hoskins, L. and Hamlett, J. (2012) '"A bright and cheerful aspect": wall decoration and the treatment of mental illness in the nineteenth and early twentieth centuries', *Wallpaper History Review* 11, pp.42-45.

Huey, P. R. (2001) 'The almshouse in Dutch and English colonial North America and its precedent in the old world: Historical and archaeological evidence', *International Journal of Historical Archeology*, 5(2), pp. 123–154.

Hume, I. N. (1964) 'Archaeology: Handmaiden to history', *The North Carolina Historical Review.*, 41, pp. 214–225.

Huxley, M. (2006) 'Spatial rationalities: order, environment, evolution and government', *Social & Cultural Geography*, 7(5), pp. 771–787.

Jackson, M. (2000) *The borderland of imbecility: medicine, society and the fabrication of the feeble mind in late Victorian and Edwardian England*. Manchester: Manchester University Press.

Jetter, D. (1971) *Geschichte des Hospitals. 2. Zur Typologie des Irrenhauses in Frankreich und Deutschland (1780-1840)*. Wiesbaden: Steiner.

Jetter, D. (1981) *Grundzüge der Geschichte des Irrenhauses*, Darmstadt: Wissenschaftliche Buchgesellschaft.

Jetter, D. (1981) 'Projects for a better insane asylum replacing the "wiener narrenthurm"', *Fortschritte der Neurologie-Psychiatrie*, 49(2), pp. 43–52.

Johnson, M. (2010) *English Houses 1300-1800: Vernacular achitecture, social life*. Harlow: Pearson Education.

Jones, K. (1993) *Asylums and after: a revised history of the mental health services: from the early 18th century to the 1990s*. London: Athlone Press.

Kelly, S. (2012) *A Grand Old Lady: the life and times of Downshire Hospital*. Dundonald: South Eastern Health and Social Services Trust.

Kisacky, J. (2000) *An Architecture of Light and Air: Theories of Hygiene and the Building of the New York Hospital, 1771--1932*. Ithaca: Cornell University Press.

Koppelkamm, S. (1981) *Glasshouses and wintergardens of the nineteenth century*. London: Granada.

Lawrence, W. J. C. (1963) *Science and the glasshouse*. Edinburgh: Oliver and Boyd.

Ledger, S. and Luckhurst, R. (2000) *The fin de siècle: A Reader in Cultural History, c. 1880-1900*. Oxford and New York: Oxford University Press.

Leech, R. H. (2006) 'Buildings Archaeology: Context and points of convergence', in Arnold, D., Ergut, E. A., and Ozkaya, B. T. (eds) *Rethinking Architectural Historiography*. Abingdon and New York: Routledge, pp. 24–35.

Lefebvre, H. (1991). *The production of space*. Oxford: Blackwell.

Lindauer, O. (1996) *Historical archaeology of the United States Industrial Indian School at Phoenix:*

Investigations of a turn of the century trash dump. Anthropological field studies number 42. Tempe: Arizona State University.

Livingstone, D. N. (2003) *Putting science in its place. Geographies of scientific knowledge*. Chicago: University of Chicago Press.

Longhurst, P. (2015) 'Institutional non-correspondence: materiality and ideology in the mental institutions of New South Wales', *Post-Medieval Archaeology*, 49(2), pp. 220–237.

Longhurst, P. (2017) 'Madness and the Material Environment: An Archaeology of Reform in and of the Asylum', *International Journal of Historical Archaeology*, 21 (4) pp. 848-866.

Louw, J., & Swartz, S. (2001). An English Asylum in Africa: Space and order in Valkenberg Asylum. *History of Psychology*, *4*(1), 3–24.

Lucas, G. (1999) 'The archaeology of the workhouse: The changing uses of the workhouse buildings at St Mary's, Southampton', in S. Tarlow and S West (eds), *The Familiar Past*, London and New York: Routledge, pp. 125–139.

Luckin, B. (2006) 'Revisiting the idea of degeneration in urban Britain, 1830–1900', *Urban History*, 33(2), pp. 234–252.

Malcolm, E. (2009). Australian Asylum Architecture through German Eyes: Kew, Melbourne, 1867. *Health and History*, *11*(1), 46–64.

Markus, T. A. (1993) *Buildings & power: Freedom and control in the origin of modern building types*. London: Routledge..

McCandless, P. (1979). "Build! Build!" The controversy over the care of the chronically insane in England, 1855-1870. *Bulletin of the History of Medicine*, *53*(4), 553–574.

McEwan, B. (2002) 'San Luis, Florida, USA', in Orser, C. (ed.) *Encyclopedia of Historical Archaeology*. London: Routledge, pp. 295–321.

McLaughlan, R. (2016). Corrupting the Asylum: The Diminishing Role of the Architect in the Design of Curative Environments for Mental Illness in New Zealand. *Architectural Theory Review*, July, pp.1-22.

McManus, R. (2011) 'Suburban and urban housing in the twentieth century', *Proceedings of the Royal Irish Academy*, Section C, 111C, pp. 253–286.

Miller, M. (1989) 'Letchworth Garden City: an architectural view' in *Garden Cities and New Towns*, Hertford: Hertfordshire Publications, pp.48-87.

Morrison, K. (1998) 'Cottage Home Villages', *Transactions of the Ancient Monuments Society*, 42, pp. 81–102.

Morrison, K. (1999) *The Workhouse: a study of poor-law buildings in England*. Swindon: Royal Commission on the Historical Monuments of England.

Müller, N. (1997) 'Historische und aktuelle Bauprinzipien psychiatrischer Kliniken', *Nervenarzt*, 68 (3), pp. 184–195.

Myers, A. and Moshenska, G.(eds) (2011) *Archaeologies of Internment*. New York, NY: Springer.

Mytum, H. and Carr, G. (eds) (2012) *Prisoners of war: archaeology, memory, and heritage of 19th-and 20th-century mass internment*. New York: Springer

Newman, C. (2013a) 'An archaeology of poverty: architectural innovation and pauper experience at Madeley Union Workhouse, Shropshire', *Post-Medieval Archaeology*. 47(2), pp. 359–377.

Newman, C. (2013b) 'To Punish or Protect: The New Poor Law and the English Workhouse', *International Journal of Historical Archaeology*. 18(1), pp. 122–145.

Newman, C. (2015) 'A mansion for the mad: an archaeology of Brooke House, Hackney', *Post-Medieval Archaeology*, 49(1), pp. 156–174.

O'Dwyer, F. (2000) 'The architecture of John Skipton Mulvany', *Irish Architectural and Decorative Studies*, 3, pp. 65–66.

Orser, C. (ed.) (2002) *Encyclopedia of Historical Archaeology*. New York: Routledge.

Osborne, T. and Rose, N. (1999) 'Governing cities: Notes on the spatialisation of virtue', *Environment and Planning D: Society and Space*, 17(6), pp. 737–760.

Otter, C. (2008) *The Victorian eye: A political history of light and vision in Britain, 1800-1910*. Chicago: University of Chicago Press.

Overy, P. (2008) *Light, air and openness: modern architecture between the wars*. London: Thames and Hudson Ltd.

Pechenick, E. A. *et al.* (2015) 'Characterizing the Google Books Corpus: Strong Limits to Inferences of Socio-Cultural and Linguistic Evolution', *PLOS ONE.*, 10(10), pp.1-24.

Philo, C. (1987). '"Fit localities for an asylum": the historical geography of the nineteenth-century "mad business" in England as viewed through the pages of the asylum journal.' *Journal of Historical Geography*, *13*(4), 398–415.

Philo, C. (1989) 'Enough to drive one mad: the organisation of space in nineteenth-century lunatic asylums', in Wolch, J. and Dear, M. (eds) *The Power of Geography: How territory shapes social life*. Boston, London, Sydney, Wellington: Unwin Hyman, pp. 258–290.

Philo, C. (2004) *A Geographical History of Institutional Provision for the Insane from Medieval Times to the 1860's in England and Wales*. New York: Edwin Mellen Press.

Piddock, S. (2001) 'Convicts and the free: nineteenth-century lunatic asylums in South Australia and Tasmania.', *Australasian historical archaeology: journal of the Australasian Society for Historical Archaeology*, 19(2001), pp. 84–96.

Piddock, S. (2007) *A Space of Their Own : The Archaeology of Nineteenth Century Lunatic Asylums in Britain , South Australia and Tasmania*. New York: Springer.

Piddock, S. (2011) 'To each a space: class, classification and gender in colonial South Australian institutions', *Historical Archaeology*, 45(3), pp. 89–105.

Piddock, S. (2016) 'A Place for Convicts: The Fremantle Lunatic Asylum, Western Australia and John Conolly's "Ideal" Asylum', *International Journal of Historical Archaeology*, 20(3), pp. 562–573.

Pietikäinen, P. (2015) *Madness: A History*. Abingdon, New York: Routledge.

Porter, R. (1990) 'Foucault's great confinement', *History of the Human Sciences*, 3(1), pp.47-54.

Porter, R. (1996) 'Mental Illness', in Porter, R. (ed.) *Cambridge Illustrated History of Medicine*. Cambridge, New York, Melbourne: Cambridge University Press, pp. 278–303.

Porter, R. (2002) *Madness: a brief history*. Oxford University Press, USA.

Porter, R. and Wright, D. (2003) *The confinement of the insane: International perspectives, 1800-1965*. Cambridge and New York: Cambridge University Press.

Quinn, K. (2011) 'From Asylum to Hospital 1886-96: the work of Dr William Graham', *History Armagh*, 2(3), pp. 29–30.

Radford, J. P. (1991). Sterilization versus segregation: control of the "feebleminded", 1900-1938. *Social Science & Medicine*, *33*(4), 449–458.

Radford, J. P., & Park, D. C. (1995). The Eugenic Legacy. *Focus on History of Disabilities, 4*(1), 63–74.

Rafferty, A. M. (1996) *The politics of nursing knowledge*. London and New York: Routledge.

Renvoize, E. (1991) 'The Association of Medical Officers of Asylums and Hospitals for the Insane, the Medico-Psychological Association, and their Presidents', in H. Freeman and G. Berrios (eds),*150 years of British Psychiatry, 1841-1891*. London: Gaskell, pp. 29–78.

Reuber, M. (1996) 'The architecture of psychological management: the Irish asylums (1801-1922)', *Psychological medicine,* 26(6), pp. 1179–1190.

Richardson, H. (1991) 'A continental solution to the planning of lunatic asylums 1900-1940', in Frew, J. and Jones, D. (eds) *Scotland and Europe: Architecture and*

Design 1850-1940 (St Andrews Studies in the History of Scottish Architecture and Design, Proceedings of a Symposium held at the University, St Andrews May 19th 1990), pp. 67–79.

Richardson, H. (ed) (1998) *English Hospitals 1660-1948: A survey of their architecture and design*. Swindon: Royal Commission on the Historical Monuments of England.

Richardson, H. and MacInnes, R. (2010) *Building up our Health: the architecture of Scotland's historic hospitals*. Edinburgh: Historic Scotland.

Robins, J. (1986) *Fools and mad: A history of the insane in Ireland*. Dublin: Institute of Public Administration.

Rose, G. (2011) *Visual methodologies: An introduction to researching with visual materials*. London: Sage Publications.

Rose, N. (1985) *The Psychological Complex: Psychology, Politics and Society in England 1869-1939*. London, Boston, Melbourne and Henley: Routledge & Kegan Paul.

Rutherford, S. (2004) 'Victorian and Edwardian Institutional Landscapes in England', *Landscapes*, 5(2), pp. 25–41.

Rutherford, S. (2005) 'Landscapers for the Mind: English Asylum Designers, 1845-1914', *Garden History*, 33(1), pp. 61–86.

Scull, A. (1979) *Museums of madness: The social organization of insanity in nineteenth-century England*. London: Allen Lane.

Scull, A. (1980) 'A convenient place to get rid of inconvenient people: the Victorian lunatic asylum', in King, A. (ed.) *Buildings and Society*. London: Routledge & Kegan Paul.

Scull, A. (1983) 'The domestication of madness', *Medical history*, 27, pp. 233–248.

Scull, A. (1985) 'A Victorian alienist: John Conolly FRCP, DCL (1794-1866)', in Bynum, W., Porter, R., and Shepherd, M. (eds) *The Anatomy of Madness: Essays in the History of Psychiatry, Volume I, People and Ideas*. London and New York: Tavistock Publications.

Scull, A. (1993) *The Most Solitary of Afflictions: Madness and Society 1700–1900*. New Haven and London: Yale University Press.

Scull, A. (2015) *Madness in Civilization, a cultural history of insanity from the Bible to Freud, from the Madhouse to Modern Medicine*. London: Thames and Hudson.

Scull, A. (2017) 'The asylum, hospital and clinic', in G Eghigian (ed), *The Routledge history of madness and mental health*. Abingdon and New York: Routledge, pp. 101–114.

Sedgwick, P. (1981) 'Michael Foucault: the anti-history of Psychiatry', *Psychological medicine*, 11, pp. 235–248.

Shorter, E. (1997) *A history of psychiatry: From the era of the asylum to the age of Prozac*. New York: John Wiley & Sons.

Shorter, E. (2007) 'The Historical Development of mental health services in Europe', in E Mossialos, G Thornicroft, M Knapp, D McDaid (eds) *Mental Health Policy and Practice across Europe*. Milton Keynes: Open University Press, pp. 15–33.

Skålevåg, S. A. (2002). Constructing curative instruments: psychiatric architecture in Norway, 1820-1920. *History of Psychiatry*, 13(49), 51.

Skultans, V. (1979) *English madness: ideas on insanity, 1580-1890*. Routledge & K. Paul.

Smith, L. D. (1999) *Cure, Comfort and Safe Custody: public lunatic asylums in early nineteenth-century England*. Leicester: Leicester University Press.

Smith, L. D. (2007). The architecture of confinement: Urban public asylums in England, 1750-1820. In L. Topp, J. E. Moran, & J. Andrews (Eds.), *Madness, architecture and the built environment. Psychiatric spaces in historical context*. (pp. 41–62). New York and Abingdon: Routledge.

Snelders, S., Meijman, F. J., & Pieters, T. (2007). Heredity and Alcoholism in the Medical Sphere: The Netherlands, 1850-1900. *Medical History*, 51, 219–236.

Spencer-Wood, S. M. (2001). Views and commentaries: What difference does feminist theory make? *International Journal of Historical Archeology*, 5(1), 97–114.

Spencer-Wood, S. M. (2009). 'A feminist approach to European ideologies of poverty and the institutionalization of the poor in Falmouth, Massachusetts.' in A. M. Beisaw & J. G. Gibb (eds.), *The Archaeology of Institutional Life*, University of Alabama Press, Tuscaloosa.

Spencer-Wood, S. M. and Baugher, S. (2001) 'Introduction and historical context for the archaeology of institutions of reform. Part I: Asylums', *International Journal of Historical Archeology*, 5(1), pp. 3–17.

Springate, M. E. (2017) 'Connecting the Threads: Archaeology of Reform / Archaeology as Reform', *International Journal of Historical Archaeology*, 21(4), pp.773-784.

Stamp, G. (1980) *The English House 1860 - 1914*. London: International Architect and the Building Centre Trust.

Stell, G., Shaw, J. and Storrier, S. (2003) *Scottish Life and Society, A Compendium of Scottish Ethnology, Volume 3: Scotland's Buildings*. East Lothian: Tuckwell Press.

Stevenson, C. (1997) 'The Architecture of Bethlem at Moorfields', in J Andrews, A Briggs, R Porter, P Tucker and K Waddington, *The History of Bethlem*. London: Routledge, pp. 230–259.

Stevenson, C. (2000) *Medicine and magnificence: British hospital and asylum architecture, 1660-1815*. New Haven: Yale University Press.

Stone, M. H. (1998) *Healing the Mind. A history of psychiatry from antiquity to the present.* London: Pimlico.

Storper, M. (1985) 'The spatial and temporal constitution of social action', *Environment and Planning D: Society and Space*, (3), pp. 407–424.

Sturdy, H. and Parry-Jones, W. (1999) 'Boarding-out insane patients: the significance of the Scottish system 1857-1913', in Bartlett, P. and Wright, D. (eds) *Outside the walls of the asylum: the history of care in the community, 1750–2000*. London: Athlone, pp. 86–114.

Suzuki, A. (1995) 'The politics and ideology of non-restraint: the case of the Hanwell Asylum', *Medical history*, 39, pp.1-17.

Szasz, T. S. (1961) *The myth of mental illness*. New York: Dell.

Tarlow, S. (2007) *The Archaeology of Improvement in Britain, 1750-1850*. Cambridge: Cambridge University Press.

Taylor, J. (1991) *Hospital and asylum architecture in England, 1840-1914 : building for health care*. London: Mansell.

Taylor, J. (2007) 'The architect and the pauper asylum in late nineteenth-century England: G T Hine's 1901 review of asylum space and planning', in Topp, L., Moran, J. E., and Andrews, J. (eds) *Madness, architecture and the built environment. Psychiatric spaces in historical context*. New York and Abingdon: Routledge, pp. 263–284.

The Climate of Northern Ireland (1983). Bracknell, Berkshire: Meteorological Office.

Thomas, D. H. (1993) 'The architecture of Mission Santa Catalina de Guale: our first 15 years', in McEwan, B. G. (ed.) *The Spanish missions of La Florida*. Gainesville: University of Florida.

Thomas, L. (2013) 'The Evolving Moral and Physical Geometry of Childhood in Ulster Workhouses, 1838-55', *Childhood in the Past: An International Journal*, 6(1), pp. 22–51.

Thomas, L. (2017) 'Manifestations of Institutional Reform and Resistance to Reform in Ulster Workhouses, Ireland, 1838-1855', *International Journal of Historical Archaeology*, 21 (4), pp. 867-900.

Thompson, J. D. and Goldin, G. (1975) *The Hospital: a Social and Architectural History*. New Haven and London: Yale University Press.

Topp, L. (1997). An Architecture for Modern Nerves: Josef Hoffmann's Purkersdorf Sanatorium. *The Journal of the Society of Architectural Historians*, 56 (4), pp. 414–437.

Topp, L. E. (2004). *Architecture and Truth in Fin-de-siècle Vienna*. Cambridge University Press.

Topp, L. (2005). Otto Wagner and the Steinhof Psychiatric Hospital: Architecture as Misunderstanding. *The Art Bulletin*, 87(1), 130–156.

Topp, L. (2007) 'Psychiatric institutions, their architecture, and the politics of regional autonomy in the Austro-Hungarian monarchy', *Studies in History and Philosophy of Science Part C: Studies in History and Philosophy of Biological and Biomedical Sciences*, 38(4), pp. 733–755.

Topp, L. (2009). Architecture, Language, and Representation. *Oxford Art Journal*, 32(2), 321–324.

Topp, L. (2012). Complexity and Coherence : The Challenge of the Asylum Mortuary in Central Europe 1898-1908. *Journal of the Society of Architectural Historians*, 71(1), 8–41.

Topp, L. (2017) *Freedom and the cage: modern architecture and psychiatry in Central Europe, 1890-1914*. University Park, Pennsylvania: Pennsylvania State University Press.

Topp, L., Moran, J. E. and Andrews, J. (2007) *Madness, Architecture and the Built Environment: Psychiatric Spaces in Historical Context*. Abingdon, New York: Routledge.

Topp, L. and Wieber, S. (2009) 'Architecture, Psychiatry, and Lebensreform at an Agricultural Colony of the Insane—Lower Austria, 1903', *Central Europe*, 7(2), pp. 125–149.

Townsend, G. (1989) 'Airborne toxins and the American house, 1865-1895.', *Winterthur portfolio*, 24(1), pp. 29–42.

Waddington, K. (2011) *An introduction to the social history of medicine: Europe since 1500*. London: Palgrave Macmillan.

Wallace, E. R. and Gach, J. (eds) (2008) *History of Psychiatry and Medical Psychology*. New York: Springer.

Weiner, D. B. (1994) '"Le geste de Pinel": the history of a psychiatric myth', in Micale, M. S. and Porter, R. (eds) *Discovering the History of Psychiatry*. Oxford and New York: Oxford University Press, pp. 232-247

Whatley, C. A. (2000). *Scottish Society 1707-1830 Beyond Jacobitism, towards industrialisation*. Manchester: Manchester University Press.

Whitehand, J. W. R. (2001) 'British urban morphology: the Conzenian tradition', *Urban Morphology*, 5(2), pp. 103–109.

Whyte, W. (2006) 'How do buildings mean? Some issues of interpretation in the history of architecture', *History and Theory*, 45(2), pp. 153–177.

Wood, J. and Chitty, G. (1994) *Buildings archaeology: applications in practice*. Oxford: Oxbow Books in

assocation with the Institute of Field Archaeologists
Buildings Special Interest Group.

Worboys, M. (2000) *Spreading Germs: Disease theories
and medical practice in Britain, 1865-1900*. Cambridge,
New York, Melbourne, Madrid: Cambridge University
Press.

Wright, D. (2001) *Mental Disability in Victorian England:
The Earlswood Asylum 1847-1901*. Oxford, New York:
Clarendon Press.

Yanni, C. (2007) *The architecture of madness: Insane
asylums in the United States*. Minneapolis and London:
University of Minnesota Press.

Online Sources

Canmore, National Record of the Historic Environment
Scotland (https://canmore.org.uk/)

County Asylums (Images) (www.countyasylums.co.uk)

Deutsche Wetterdienst (www.dwd.de)

Dictionary of Irish Architects (www.dia.ie)

Dictionary of Scottish Architects (www.scottisharchitects.
org.uk)

EDINA Digimap (http://digimap.edina.ac.uk/)

Epsom and Ewell History Explorer (http://www.
epsomandewellhistoryexplorer.org.uk)

Historic England (https://historicengland.co.uk)(www.
pastscape.org.uk)

Historic Environment Viewer (Republic of Ireland) (http://
webgis.archaeology.ie/historicenvironment)

Historic Environment Map Viewer (Northern Ireland)
(https://dfcgis.maps.arcgis.com)

Historic Hospitals (https://historic-hospitals.com/mental-
hospitals-in-britain-and-ireland/)

Index of Lunatic Asylums and Mental Hospitals (http://
studymore.org.uk)

Meteorological office (https://www.metoffice.gov.uk/
public/weather/climate

National Inventory of Architectural Heritage (www.
buildingsofireland.ie)

National Library of Ireland (images) (http://catalogue.nli.ie)

National Library of Scotland (map images) (http://maps.
nls.uk)

The Time Chamber (The Asylums List)(http://
thetimechamber.co.uk)

Topographic maps (http://en-gb.topographic-map.com/)

US National Library of Medicine (images) (https://openi.
nlm.nih.gov)

Wellcome Collection (images) (https://wellcomecollection.
org)

CPSIA information can be obtained
at www.ICGtesting.com
Printed in the USA
LVHW070221230323
742314LV00039B/1104